KETO VEGETARIAN COOKBOOK 2019-2020

~ 600+ ~

Low-Carb Vegetarian Recipes, 1000-Day Diet Plan, and 10 Tips for Success- Lose Up to 20 Pounds in 3 Weeks

Anthony James William

Table of Contents

DESCRIPTION 1
INTRODUCTION 1
BREAKFAST 2
    01. Pear Oatmeal 2
    02. Pumpkin Oatmeal 2
    03. Veggie Burrito 2
    04. Apple Steel Cut Oats 2
    05. Tofu Casserole 3
    06. Carrot Mix 3
    07. Blueberries Oats 3
    08. Apple and Pears Mix 3
    09. Bell Pepper Oatmeal 4
    10. Banana and Walnuts Oats 4
    11. Simple Granola 4
    12. Zucchini Oatmeal 4
    13. Cranberry Coconut Quinoa 5
    14. Sweet Quinoa Mix 5
    15. Chia Pudding 5
    16. Simple Creamy Breakfast Potatoes 5
    17. Sweet Potatoes Mix 6
    18. Breakfast Bowls 6
    19. Mediterranean Chickpeas Breakfast 6
    20. Pumpkin Breakfast Muffins 6
    21. Delicious Porridge 7
    22. Strawberry Quinoa 7
    23. Breakfast Broccoli and Tofu Bowls 7
    24. Cool Tofu Breakfast Mix 7
    25. Cinnamon Oatmeal 8
    26. Coconut Rice 8
    27. Blackberry Pudding 8
    28. Parsley Quiche 8
    29. Coconut muffin 8
    30. Orange delight 9
    31. Egg mayonnaise 9
    32. Strawberry Choco shake 9
    33. Lemon jelly 9
    34. Strawberry mug cake 9
    35. Fluffy cinnamon muffin 10
    36. Cappuccino Shake 10
    37. Lemon Cheese Smoothie 10
    38.. Zucchini tasty chips 10
    39. Blackberry avocmado Mousse 10
    40. Queso crunch 11
    41. Cocoa butter balls 11
    42. Choco Cheese Mousse 11
    43. Hot cheese crackers 11
    44. Cinnamon pudding 12
    45. Saffron avocado paste 12
LUNCH 13
    46. Rich Chickpeas And Lentils Soup 13
    47. Chard And Sweet Potato Soup 13
    48. Chinese Soup And Ginger Sauce 13
    49. Corn Cream Soup 14

50. Veggie Medley 14
51. Lentils Curry 14
52. Lentils Dal 15
53. Rich Jackfruit Dish 15
54. Vegan Gumbo 15
55. Eggplant Salad 15
56. Corn And Cabbage Soup 16
57. Okra Soup 16
58. Carrot Soup 16
59. Baby Carrots And Coconut Soup 16
60. Chinese Carrot Cream 17
61. Seitan Stew 17
62. Spicy Carrot Stew 17
63. Tomato Soup 18
64. Classic Tomato Soup 18
65. Collard Greens Mix 18
66. Colored Collard Greens Dish 18
67. Chinese Collard Greens Mix 19
68. Fresh Collard Greens Mix 19
69. Artichoke Soup 19
70. Intense Beet Soup 19
71. Brussels Sprouts Delight 20
72. Mushroom Soup 20
73. Beets And Capers Mix 20
74. Asparagus Soup 20
75. Fennel Soup 21
76. Endives Soup 21
77. Special Minestrone Soup 21
78. Green Chili Soup 21
79. Caribbean Dish 22
80. Mediterranean Stew 22
81. Chickpeas Delight 22
82. Mexican Quinoa Dish 23
83. Sweet Potato Soup 23
84. White Beans Stew 23
85. Spaghetti Squash Bowls 23
86. Italian Cauliflower Mix 24
87. Mushroom Delight 24
88. Quinoa And Veggie Mix 24
89. Bulgur Chili 24
90. Cauliflower Chili 25
91. Quinoa Chili 25
92. Pumpkin Chili 25
93. 3 Bean Chili 26
94. Root Vegetable Chili 26
95. Brown Rice Soup 26
96. Butternut Squash Soup 27
97. Green Beans Soup 27
98. Vegan Sandwich with Tofu & Lettuce Slaw ... 27
99. Southern Collard Greens 28
100. Nicely Flavored Swiss Chard 28
101. American Style Kale 28
102. Sweet & Sour Kale 29
103. Super-Food Casserole 29

Table of Contents

104. Traditional Indian Spinach 29
105. Holiday Gathering Casserole 30
106. Simple Steamed Asparagus 30
107. Buttered Asparagus 30
108. Zesty Artichokes 31
109. Loveable Brussels Sprouts 31
110. Chinese Brussels Sprouts 31
111. Garlicky Green Beans 32
112. Southern Green Beans 32
113. Holiday Dinner Table Casserole 32
114. Mexican Style Mushrooms 33
115. Aromatic Mushrooms 33
116. Thanksgiving Side Dish 33
117. Authentic Sri Lankan Cabbage 34
118. Bright Carrot Mash 34
119. Delish Carrots 34
120. Glazed Carrots 35
121. Sweet & Spicy Carrots 35
122. Bell Pepper Gumbo 35
123. Italian Bell Pepper Platter......................... 36

DINNER 37
124. 2-Minutes Broccoli.................................... 37
125. Brilliant Cheesy Broccoli 37
126. Easy-to-Prepare Broccoli.......................... 37
127. Luscious Broccoli Casserole 38
128. Better-Than-Real Mash 38
129. Spicy Cauliflower....................................... 38
130. Veggie Mac and Cheese 39
131. Keto Soufflé 39
132. Indian Veggie Platter 40
133. French Veggie Combo 40
134. Provincial Ratatouille 41
135. South-East Asian Curry 41
136. Summery Veggie Curry 41
137. eritable Feast Curry.................................. 42
138. Italian Veggie Stew.................................... 42
139. Spaghetti Squash.. 43
140. Chili & Blue Cheese Stuffed Mushrooms 43
141. Fresh Coconut Milk Shake with Blackberries 43
142. Burritos Wraps with Avocado & Cauliflower 43
143. Pizza Bianca with Mushrooms 44
144. Hot Pizza with Tomatoes, Cheese & Olives 44
145. Spicy Vegetarian Burgers with Fried Eggs 44
146. Grilled Cauliflower Steaks with Haricots Vert.... 45
147. Tofu & Vegetable Stir-Fry......................... 45
148. Chili Lover's Frittata with Spinach & Cheese 45
149. Spicy Cauliflower Falafel 46
150. Mediterranean Eggplant Squash Pasta 46
151. Spiral Zucchini Noodles with Cheesy Sauce 46
152. Cajun Flavored Stuffed Mushrooms.................. 46
153. Keto Tortilla Wraps with Vegetables................. 47
154. Roasted Cauliflower Gratin 47
155. Basil Spinach & Zucchini Lasagna 47
156. Broccoli & Asparagus Flan 48
157. Grilled Vegetables & Tempeh Shish Kebab........ 48

158. Grilled Tofu Kabobs with Arugula Salad 48
159. Sticky Tofu with Cucumber & Tomato Salad 49
160. Stewed Vegetables 49
161. Grilled Halloumi with Cauli-Rice & Almonds ... 49
162. Portobello Bun Mushroom Burgers 50
163. Soy Chorizo & Cabbage Bake.................. 50
164. One-Pot Mushroom Stroganoff............... 50
165. Vegetable Stew... 51
166. Sautéed Tofu with Pistachios................... 51
167. Zucchini Spaghetti with Avocado & Capers...... 51
168. Mushroom & Cheese Cauliflower Risotto 51
169. Avocado Boats 52
170. Basil Tofu with Cashew Nuts 52
171. Stuffed Mushrooms 52
172. Steamed Bok Choy with Thyme & Garlic........... 52
173. Stir-Fried Brussels Sprouts with Tofu & Leeks... 53
174. Colorful Peppers Stuffed with Mushrooms & "Rice" 53
175. Fennel & Celeriac with Chili Tomato Sauce 53
176. Steamed Asparagus with Feta 54
177. Roasted Pumpkin with Almonds & Cheddar 54
178. Smoked Vegetable Bake with Parmesan.............. 54
179. Sauteed Spinach with Spicy Tofu 54
180. Traditional Greek Eggplant Casserole 55
Poppy Seed Coleslaw.. 55
182. Tofu & Hazelnut Loaded Zucchini 56
183. Parsnip & Carrot Strips with Walnut Sauce 56
184. Cauliflower & Celery Bisque 56
185. Balsamic Roasted Vegetables with Feta & Almonds 56
186. Cauliflower-Kale Dip................................ 57
187. Tofu & Vegetable Casserole..................... 57
188. Cauliflower-Based Waffles with Zucchini & Cheese 57
189. Pumpkin & Bell Pepper Noodles with Avocado Sauce 58
190. Curried Cauliflower & Mushrooms Traybake 58
191. Tasty Tofu & Swiss Chard Dip 58
192. One-Pot Ratatouille with Pecans 59
193. Baked Parsnip Chips with Yogurt Dip..... 59
194. Roasted Cauliflower with Bell Peppers & Onion 59
195. Oven-Roasted Asparagus with Romesco Sauce .. 59
196. Parmesan Brussels Sprouts with Onion................ 60
197. Chocolate Nut Granola............................. 60
198. Mozzarella & Bell Pepper Avocado Cups 60
199. Green Mac and Cheese 61
200. Roasted Tomatoes with Vegan Cheese Crust...... 61

SIDES...62
201. Mashed Cauliflower 62
202. Fragrant Cauliflower Steaks..................... 62
203. Fried Cheese 62
204. Cabbage Salad 62
205. Hummus.. 63
206. Roasted Halloumi 63
207. Roasted Cabbage 63
208. Deviled Eggs 63

#	Recipe	Page
209.	Fried Broccoli	63
210.	Brussel Sprouts with Nuts	64
211.	Zucchini Pasta	64
212.	Shirataki Noodles	64
213.	Low Carb Baked Vegetables	64
214.	Rutabaga Swirls	65
215.	Fettuccine	65
216.	French Fries	65
217.	Broccoli Fritters	66
218.	Spinach in Cream	66
219.	Dill Radish	66
220.	Curry Rice	66
221.	Garlic Artichokes	66
222.	Turnip Slaw	67
223.	Sauteed Cabbage	67
224.	Spiced Rutabaga	67
225.	Swiss Chard	67
226.	Broccoli Cream	68
227.	Cauliflower and Tomatoes Mix	68
228.	Shallots and Kale Soup	68
229.	Hot Kale Pan	68
230.	Baked Broccoli	69
231.	Leeks Cream	69
232.	Fennel Soup	69
233.	Cauliflower and Green Beans	69
234.	Bok Choy Soup	69
235.	Cabbage Sauté	70
236.	Mustard Greens Sauté	70
237.	Bok Choy and Tomatoes	70
238.	Sesame Savoy Cabbage	70
239.	Chili Collard Greens	71
240.	Artichokes Soup	71
241.	Ginger and Bok Choy Soup	71
242.	Spinach Soup	71
243.	Asparagus Soup	72
244.	Baked Endives	72
245.	Baked Asparagus	72
246.	Asparagus and Tomatoes	72
247.	Endives and Mustard Sauce	73
248.	Mexican Peppers Mix	73
249.	Garlic Eggplants	73
250.	Broccoli and Mushrooms Mix	73
251.	Green Beans Side Salad	74
252.	Red Potatoes and Green Beans	74
253.	Baby Potatoes Salad	74
254.	Arabic Plums Mix	74
255.	Lemony Baby Potatoes	75
256.	White Mushrooms Mix	75
257.	Gold Potatoes and Bell Pepper Mix	75
258.	Delicious Potato Mix	75
259.	Chinese Long Beans Mix	76
260.	Easy Portobello Mushrooms	76
261.	Summer Squash Mix	76
262.	Corn Side Salad	76
263.	Colored Veggie Mix	76
264.	Leeks Medley	77
265.	Corn and Tomatoes	77
266.	Broccoli, Tomatoes and Carrots	77
267.	Oregano Bell Peppers	77
268.	Yellow Lentils Mix	78
269.	Creamy Zucchini and Sweet Potatoes	78
270.	Baked Brussels Sprouts	78
271.	Roasted Tomatoes	79
272.	Brussels Sprouts and Green Beans	79
273.	Crispy Radishes	79
274.	Creamy Radishes	79
275.	Radish Soup	79
276.	Tasty Avocado Salad	80
277.	Avocado And Egg Salad	80
278.	Avocado And Cucumber Salad	80
279.	Delicious Avocado Soup	80
280.	Delicious Avocado And Bacon Soup	81
281.	Thai Avocado Soup	81
282.	Simple Arugula Salad	81
283.	Arugula Soup	82
284.	Arugula And Broccoli Soup	82
285.	Delicious Zucchini Cream	82
286.	Zucchini And Avocado Soup	82
287.	Swiss Chard Pie	83
288.	Swiss Chard Salad	83
289.	Green Salad	83
290.	Catalan Style Greens	84
291.	Swiss Chard Soup	84
292.	Special Swiss Chard Soup	84
293.	Roasted Tomato Cream	85
294.	Eggplant Soup	85
295.	Eggplant Stew	85
296.	Roasted Bell Peppers Soup	86
297.	Delicious Cabbage Soup	86

SOUP RECIPES 87

#	Recipe	Page
298.	Creamy Cauliflower Mushroom Soup	87
299.	Avocado Broccoli Soup	87
300.	Healthy Zucchini Soup	87
301.	Coconut Leek Cauliflower Soup	87
302.	Chilled Mint Avocado Soup	88
303.	Pumpkin Tomato Soup	88
304.	Delicious Tomato Herb Soup	88
305.	Healthy Spinach Kale Soup	89
306.	Simple Celery Soup	89
307.	Broccoli Cheddar Soup	89
398.	Onion Mushroom Clear Soup	89
309.	Lemon Garlic Asparagus Soup	90
310.	Smooth Spinach Cauliflower Soup	90
311.	EZucchini Asparagus Soup	90
312.	Cholesterol 0 mg.	91
313.	Yummy Carrot Tomato Soup	91
314.	Garbanzo Bean Tortilla Soup	91
315.	Black Bean and Annatto Seed Tortilla Soup	91
316.	Navy Bean Taco Soup	92
317.	Habanero Garbanzo Taco Soup	92
318.	Jalapeno Taco Soup	92

Table of Contents

- 319. Black Bean Pepper Soup 93
- 320. Garbanzo and Jalapeno Pepper Soup 93
- 321. Carrot and Chili Soup 93
- 322. Oriental Carrot Soup 93
- 323. Vietnamese Carrot Soup 94
- 324. Italian Carrot Soup 94
- 325. Potato and Parsnip Soup 94
- 526. Jalapeno Carrot Soup 94
- 327. Mexican Potato and Onion Soup 94
- 328. Japanese Sweet Potato Soup 95
- 329. Creamy Poblano Pepper Soup 95
- 330. Middle Eastern Inspired Creamy Potato Soup ... 95
- 331. Lebanese Inspired Potato Soup 96
- 332. Habanero and Ancho Chili Potato Soup 96
- 333. Thai and Mexican Fusion Potato Soup 96
- 334. Spanish Potato and Poblano Pepper Soup 97
- 335. Creamy Nutty Potato Soup 97
- 336. Squash, Lentil and Fenugreek Soup 98
- 337. Sichuan Lentil and Squash Soup 98
- 338. Squash Curry Soup 98
- 339. Squash and Ginger Soup 98
- 340. Squash and Kidney Bean Soup 99
- 341. Simple Squash and Lentil Soup 99
- Carrot and Tarragon Soup 99
- 343. Creamy Almond Carrot and Celery Soup 99
- 344. Thai Carrot and Celery Soup 100
- 345. Creamy French Carrot Soup 100
- 346. Creamy Lemon Garlic Carrot Soup 100
- 347. Italian Carrot Soup 100
- 348. Spicy Red Onion Soup 101
- 349. Hungarian Red Onion Soup 101
- 350. Simple French Red Soup 101
- 351. Spanish Vegan Chorizo Onion Soup 101

SOUPS **102**
- 352. Sun-dried Tomato Navy Bean Soup 102
- 353. Vegan Chorizo and Potato Soup 102
- 354. Asian Spinach and Mung Bean Soup 102
- 355. Potato and White Bean Soup 102

BEAN & GRAIN MAINS **104**
- 356. Kidney Bean Dinner 104
- 357. Rice Lentil Meal 104
- 358. Mushroom Quinoa Pilaf 104
- 359. Cabbage Rice Treat 105
- 360. Almond Quinoa Pilaf 106
- 361. Bean Pepper Salad 106
- 362. Lentils Tomato Bowl 106
- 363. Squash Barley Meal 107
- 364. Creamed Peas & Rice 107
- 365. Cornmeal Onion Polenta 108

GRILLED RECIPES **109**
- 366. Grilled Zucchinis and Button Mushrooms 109
- 367. Grilled Zucchini and Cremini Mushrooms with Balsamic Glaze 109
- 368. Grilled Asparagus Green Pepper and Squash ... 109
- 369. Simple Grilled Zucchini and Red Onions 109
- 370. Simple Grilled Corns and Portobello 110
- 371. Grilled Marinated Eggplant and Zucchini 110
- 372. Grilled Bell Pepper and Broccolini 110
- 373. Grilled Cauliflower and Brussel Sprouts 110
- 374. Grilled Corn and Crimini Mushrooms 110
- Grilled Eggplant, Zucchini and Corn 110
- 376. Grilled Zucchini and Pineapple 111
- 377. Grilled Portobello and Asparagus 111
- 378. Simple Grilled Vegetables Recipe 111
- 379. Grilled Japanese Eggplant and Shitake Mushroom 111
- 380. Grilled Japanese Eggplant and Broccolini 111
- 381. Grilled Cauliflower and Brussel Sprouts 112
- 382. Grilled Japanese and Cauliflower Recipe with Balsamic Glaze 112
- 383. Simple Grilled Vegetables Recipe 112
- 384. Grilled Eggplant and Green Bell Peppers 112
- 385. Grilled Portobello Asparagus and Green Beans with Apple Cider Vinaigrette 112
- 386. Grilled Beans and Portobello Mushrooms 112
- 387. Brussel Sprouts and Green Beans 113
- 388. Zucchini and Onion in Ranch Dressing 113
- 389. Grilled Green Bean and Pineapple in Balsamic Vinaigrette 113
- 390. Grilled Broccolini and Eggplants 113
- 391. Grilled Broccolini and Green Bell Peppers 113
- 392. Grilled Zucchini and Carrots 113
- 393. Grilled Portobello Mushrooms in Apple Cider Vinaigrette 114
- 394. Grilled Carrots with Brussel Sprouts 114
- 395. Grilled Parsnip and Zucchini Recipe 114
- 396. Grilled Turnip in Oriental Vinaigrette 114
- 397. Grilled Carrot, Turnip and Portobello with Balsamic Glaze 114
- 398. Grilled Zucchinis and Mangoes 115
- 399. Grilled Baby Corn and Green Beans 115
- 400. Grilled Artichoke Hearts and Brussel Sprouts .. 115
- 401. Grilles Bell Peppers Broccolini and Brussel Sprouts with Honey Apple Cider Glaze 115
- 402. Grilled Assorted Bell Peppers with Broccolini Florets Recipe 115
- 403. Grilled Eggplant, Zucchini with Assorted Bell Peppers 115
- 404. Grilled Portobello and Red Onion 116
- 405. Grilled Corn and Red Onions 116

ROASTED RECIPES **117**
- 406. Roasted Napa Cabbage Baby Carrots and Spinach 117
- 407. Roasted Spinach Watercress and Carrots 117
- 408. Roasted Artichoke Hearts and Red Cabbage 117
- 409. Roasted kale and Red Cabbage 117
- 410. Roasted Napa Cabbage and Kale 117
- 411. Roasted Butterbeans and Butternut Squash 118
- 412. Roasted Black Bean and Squash 118
- 413. Roasted Kidney Beans and Potato 118
- 414. Roasted Potato and Parsnips 119
- 415. Oriental Roasted Butterbeans and Butternut Squash

.... 119
416. Smoky Roasted Kidney Beans and Potatoes 120
417. Roasted Mushrooms and Potatoes 120
418. Roasted Potatoes and Sweet Potato 120
419. Roasted Butterbeans and Butternut Squash 121
420. Roasted Tomatoes and Bean Sprouts 121
421. Roasted Carrot Turnip and Parsnips 121
422. Roasted Aromatic Tomatoes 122
423, Oriental Roasted Bean Sprouts and Broccoli 122
424. Roasted Broccoli and Onion 122
425. Roasted Brussel Sprouts and Bean Sprouts 123
426. Roasted Butterbeans and Broccoli 123
427. Lemon Garlic Roasted Potatoes 123
428. Buttery Roasted Broccoli 124
429. Roasted Broccoli and Bean Sprouts 124
430. Simple and Easy Roasted Parsnips and Potato . 124
431. Baked Beets and Potato 125
432. Roasted Carrots and Sweet Potato 125
433. Roasted Broccoli and Red Beets 125
434. Roasted Cauliflower and Parsnip 126
435. Roasted Carrot and Beets 126
436. Roasted Cabbage and Beets 126

VEGAN 127
437. Vegan Tzatziki Tofu 127
438. Avocado with Low-carb Mushrooms 127
439. Stir-Fried Tofu and Peppers 127
440. Pecans-Spiced Cubed Tofu 127
441. Kale Dip with Crudités Platter 128
442. Stuffed Mushrooms topped with Vegan Parmesan
.... 128
443. Healthy Zucchini Avocado Soup 128
444. Sautéed Stuffed Mushrooms 129
445. Dark Chocolate Almond Butter Smoothie 129
446. Chanterelle Leek Stew 129
447. Parmesan Tomato Chips Bakes 130
448. Roasted Asparagus topped Baba Ghanoush 130
449. Homemade Creamy Broccoli Soup 130
450. Orange Pecans Stuffed Avocado 131
451. Pepper-Spiced Roasted Curried Cauliflower 131
452. Cashew Nuts Baked Tofu Stuffed Zucchini 131
453. Garlic-Avocado Spinach Chips 132
454. Brussels Sprouts and Tempeh Hash with Soy Dressing 132
455. Spicy Garam Masala Broccoli 132
456. Cashew Parmesan Zoodles 132
457. Summer Salad dressed with Sunflower Seed. 133
458. Cozy Rainbow Vegan Soup 133
459. Protein Quickie Smoothie 134
460. Africana Carrot Salad 134
461. Sesame-Spiced Roasted Cabbage 134
462. Low-Carb Winter Mushroom Stew 134
463. Garlic-Spiced Sautéed Savoy Cabbage 135
464. Tasty Noodles with Avocado Sauce 135
465. Creamy Sautéed Cauliflower Soup 135
466. Ethiopian Stewed Cauliflower Rice 135
467. Cauliflower and Almond Soup 136
468. Crisp Vegan Tofu 136
469. Low fat Chocolate berry Smoothie 136
470. Healthy Granola 137
471. Cauliflower Salad Delight 137
472. Strawberry Overnight Oats 137
473. 10 minutes Nuts "Cereals" 137
474. Fresh and Authentic Guacamole 138
475. Healthy homemade Granola 138
476. Baked Tofu with Asian Tomato Sauce 138
477. Plums and Chia Pudding 139
478. Sautéed Fennel with Tomato Basil Sauce 139
479. Oven-Roasted Autumn Vegetables 139
480. Creamy Eggplant Cashew Soup 140
481. Chocolate Butternut Squash Smoothie 140
482. Peanut Butter Raspberry Smoothie 140
483. Roasted Cremini Mushroom and Broccoli 140
484. Crisp Topped Vegetable Bake 141
485. Stir Fry Artichoke Tofu 141

SMOOTHIES & JUICE 142
486. Almonds & Blueberries Smoothie 142
487. Almonds and Zucchini Smoothie 142
488. bAvocado with Walnut Butter Smoothie 142
489. Baby Spinach and Dill Smoothie 142
490. Blueberries and Coconut Smoothie 142
491. Chocolate Lettuce Salad Smoothie 143
492. Collard Greens, Peppermint and Cucumber Smoothie 143
493. Creamy Dandelion Greens and Celery Smoothie 143
494. Dark Turnip Greens Smoothie 143
495. Ever Butter Pecan and Coconut Smoothie 144
496. Fresh Cucumber, Kale and Raspberry Smoothie 144
497. Fresh Lettuce and Cucumber-Lemon Smoothie 144
498. Green Coconut Smoothie 144
Instant Coffee Smoothie 145
500. Keto Blood Sugar Adjuster Smoothie 145
501. Lime Spinach Smoothie 145
502. Protein Coconut Smoothie 145
503. Strong Spinach and Hemp Smoothie 145
304. Total Almond Smoothie 146
505. Ultimate Green Mix Smoothie 146

SNACKS 147
506. Chipotle Tacos 147
507. Tasty Spinach Dip 147
508. Candied Almonds 147
509. Eggplant Tapenade 147
510. Almond and Beans Fondue 148
511. Beans in Rich Tomato Sauce 148
512. Tasty Onion Dip 148
513. Special Beans Dip 148
514. Sweet and Spicy Nuts 149
515. Delicious Corn Dip 149
516. Butternut Squash Spread 149
517. Cashew And White Bean Spread 150
518. Artichoke Spread 150
519. Olives and Eggplant Dip 150

Table of Contents

- 520. Veggie Cakes ... 150
- 521. Tomatoes Salsa ... 151
- 522. Chard Party Spread ... 151
- 523. Tomato and Bell Pepper Dip ... 151
- 524., Apple Dip ... 151
- 525. Orange and Cranberry Spread ... 152
- 526. Mexican Chili Dip ... 152
- 527. Hot Tomato and Plums Dip ... 152
- 528. Carrots and Beets Dip ... 152
- 529. Creamy Cauliflower Spread ... 153
- 530. Mango Dip ... 153
- 531. Easy Tomato Chutney ... 153
- 532. Turkish Tomato Dip ... 153
- 533. Green Tomato and Currants Dip ... 154
- 534. Plum Spread ... 154
- 535. Broccoli Dip ... 154
- 536. Easy Carrot Dip ... 154
- 537. Fennel and Cherry Tomatoes Spread ... 155
- 538. Leeks Spread ... 155
- 539. Vegan Rolls ... 155
- 540. Eggplant Appetizer ... 155
- 541. Vegan Veggie Dip ... 156
- 542. Great Bolognese Dip ... 156
- 543. Black Eyed Peas Pate ... 156
- 544. Tofu Appetizer ... 156
- 545. Hummus ... 157
- 546. Vegan Cashew Spread ... 157
- 547. Spinach Dip ... 157
- 548. Chowder ... 157
- 549. Appetizer Potato Salad ... 158
- 550. Veggie Appetizer ... 158
- 551. Black Bean Appetizer Salad ... 158
- 552. Colored Stuffed Bell Peppers ... 158
- 553. Corn Dip ... 159
- 554. Artichoke Spread ... 159
- 555. Mushroom Spread ... 159
- 556, Three Bean Dip ... 159

DESSERTS ... 161
- 557. Stewed Rhubarb ... 161
- 558. Pudding Cake ... 161
- 559. Sweet Peanut Butter Cake ... 161
- 560. Blueberry Cake ... 161
- 561. Peach Cobbler ... 162
- 562. Apple Mix ... 162
- 563. Pears And Dried Fruits Bowls ... 162
- 564, Strawberry Stew ... 162
- 565. Poached Plums ... 163
- 566, Bananas And Agave Sauce ... 163
- 567. Orange Cake ... 163
- 568. Stewed Apples ... 163
- 569. Pears And Orange Sauce ... 164
- 570. Almond Cookies ... 164
- 571. Pumpkin Cake ... 164
- 572. Strawberries Jam ... 164
- 573. Lemon Jam ... 165
- 574. Strawberries And Rhubarb Marmalade ... 165
- 575. Sweet Potatoes Pudding ... 165
- 576. Cherry Marmalade ... 165
- 577. Rice Pudding ... 165
- 578. Cinnamon Rice ... 166
- 579. Cranberry Pudding ... 166
- 580. Chocolate and Coconut Bars ... 166
- 581. Raspberry Bars ... 166
- 582. Vanilla and Blueberry Squares ... 167
- 583. Cocoa Brownies ... 167
- 584. Easy Blackberries Scones ... 167
- 585. Easy Buns ... 167
- 586. Lemon Cream ... 168
- 587. Cocoa Berries Cream ... 168
- 588. Easy Cocoa Pudding ... 168
- 589. Blueberry Crackers ... 168
- 590. Zucchini Bread ... 168
- 591. Pear Pudding ... 169
- 592. Cauliflower Pudding ... 169
- 593. Sweet Cauliflower Rice ... 169
- 594. Espresso Vanilla Dessert ... 169
- 595. Sweet Rhubarb ... 170
- 596. Pineapple and Apricots Delight ... 170
- 597. Tantalizing Apple Pie Bites ... 170
- 598. Vegan Compliant Protein Balls ... 170
- T" ... 171
- he Keto Lovers "Magical" Grain Free Granola ... 171
- 600. Pumpkin Butter Nut Cup ... 171
- 601 Unique Gingerbread Muffins ... 171
- 602. The Vegan Pumpkin Spicy Fat Bombs ... 172
- 603. The Low Carb "Matcha" Bombs ... 172
- 604. The No-Bake Keto Cheese Cake ... 172
- 695. Raspberry Chocolate Cups ... 173
- 606. Exuberant Pumpkin Fudge ... 173

1000 DAY DIET PLAN ... 174

10-TIPS FOR SUCCESS ... 197

CONCLUSION ... 198

DESCRIPTION

Sometimes, it can be difficult to eat a vegan/vegetarian diet in a modern food industry that doesn't entirely focus on making sure we're supplied with the right amounts of vitamins and minerals. With a few small changes, you can make sure that your vegan diet is the healthiest and most balanced it can be before you embark on Keto. It's probably been up to you for a while now to figure out which supplementary vitamins your body needs when you're eating vegan. Not all vegans and vegetarians get the right information about supplementing their diet, however, because not all people get the right information about supplementing their diet. Most of us are deficient in more than a few vitamins and minerals even without the healthier profile of a vegan diet. All regular diets aside, there are five important supplements that vegans across the board should take. While there are certain amounts of scientific research on which plants can offer you these same vitamins, it isn't usually in a dose high enough to make up for your body's deficit. Vitamins and supplements can also never hurt you, and you're welcome to take more than these recommended five (although, you should never raise your dosages). While you should always consult with a doctor or knowledgeable medical professional before adding new medications to your routine, each supplement here is already something your body needs.

With the help of this book, you will be able to prepare over 600 ketogenic vegetarian recipes, you also have a 1000-day meal plan for easier planning.

Happy Cooking!!!

INTRODUCTION

Being a vegetarian is not a walk in the park, and you can bet that Keto vegetarian is twice as hard as that. Very few individuals lead healthy enough lives to slide effortlessly into a vegan diet without side effects, and even fewer individuals can take on a full Keto diet without experiencing such bad side effects to the point that they're driven to quit. Although we've touched a little bit on the importance of drinking water to maintain your best possible body function, your sleep routine, exercise routine, the implication of intermittent fasting, and "Keto coffee" are all best-kept secrets to helping you stay dedicated to a Keto vegetarian diet. No matter what life changes that you're thinking about making, when it comes to relatively extreme dieting, the best thing to do first is consult with your doctor.

Let's Cook!

BREAKFAST

01. Pear Oatmeal

Preparation time: 10 minutes
Cooking time: 15 minutes
Servings: 3

Ingredients:

- 2 cups coconut milk
- ½ cup steel cut oats
- ½ teaspoon vanilla extract
- 1 pear, chopped
- ½ teaspoon maple extract
- 1 tablespoon stevia

Directions:

1. In your air fryer's pan, mix coconut milk with oats, vanilla, pear, maple extract and stevia, stir, cover and cook at 360 degrees F for 15 minutes.
2. Divide into bowls and serve for breakfast.
3. Enjoy!

Nutrition Value: calories 200, fat 5, fiber 7, carbs 14, protein 4

02. Pumpkin Oatmeal

Preparation time: 10 minutes
Cooking time: 20 minutes
Servings: 4

Ingredients:

- 1 and ½ cups water
- ½ cup pumpkin puree
- 1 teaspoon pumpkin pie spice
- 3 tablespoons stevia
- ½ cup steel cut oats

Directions:

1. In your air fryer's pan, mix water with oats, pumpkin puree, pumpkin spice and stevia, stir, cover and cook at 360 degrees F for 20 minutes
2. Divide into bowls and serve for breakfast.
3. Enjoy!

Nutrition Value: calories 211, fat 4, fiber 7, carbs 8, protein 3

03. Veggie Burrito

Preparation time: 10 minutes
Cooking time: 15 minutes
Servings: 8

Ingredients:

- 16 ounces tofu, crumbled
- 1 green bell pepper, chopped
- ¼ cup scallions, chopped
- 15 ounces canned black beans, drained
- 1 cup vegan salsa
- ½ cup water
- ¼ teaspoon cumin, ground
- ½ teaspoon turmeric powder
- ½ teaspoon smoked paprika
- A pinch of salt and black pepper
- ¼ teaspoon chili powder
- 3 cups spinach leaves, torn
- 8 vegan tortillas for serving

Directions:

1. In your air fryer, mix tofu with bell pepper, scallions, black beans, salsa, water, cumin, turmeric, paprika, salt, pepper and chili powder, stir, cover and cook at 370 degrees F for 20 minutes
2. Add spinach, toss well, divide this on your vegan tortillas, roll, wrap them and serve for breakfast.
3. Enjoy!

Nutrition Value: calories 211, fat 4, fiber 7, carbs 14, protein 4

04. Apple Steel Cut Oats

Preparation time: 10 minutes
Cooking time: 15 minutes
Servings: 6

Ingredients:

- 1 and ½ cups water
- 1 and ½ cups coconut milk
- 2 apples, cored, peeled and chopped
- 1 cup steel cut oats
- ½ teaspoon cinnamon powder
- ¼ teaspoon nutmeg, ground
- ¼ teaspoon allspice, ground
- ¼ teaspoon ginger powder
- ¼ teaspoon cardamom, ground
- 1 tablespoon flaxseed, ground
- 2 teaspoons vanilla extract
- 2 teaspoons stevia
- Cooking spray

Directions:

1. Spray your air fryer with cooking spray, add

apples, milk, water, cinnamon, oats, allspice, nutmeg, cardamom, ginger, vanilla, flaxseeds and stevia, stir, cover and cook at 360 degrees F for 15 minutes
2. Divide into bowls and serve for breakfast.
3. Enjoy!

Nutrition Value: calories 172, fat 3, fiber 7, carbs 8, protein 5

05. Tofu Casserole

Preparation time: 10 minutes
Cooking time: 20 minutes
Servings: 4

Ingredients:

- 1 teaspoon lemon zest, grated
- 14 ounces tofu, cubed
- 1 tablespoon lemon juice
- 2 tablespoons nutritional yeast
- 1 tablespoon apple cider vinegar
- 1 tablespoon olive oil
- 2 garlic cloves, minced
- 10 ounces spinach, torn
- ½ cup yellow onion, chopped
- ½ teaspoon basil, dried
- 8 ounces mushrooms, sliced
- Salt and black pepper to the taste
- ¼ teaspoon red pepper flakes
- Cooking spray

Directions:

1. Spray your air fryer with some cooking spray, arrange tofu cubes on the bottom, add lemon zest, lemon juice, yeast, vinegar, olive oil, garlic, spinach, onion, basil, mushrooms, salt, pepper and pepper flakes, toss, cover and cook at 365 degrees F for 20 minutes.
2. Divide between plates and serve for breakfast.
3. Enjoy!

Nutrition Value: calories 246, fat 6, fiber 8, carbs 12, protein 4

06. Carrot Mix

Preparation time: 10 minutes
Cooking time: 15 minutes
Servings: 4

Ingredients:

- 2 cups coconut milk
- ½ cup steel cut oats
- 1 cup carrots, shredded
- 1 teaspoon cardamom, ground
- ½ teaspoon agave nectar
- A pinch of saffron
- Cooking spray

Directions:

1. Spray your air fryer with cooking spray, add milk, oats, carrots, cardamom and agave nectar, stir, cover and cook at 365 degrees F for 15 minutes
2. Divide into bowls, sprinkle saffron on top and serve for breakfast.
3. Enjoy!

Nutrition Value: calories 202, fat 7, fiber 4, carbs 8, protein 3

07. Blueberries Oats

Preparation time: 10 minutes
Cooking time: 15 minutes
Servings: 4

Ingredients:

- 1 cup blueberries
- 1 cup steel cut oats
- 1 cup coconut milk
- 2 tablespoons agave nectar
- ½ teaspoon vanilla extract
- Cooking spray

Directions:

1. Spray your air fryer with cooking spray, add oats, milk, agave nectar, vanilla and blueberries, toss, cover and cook at 365 degrees F for 10 minutes.
2. Divide into bowls and serve for breakfast.
3. Enjoy!

Nutrition Value: calories 202, fat 6, fiber 8, carbs 9, protein 6

08. Apple and Pears Mix

Preparation time: 10 minutes
Cooking time: 15 minutes
Servings: 6

Ingredients:

- 4 apples, cored, peeled and cut into medium chunks
- 1 teaspoon lemon juice
- 4 pears, cored, peeled and cut into medium chunks
- 5 teaspoons stevia
- 1 teaspoon cinnamon powder
- 1 teaspoon vanilla extract
- ½ teaspoon ginger, ground
- ½ teaspoon cloves, ground
- ½ teaspoon cardamom, ground

Directions:
1. In your air fryer,, mix apples with pears, lemon juice, stevia, cinnamon, vanilla extract, ginger, cloves and cardamom, stir, cover, cook at 360 degrees F for 15 minutes
2. Divide into bowls and serve for breakfast.
3. Enjoy!

Nutrition Value: calories 161, fat 3, fiber 7, carbs 9, protein 4

09. Bell Pepper Oatmeal
Preparation time: 10 minutes
Cooking time: 15 minutes
Servings: 2

Ingredients:
- 1 cup steel cut oats
- 2 tablespoons canned kidney beans, drained
- 2 red bell peppers, chopped
- 4 tablespoons coconut cream
- A pinch of sweet paprika
- Salt and black pepper to the taste
- ¼ teaspoon cumin, ground

Directions:
1. Heat up your air fryer at 360 degrees F, add oats, beans, bell peppers, coconut cream, paprika, salt, pepper and cumin, stir, cover and cook for 16 minutes.
2. Divide into bowls and serve for breakfast.
3. Enjoy!

Nutrition Value: calories 173, fat 4, fiber 6, carbs 12, protein 4

10. Banana and Walnuts Oats
Preparation time: 10 minutes
Cooking time: 15 minutes
Servings: 4

Ingredients:
- 1 banana, peeled and mashed
- 1 cup steel cut oats
- 2 cups almond milk
- 2 cups water
- ¼ cup walnuts, chopped
- 2 tablespoons flaxseed meal
- 2 teaspoons cinnamon powder
- 1 teaspoon vanilla extract
- ½ teaspoon nutmeg, ground

Directions:
1. In your air fryer mix oats with almond milk, water, walnuts, flaxseed meal, cinnamon, vanilla and nutmeg, stir, cover and cook at 360 degrees F for 15 minutes.
2. Divide into bowls and serve for breakfast.
3. Enjoy!

Nutrition Value: calories 181, fat 7, fiber 6, carbs 12, protein 11

11. Simple Granola
Preparation time: 10 minutes
Cooking time: 15 minutes
Servings: 3

Ingredients:
- ½ cup granola
- ½ cup bran flakes
- 2 green apples, cored, peeled and roughly chopped
- ¼ cup apple juice
- 1/8 cup maple syrup
- 2 tablespoons cashew butter
- 1 teaspoon cinnamon powder
- ½ teaspoon nutmeg, ground

Directions:
1. In your air fryer, mix granola with bran flakes, apples, apple juice, maple syrup, cashew butter, cinnamon and nutmeg, toss, cover and cook at 365 degrees F for 15 minutes
2. Divide into bowls and serve for breakfast.
3. Enjoy!

Nutrition Value: calories 188, fat 6, fiber 9, carbs 11, protein 6

12. Zucchini Oatmeal
Preparation time: 10 minutes
Cooking time: 15 minutes
Servings: 4

Ingredients:
- ½ cup steel cut oats
- 1 carrot, grated
- 1 and ½ cups almond milk
- ¼ zucchini, grated
- ¼ teaspoon nutmeg, ground
- ¼ teaspoon cloves, ground
- ½ teaspoon cinnamon powder
- 2 tablespoons maple syrup
- ¼ cup pecans, chopped
- 1 teaspoon vanilla extract

Directions:
1. In your air fryer, mix oats with carrot, zucchini, almond milk, cloves, nutmeg, cinnamon, maple syrup, pecans and vanilla extract, stir, cover and

Breakfast

  2. Divide into bowls and serve.
  3. Enjoy!

Nutrition Value: calories 175, fat 4, fiber 7, carbs 12, protein 7

13. Cranberry Coconut Quinoa

Preparation time: 10 minutes
Cooking time: 13 minutes
Servings: 4

Ingredients:

- 1 cup quinoa
- 3 cups coconut water
- 1 teaspoon vanilla extract
- 3 teaspoons stevia
- 1/8 cup coconut flakes
- ¼ cup cranberries, dried
- 1/8 cup almonds, chopped

Directions:

1. In your air fryer, mix quinoa with coconut water, vanilla, stevia, coconut flakes, almonds and cranberries, toss, cover and cook at 365 degrees F for 13 minutes.
2. Divide into bowls and serve for breakfast.
3. Enjoy!

Nutrition Value: calories 146, fat 5, fiber 5, carbs 10, protein 7

14. Sweet Quinoa Mix

Preparation time: 10 minutes
Cooking time: 14 minutes
Servings: 6

Ingredients:

- ½ cup quinoa
- 1 and ½ cups steel cut oats
- 4 tablespoons stevia
- 4 and ½ cups almond milk
- 2 tablespoons maple syrup
- 1 and ½ teaspoons vanilla extract
- Strawberries, halved for serving
- Cooking spray

Directions:

1. Spray your air fryer with cooking spray, add oats, quinoa, stevia, almond milk, maple syrup and vanilla extract, toss, cover and cook at 365 degrees F for 14 minutes
2. Divide into bowls, add strawberries on top and serve for breakfast.
3. Enjoy!

Nutrition Value: calories 207, fat 5, fiber 8, carbs 14, protein 5

15. Chia Pudding

Preparation time: 10 minutes
Cooking time: 15 minutes
Servings: 4

Ingredients:

- 1 cup chia seeds
- 2 cups coconut milk
- 2 tablespoons coconut, shredded and unsweetened
- ¼ cup maple syrup
- ½ teaspoon cinnamon powder
- 2 teaspoons cocoa powder
- ½ teaspoon vanilla extract

Directions:

1. In your air fryer, mix chia seeds, coconut milk, coconut, maple syrup, cinnamon, cocoa powder and vanilla, toss, cover and cook at 365 degrees F for 15 minutes
2. Divide chia pudding into bowls and serve for breakfast.
3. Enjoy!

Nutrition Value: calories 261, fat 4, fiber 8, carbs 10, protein 4

16. Simple Creamy Breakfast Potatoes

Preparation time: 10 minutes
Cooking time: 20 minutes
Servings: 8

Ingredients:

- Cooking spray
- 2 pounds gold potatoes, halved and sliced
- 1 yellow onion, cut into medium wedges
- 10 ounces canned vegan potato cream soup
- 8 ounces coconut milk
- 1 cup tofu, crumbled
- ½ cup veggie stock
- Salt and black pepper to the taste

Directions:

1. Grease your air fryer's pan with cooking spray and arrange half of the potatoes on the bottom.
2. Layer onion wedges, half of the vegan cream soup, coconut milk, tofu, stock, salt and pepper.
3. Add the rest of the potatoes, onion wedges, cream, coconut milk, tofu and stock, cover and cook at 365 degrees F for 20 minutes.
4. Divide between plates and serve.

5. Enjoy!

Nutrition Value: calories 206, fat 14, fiber 4, carbs 10, protein 12

17. Sweet Potatoes Mix

Preparation time: 10 minutes
Cooking time: 20 minutes
Servings: 10

Ingredients:

- 4 pounds sweet potatoes, thinly sliced
- 3 tablespoons stevia
- ½ cup orange juice
- Salt and black pepper to the taste
- ½ teaspoon thyme, dried
- ½ teaspoon sage, dried
- 2 tablespoons olive oil

Directions:

1. Arrange potato slices on the bottom of your air fryer's pan.
2. In a bowl, mix orange juice with salt, pepper, stevia, thyme, sage and oil and whisk well.
3. Add this over potatoes, cover and cook at 365 degrees F for 20 minutes
4. Divide between plates and serve for breakfast
5. Enjoy!

Nutrition Value: calories 189, fat 4, fiber 4, carbs 16, protein 4

18. Breakfast Bowls

Preparation time: 10 minutes
Cooking time: 15 minutes
Servings: 4

Ingredients:

- 1 block firm tofu, cut into thin strips
- 1 teaspoon turmeric powder
- ¼ cup coconut aminos
- ½ teaspoon onion powder
- ½ cup nutritional yeast
- 2 tablespoons olive oil
- 1 avocado, peeled, cored and sliced
- A handful cherry tomatoes, halved
- 2 green onions, chopped
- Salt and black pepper to the taste

Directions:

1. In a bowl, mix tofu strips with turmeric, coconut aminos, onion powder, half of the oil and yeast and toss.
2. Transfer this to your preheated air fryer at 370 degrees F and cook for 15 minutes.
3. In a large bowl, mix tomatoes with green onions, salt and pepper and toss.
4. Add tofu and the rest of the oil, toss, divide between plates and serve for breakfast.
5. Enjoy!

Nutrition Value: calories 200, fat 4, fiber 6, carbs 14, protein 5

19. Mediterranean Chickpeas Breakfast

Preparation time: 10 minutes
Cooking time: 12 minutes
Servings: 2

Ingredients:

- Cooking spray
- 3 shallots, chopped
- 2 garlic cloves, minced
- ½ teaspoon sweet paprika
- ½ teaspoon smoked paprika
- ½ teaspoon cinnamon powder
- Salt and black pepper to the taste
- 2 tomatoes, chopped
- 2 cup chickpeas, cooked
- 1 tablespoon parsley, chopped

Directions:

1. Spray your air fryer with cooking spray and preheat it to 365 degrees F.
2. Add shallots, garlic, sweet and smoked paprika, cinnamon, salt, pepper, tomatoes, parsley and chickpeas, toss, cover and cook for 12 minutes.
3. Divide into bowls and serve for breakfast.
4. Enjoy!

Nutrition Value: calories 200, fat 4, fiber 6, carbs 12, protein 5

20. Pumpkin Breakfast Muffins

Preparation time: 10 minutes
Cooking time: 10 minutes
Servings: 2

Ingredients:

- 1 and ½ cups rolled oats
- ½ cup pumpkin, peeled and cubed
- ¼ cup maple syrup
- 1 teaspoon cinnamon powder
- ¼ teaspoon nutmeg, ground
- ¼ teaspoon ginger powder
- 1/3 cup cranberries

Directions:

1. In your blender, mix oats with pumpkin, maple

syrup, cinnamon, ginger and nutmeg and pulse well.
2. Fold cranberries into the mix, spoon the whole mix into muffin cups, place them in your air fryer's basket, cover and cook at 360 degrees F for 10 minutes.
3. Serve them for breakfast.
4. Enjoy!

Nutrition Value: calories 192, fat 4, fiber 5, carbs 14, protein 2

21. Delicious Porridge
Preparation time: 10 minutes
Cooking time: 16 minutes
Servings: 4

Ingredients:

- 3 cups brown rice, cooked
- 1 and ¾ cups almond milk
- 2 tablespoons coconut sugar
- 2 tablespoons flaxseed meal
- 2 tablespoons raisins
- ¼ teaspoon cinnamon powder
- ¼ teaspoon vanilla extract

Directions:

1. In your air fryer, mix rice, milk, sugar, flax meal, raisins, cinnamon and vanilla, stir, cover and cook at 360 degrees F for 16 minutes.
2. Stir porridge again, divide into bowls and serve for breakfast.
3. Enjoy!

Nutrition Value: calories 221, fat 4, fiber 6, carbs 11, protein 4

22. Strawberry Quinoa
Preparation time: 10 minutes
Cooking time: 10 minutes
Servings: 1

Ingredients:

- ¾ cup water
- 1 cup strawberries, halved
- ¼ cup cashews
- 1 stevia packet
- 1 cup quinoa

Directions:

1. In your air fryer's pan, mix water with cashews, quinoa and stevia, stir, cover and cook at 400 degrees F for 10 minutes.
2. Add strawberries, stir, divide into bowls and serve for breakfast.
3. Enjoy!

Nutrition Value: calories 177, fat 2, fiber 5, carbs 10, protein 4

23. Breakfast Broccoli and Tofu Bowls
Preparation time: 10 minutes
Cooking time: 15 minutes
Servings: 4

Ingredients:

- 1 block firm tofu, pressed and cubed
- 1 teaspoon rice vinegar
- 2 tablespoons coconut aminos
- 1 tablespoon olive oil
- 1 cup quinoa, cooked
- 4 cups broccoli florets
- 2 tablespoons vegan avocado pesto

1. **Directions:**
2. In a bowl, mix tofu cubes with vinegar, coconut aminos, oil and broccoli, toss and leave aside for 10 minutes.
3. Transfer tofu to your air fryer's basket and cook at 400 degrees F for 10 minutes.
4. Add broccoli, cover fryer again and cook for 5 minutes more.
5. Divide quinoa into bowls, add tofu and broccoli, top with avocado pesto and serve for breakfast.
6. Enjoy!

Nutrition Value: calories 188, fat 3, fiber 5, carbs 8, protein 2

24. Cool Tofu Breakfast Mix
Preparation time: 10 minutes
Cooking time: 10 minutes
Servings: 1

Ingredients:

- 3 ounces firm tofu, pressed and crumbled
- 1 cup kale, torn
- ½ cup broccoli florets
- ½ cup mushrooms, halved
- ¼ cup cherry tomatoes, halved
- ½ cup carrot, grated
- ¼ teaspoon garlic powder
- ¼ teaspoon onion powder
- ½ teaspoon yellow curry powder
- ¼ teaspoon sweet paprika
- Salt and black pepper to the taste
- Cooking spray
- ¼ cup micro greens

Directions:

1. Heat up your air fryer at 380 degrees F, grease its pan with cooking spray, add tofu, kale, broccoli, mushrooms, tomatoes, carrot, garlic powder, onion powder, curry powder, paprika, salt and pepper, toss, cover and cook for 10 minutes.
2. Divide between plates, add micro greens, toss and serve.
3. Enjoy!

Nutrition Value: calories 199, fat 2, fiber 5, carbs 12, protein 3

25. Cinnamon Oatmeal

Preparation time: 10 minutes
Cooking time: 15 minutes
Servings: 3

Ingredients:

- 3 cups water
- 1 cup steel cut oats
- 1 apple, cored and chopped
- 1 tablespoon cinnamon powder

Directions:

In your air fryer, mix water with oats, cinnamon and apple, stir, cover and cook at 365 degrees F for 15 minutes.
Stir again, divide into bowls and serve for breakfast.
Enjoy!

Nutrition Value: calories 200, fat 1, fiber 7, carbs 12, protein 10

26. Coconut Rice

Preparation time: 10 minutes
Cooking time: 15 minutes
Servings: 4

Ingredients:

- 1 cup Arborio rice
- 2 cups almond milk
- 1 cup coconut milk
- 1/3 cup agave nectar
- 2 teaspoons vanilla extract
- ¼ cup coconut flakes, toasted

Directions:

1. In your air fryer, mix rice with almond milk, coconut milk, agave nectar, vanilla extract and coconut flakes, cover and cook at 360 degrees F for 15 minutes.
2. Divide into bowls and serve warm.
3. Enjoy!

Nutrition Value: calories 192, fat 1, fiber 1, carbs 20, protein 4

27. Blackberry Pudding

Servings: 1

Ingredients:

- ½ cup unsweetened almond milk
- 1 tablespoon chia seeds
- 2 tablespoons of cocoa butter, softened at room temperature
- 1 teaspoon stevia
- 1 drop of vanilla extract
- ¼ cup fresh or frozen blackberries, chopped

Directions:

1. In medium bowl, combine chia seeds into the almond milk and cocoa butter
2. Add stevia, vanilla extract, and blackberries
3. Mix all ingredients well
4. Stir every 5 minutes for the next 15 minutes
5. Chill in a bowl for at least 4 hours or overnight

Nutrition Value: Calories: 418 Kcal, Fat: 29,8 gr, Total carbs: 10.8, Net carbs: 3, Protein 4.4 g

28. Parsley Quiche

Servings: 1

Ingredients:

- 1 tablespoon of ghee
- ½ tablespoon freshly chopped basil
- 2 medium eggs
- 1 tablespoon of Parmesan cheese, shredded
- 1 pinch of salt
- 1 pinch of paprika
- 2 tablespoons of heavy whipping cream

Directions:

1. Preheat the oven to 175 degrees and grate the cheese
2. Whisk the eggs with Parmesan, salt, paprika, ghee, and cream
3. Coat 3 small cup muffin tins with a little spray oil. Scatter basil over the bottom of each cup
4. Evenly distribute the egg mixture in the cups
5. Bake until the quiches are browned and puffed on top, for 20-30 minutes, rotating the tray halfway through
6. Let them cool for a few minutes. Eat immediately, or store in the fridge for up to 4 days.

Nutrition Value: Calories -per serving, 3 mini quiches: 397 Kcal, Fat: 31.9 gr, Total carbs: 3.8, Net carbs: 3, Protein 15.4 g

29. Coconut muffin

Servings: 1

Ingredients:

- 1 large egg
- 2 tablespoons of coconut flour
- 1 pinch baking soda
- 1 teaspoon of natural Stevia powder
- 1 pinch salt
- 1 tablespoon of cocoa butter
- 1 teaspoon coconut flakes, unsweetened
- ¼ cup of whipping cream, full fat, for topping

Directions:

1. Grease a dish with some spray oil or butter
2. In a bowl, mix all the ingredients together with a fork and ensure mixture is smooth
3. Place the dough in the greased dish and cook in the microwave on 'high' for 1 minute. If you do not have a microwave, bake in the oven, at 180° C / 350 F for 14 minutes.

Nutrition Value: Calories: 265.3 Kcal, Fat: 26.75 gr, Total carbs: 10.14, Net carbs: 8.14, Protein 17.75 g

30. Orange delight

Servings: 1

Ingredients:

- ½ cup full fat plain Greek yogurt (you can also use Skyr as an alternative)
- 1 tablespoon of natural Stevia powder (always verify that the product does not contain other sweeteners by checking the label!)
- 1 tablespoon cocoa butter
- 1 tablespoon MTC oil
- 1 teaspoon orange peel, grated

Directions:

1. Soften the cocoa butter at room temperature for 15 minutes.
2. In a food processor, combine the yogurt, coconut butter, orange peel and Stevia.
3. Nutrition Value: Calories: 225.5 Kcal, Fat: 33.75 gr, Total carbs: 7.45, Net carbs: 5.45, Protein 8.05 g

31. Egg mayonnaise

Servings: 1

Ingredients:

- 1 small boiled egg
- 1 tablespoon of mayonnaise
- 1 tablespoon avocado oil
- Salt and pepper
- 1 pinch of paprika

Directions:

1. Hard boil the egg
2. In a small bowl, mash the peeled egg adding all the other ingredients
3. Season to pleasure

Nutrition Value: Calories: 456 Kcal, Fat: 42 gr, Total carbs: 0.76, Net carbs: 0.76, Protein 13.05 g

32. Strawberry Choco shake

Servings: 1

Ingredients:

- 1 cup unsweetened coconut milk
- ¼ cup strawberries, fresh or frozen
- 1 tablespoon cocoa powder, unsweetened
- 2 tablespoons cocoa butter
- 12 drops liquid Stevia
- ¼ teaspoon xanthan gum

Directions:

1. Combine all ingredients in a blender and mix on high for about 30 seconds.

Nutrition Value: Calories per serving: 297 Kcal, Fat: 34.17 gr, Total carbs: 11.7, Net carbs: 4.8, Protein 2.62 g

33. Lemon jelly

Servings: 1

Ingredients:

- 1/4 cup of coconut milk
- ½ teaspoon agar agar (gelatine can also be used)
- 1 tablespoon ghee
- 1 tablespoon cocoa butter
- Lemon aroma
- 1 teaspoon of Stevia sweetener

Directions:

1. Heat up on low flame the coconut milk with the cocoa butter, ghee, aroma, and sweetener
2. Add the agar agar and boil for 3-4 minutes
3. Put the mixture in a jelly mold and allow to cool overnight until it becomes hard. Then cut in pieces (about 4 slices)

Nutrition Value: Calories: 68 Kcal, Fat: 34.8 gr, Total carbs: 1.6, Net carbs: 1.6, Protein 0.8 g

34. Strawberry mug cake

Servings: 1

Ingredients:

- 2 tablespoons almond flour
- 1 tablespoon coconut flour
- 1/4 teaspoon baking powder
- 1 dash salt

- 1 tablespoon fresh or frozen strawberries
- 1 tablespoon coconut oil melted
- 1 tablespoon heavy cream
- 1 small egg
- 1 teaspoon natural Stevia
- 1 drop vanilla extract
- 1 drop lemon extract

Directions:
1. Mix together almond flour, coconut flour, baking powder, and salt in small bowl. Stir in strawberries
2. Melt coconut oil in a small microwaveable bowl. Stir in heavy cream, egg, sweetener, and extracts into melted coconut.
3. Mix the dry ingredients into the liquid dough with a fork and combine well
4. Divide batter in two lightly buttered ramekins
5. Microwave on high from 1 1/2 minutes to 2 minutes or until cake is no longer wet

Nutrition Value: Calories: 219 Kcal, Fat: 19.5 gr, Total carbs: 6.2, Net carbs: 3.7, Protein 5.4 g

35. Fluffy cinnamon muffin

Servings: 1

Ingredients:
- 1 large egg
- 2 tablespoons coconut flour
- 1 pinch baking soda
- 1 teaspoon of natural Stevia powder
- 1 pinch salt
- 1 teaspoon cinnamon powder

Directions:
1. Grease a muffin dish with cooking spray oil or butter
2. In a bowl, mix all the ingredients together with a fork to ensure you have a smooth mixture
3. Place the dough in the greased dish and cook in the microwave on 'high' for 1 minute. If you do not have a microwave, bake in the oven, at 180° C / 350 F for 14 minutes

Nutrition Value: Calories: 113 Kcal, Fat: 6 gr, Total carbs: 6.25, Net carbs: 2.7, Protein 7 g

36. Cappuccino Shake

Servings: 1

Ingredients:
- 1 cup of Unsweetened Almond milk
- 1 freshly brewed espresso coffee
- 1 cup of ice
- 1 tablespoon of cocoa butter
- 1 tablespoon coconut oil
- 1 teaspoon xanthan gum
- 1 teaspoon of Stevia powder
- 1 pinch of dark unsweetened cocoa for topping

Directions:
1. Pour almond milk into a blender and add ice, and the other ingredients. Blend until smooth and pour into glasses.

Nutrition Value: Calories: 269.68 Kcal, Fat: 31 gr, Total carbs: 2, Net carbs: 2, Protein 1 g

37. Lemon Cheese Smoothie

Ingredients:
- 1/3 cup of coconut milk
- 1 cup of ice
- 1 tablespoon lactose-free Mascarpone cheese
- 1 tablespoon vanilla-flavored vegan protein powder
- 1 teaspoon freshly squeezed lemon juice
- 1 tablespoon heavy whipping cream
- 1 tablespoon cocoa butter
- 1 drop of lemon zest extract
- 1 teaspoon stevia powder (optional)

Directions:
- Pour coconut milk into a blender and add all of the ingredients. Blend until smooth and pour into glass.

Nutrition Value: Calories: 374 Kcal, Fat: 31.37 gr, Total carbs: 8.54, Net carbs: 1.96, Protein 12.81 g

38.. Zucchini tasty chips

Servings: 1

Ingredients:
1 small zucchini
2 tablespoons olive oil or avocado oil
1 teaspoon apple cider vinegar or vinegar of choice
1 pinch of salt and pepper

Directions:

Slice the zucchini very thin. Use a mandoline slicer to get the shape of long chips
Remove excess moisture from slices using a paper towel
Put slices in a large bowl and toss with oil, vinegar, and salt
Place slices on parchment lined baking tray. Dry at 175°F/100°C for 3-4 hours or until crispy

Nutrition Value: Calories: 50 Kcal, Fat: 28 gr, Total carbs: 3, Net carbs: 3, Protein 0 g

39. Blackberry avocmado Mousse

Servings: 1

Ingredients:

- ½ medium avocado
- 1 tablespoon cocoa butter
- 1 tablespoon vegan protein powder, chocolate flavor
- 1 tablespoon frozen blackberries
- 1 tablespoon cream
- 1 drop pure vanilla extract
- 2 tablespoons of water
- 3 cubes of ice

Directions:

2. Mix everything with a kitchen robot, adding cubes of ice
3. Put to rest in the fridge for 1 hour to thicken it
4. If the mousse becomes too thick, mix it with a tablespoon of unsweetened soy milk

Nutrition Value: Calories: 377 Kcal, Fat: 49.2 gr, Total carbs: 15, Net carbs: 5, Protein 6.1 g

40. Queso crunch

Servings: 1

Ingredients:

For the cereal:

- 2 tablespoons Queso fresco (any Mexican frying cheese will work)
- 1 small cucumber
- 1 teaspoon of Stevia
- ½ tablespoon of butter
- 1 pinch of pepper and salt

For the Coating:

- 1 teaspoon of stevia powder

Directions:

1. Mix cheese and cucumber in a food mixer
2. Add melted butter and stevia to combine
3. Lay out the mixture onto a greased baking sheet and spread as thick as preferred. Make sure it is even to ensure even heating
4. Lay another baking sheet on top and place it in a 220° C/450 F oven for 8 minutes
5. Remove top baking sheet and bake for additional 2 minutes
6. Remove pan and gently cut the layer into square pieces. It will still be soft so be careful when cutting
7. Remove any fully cooked pieces (usually around the edge) and place back into the oven for additional 7 minutes

Nutrition Value: Calories: 108.5 Kcal, Fat: 21.5 gr, Total carbs: 4, Net carbs: 2, Protein 8 g

41. Cocoa butter balls

Servings: 1

Ingredients:

- 2 tablespoons cocoa butter
- 1 tablespoon vanilla vegan protein powder
- 2 tablespoons unsweetened flaked coconut
- 1 teaspoon sugar-free chocolate chips
- 1 pinch natural Stevia

Directions:

1. Mix all ingredients together in medium bowl until well combined
2. Scoop and form into balls about a tablespoon in size
3. Cover and store in the refrigerator for the night

Nutrition Value: Calories per serving: 3 balls: 234 Kcal, Fat: 14 gr, Total carbs: 12, Net carbs: 6, Protein 9 g

42. Choco Cheese Mousse

Servings: 1

Ingredients:

- 1/3 cup of Silk Original Unsweetened Almond milk
- 1 cup of ice
- 1 tablespoon lactose-free Mascarpone cheese
- 1 tablespoon chocolate flavor vegan protein powder
- 1 tablespoon heavy whipping cream
- 1 tablespoon cocoa butter
- 1 drop of vanilla extract
- 1 teaspoon stevia powder (optional)

Directions:

1. Pour almond milk into a blender and add ice, protein powder, cream, mascarpone, vanilla extract, and stevia powder in that order. Blend until smooth and pour into glasses.

Nutrition Value: Calories: 374 Kcal, Fat: 31.37 gr, Total carbs: 8.54, Net carbs: 1.96, Protein 15.81 g

43. Hot cheese crackers

Servings: 1

Ingredients:

- ½ cup Swiss cheese
- 1 teaspoon hot chili powder
- 1 pinch of salt and pepper

Directions:

1. Preheat the oven to 350°F/180°C and line a baking tray with baking paper
2. Cut Swiss cheese in fine strips and lay them on the baking tray

3. Sprinkle with the chili
4. Bake in the oven for 10-12 minutes until the cheese has a brown color
5. Use a paper towel to absorb the excess oil and let it cool
6. Season to taste

Nutrition Value: Calories per serving: 512 Kcal, Fat: 40.4 gr, Total carbs: 1.4, Net carbs: 1.4, Protein 34.4 g

44. Cinnamon pudding

Ingredients:
- 2 cups of coconut milk
- 2 tablespoons of erythritol
- 2 tablespoons of cocoa butter
- 1 pinch of cinnamon powder
- 2 teaspoons of glucomannan powder

Directions:
1. Combine milk with cinnamon and sweetener
2. Slowly, to avoid lumps, join glucomannan
3. Microwave for a minute and half avoiding high-temperature mode boiling.
4. Rest in the fridge for a few hours, until its cold
5. Garnish with some more cinnamon powder

Nutrition Value: Calories: 402 Kcal, Fat: 34.3 gr, Total carbs: 6.09, Net carbs: 3.47, Protein 3.25 g

45. Saffron avocado paste

Servings: 1

Ingredients:
- 1 small boiled egg
- 3 tablespoons of avocado, ripe
- 1 tablespoon of avocado oil
- Salt and pepper
- 2 pinches of saffron powder

Directions:
1. Hard boil the egg
2. In a small bowl, mash the peeled egg adding all the other ingredients
3. Season to pleasure

Nutrition Value: Calories: 422 Kcal, Fat: 46 gr, Total carbs: 1.76, Net carbs: 1.76, Protein 9.05 g

LUNCH

46. Rich Chickpeas And Lentils Soup

Preparation time: 10 minutes
Cooking time: 5 hours
Servings: 6

Ingredients:

- 1 yellow onion, chopped
- 1 tablespoon olive oil
- 1 tablespoon garlic, minced
- 1 teaspoons sweet paprika
- 1 teaspoon smoked paprika
- Salt and black pepper to the taste
- 1 cup red lentils
- 15 ounces canned chickpeas, drained
- 4 cups veggie stock
- 29 ounces canned tomatoes and juice

Directions:

1. In your slow cooker, mix onion with oil, garlic, sweet and smoked paprika, salt, pepper, lentils, chickpeas, stock and tomatoes, stir, cover and cook on High for 5 hours.
2. Ladle into bowls and serve hot.
3. Enjoy!

Nutrition Value: calories 341, fat 5, fiber 8, carbs 19, protein 3

47. Chard And Sweet Potato Soup

Preparation time: 10 minutes
Cooking time: 8 hours
Servings: 6

Ingredients:

- 1 yellow onion, chopped
- 1 tablespoon olive oil
- 1 carrot, chopped
- 1 celery stalk, chopped
- 1 bunch Swiss chard, leaves torn
- 2 garlic cloves, minced
- 4 sweet potatoes, cubed
- 1 cup brown lentils, dried
- 6 cups veggie stock
- 1 tablespoon coconut aminos
- Salt and black pepper to the taste

Directions:

- In your slow cooker, mix oil with onion, carrot, celery, chard, garlic, potatoes, lentils, stock, salt, pepper and aminos, stir, cover and cook on Low for 8 hours.
- Ladle soup into bowls and serve right away.
- Enjoy!

Nutrition Value: calories 312, fat 5, fiber 7, carbs 10, protein 5

48. Chinese Soup And Ginger Sauce

Preparation time: 10 minutes
Cooking time: 8 hours
Servings: 6

Ingredients:

- 2 celery stalks, chopped
- 1 yellow onion, chopped
- 1 cup carrot, chopped
- 8 ounces water chestnuts
- 8 ounces canned bamboo shoots, drained
- 2 teaspoons garlic, minced
- 2 teaspoons ginger paste
- ½ teaspoon red pepper flakes
- 3 tablespoons coconut aminos
- 1-quart veggie stock
- 2 bunches bok choy, chopped
- 5 ounces white mushrooms, sliced
- 8 ounces tofu, drained and cubed
- 1 ounce snow peas, cut into small pieces
- 6 scallions, chopped

For the ginger sauce:

- 1 teaspoon sesame oil
- 2 tablespoons ginger paste
- 2 tablespoons agave syrup
- 2 tablespoon coconut aminos

Directions:

1. In your slow cooker, mix onion with carrot, celery, chestnuts, bamboo shoots, garlic paste, 2 teaspoons ginger paste, pepper flakes, 3 tablespoons coconut aminos, stock, bok choy, mushrooms, tofu, snow peas and scallions, stir, cover and cook on Low for 8 hours.
2. In a bowl, mix 2 tablespoons ginger paste with agave syrup, 2 tablespoons coconut aminos and sesame oil and whisk well.
3. Ladle Chinese soup into bowls, add ginger sauce on top and serve.
4. Enjoy!

Nutrition Value: calories 300, fat 4, fiber 6, carbs 19, protein 4

49. Corn Cream Soup

Preparation time: 10 minutes
Cooking time: 8 hours and 10 minutes
Servings: 6

Ingredients:

- 1 yellow onion, chopped
- 2 tablespoons olive oil
- 1 red bell pepper, chopped
- 3 cups gold potatoes, chopped
- 4 cups corn kernels
- 4 cups veggie stock
- ½ teaspoon smoked paprika
- 1 teaspoon cumin, ground
- Salt and black pepper to the taste
- 1 cup almond milk
- 2 scallions, chopped

Directions:

1. Heat up a pan with the oil over medium high heat, add onion, stir and cook for 5-6 minutes.
2. Transfer this to your slow cooker, add bell pepper, potatoes, 3 cups corn, stock, paprika, cumin, salt and pepper, stir, cover and cook on Low for 7 hours and 30 minutes.
3. Blend soup using an immersion blender, add almond milk and blend again.
4. Add the rest of the corn, cover pot and cook on Low for 30 minutes more.
5. Ladle soup into bowls, sprinkle scallions on top and serve.
6. Enjoy!

Nutrition Value: calories 312, fat 4, fiber 6, carbs 12, protein 4

50. Veggie Medley

Preparation time: 10 minutes
Cooking time: 4 hours
Servings: 6

Ingredients:

- 1 tablespoon ginger, grated
- 3 garlic cloves, minced
- 1 date, pitted and chopped
- 1 and ½ teaspoon coriander, ground
- ½ teaspoon dry mustard
- 1 and ¼ teaspoon cumin, ground
- A pinch of salt and black pepper
- ½ teaspoon turmeric powder
- 1 tablespoon white wine vinegar
- ¼ teaspoon cardamom, ground
- 2 carrots, chopped
- 1 yellow onion, chopped
- 4 cups cauliflower florets
- 1 and ½ cups kidney beans, cooked
- 2 zucchinis, chopped
- 6 ounces tomato paste
- 1 green bell pepper, chopped
- 1 cup green peas

Directions:

1. In your slow cooker, mix ginger with garlic, date, coriander, dry mustard, cumin, salt, pepper, turmeric, vinegar, cardamom, carrots, onion, cauliflower, kidney beans, zucchinis, tomato paste, bell pepper and peas, stir, cover and cook on High for 4 hours.
2. Divide into bowls and serve hot.
3. Enjoy!

Nutrition Value: calories 165, fat 2, fiber 10, carbs 32, protein 9

51. Lentils Curry

Preparation time: 10 minutes
Cooking time: 6 hours
Servings: 8

Ingredients:

- 10 ounces spinach
- 2 cups red lentils
- 1 tablespoon garlic, minced
- 15 ounces canned tomatoes, chopped
- 2 cups cauliflower florets
- 1 teaspoon ginger, grated
- 1 yellow onion, chopped
- 4 cups veggie stock
- 2 tablespoons curry paste
- ½ teaspoon cumin, ground
- ½ teaspoon coriander, ground
- 2 teaspoons stevia
- A pinch of salt and black pepper
- ¼ cup cilantro, chopped
- 1 tablespoon lime juice

Directions:

1. In your slow cooker, mix spinach with lentils, garlic, tomatoes, cauliflower, ginger, onion, stock, curry paste, cumin, coriander, stevia, salt, pepper and lime juice, stir, cover and cook on Low for 6 hours.
2. Add cilantro, stir, divide into bowls and serve.
3. Enjoy!

Nutrition Value: calories 105, fat 1, fiber 7, carbs 22, protein 7

52. Lentils Dal

Preparation time: 10 minutes
Cooking time: 5 hours
Servings: 12

Ingredients:

- 6 cups water
- 3 cups red lentils
- 28 ounces canned tomatoes, chopped
- 1 yellow onion, chopped
- 4 garlic cloves, minced
- 1 tablespoon turmeric powder
- 2 tablespoons ginger, grated
- 3 cardamom pods
- 1 bay leaf
- 2 teaspoons mustard seeds
- 2 teaspoons onion seeds
- 2 teaspoons fenugreek seeds
- 1 teaspoon fennel seeds
- Salt and black pepper to the taste

Directions:

1. In your slow cooker, mix water with lentils, tomatoes, onion, garlic, turmeric, ginger, cardamom, bay leaf, mustard seeds, onion seeds, fenugreek seeds, fennel seeds, salt and pepper, stir, cover and cook on High for 5 hours.
2. Divide into bowls and serve.
3. Enjoy!

Nutrition Value: calories 283, fat 4, fiber 8, carbs 12, protein 4

53. Rich Jackfruit Dish

Preparation time: 10 minutes
Cooking time: 6 hours
Servings: 4

Ingredients:

- ½ cup tamari
- 40 ounces canned young jackfruit, drained
- ¼ cup coconut aminos
- 1 cup mirin
- ½ cup agave nectar
- 8 garlic cloves, minced
- 2 tablespoons ginger, grated
- 1 yellow onion, chopped
- 4 tablespoons sesame oil
- 1 green pear, cored and chopped
- ½ cup water

Directions:

1. In your slow cooker, mix tamari with jackfruit, aminos, mirin, agave nectar, garlic, ginger, onion, sesame oil, water and pear, stir, cover and cook on Low for 6 hours.
2. Divide into bowls and serve.
3. Enjoy!

Nutrition Value: calories 160, fat 4, fiber 1, carbs 20, protein 4

54. Vegan Gumbo

Preparation time: 10 minutes
Cooking time: 8 hours
Servings: 4

Ingredients:

- 2 tablespoons olive oil
- 1 green bell pepper, chopped
- 1 yellow onion, chopped
- 2 celery stalks, chopped
- 3 garlic cloves, minced
- 15 ounces canned tomatoes, chopped
- 2 cups veggie stock
- 8 ounces white mushrooms, sliced
- 15 ounces canned kidney beans, drained
- 1 zucchini, chopped
- 1 tablespoon Cajun seasoning
- Salt and black pepper to the taste

Directions:

1. In your slow cooker, mix oil with bell pepper, onion, celery, garlic, tomatoes, stock, mushrooms, beans, zucchini, Cajun seasoning, salt and pepper, stir, cover and cook on Low for 8 hours
2. Divide into bowls and serve hot.
3. Enjoy!

Nutrition Value: calories 312, fat 4, fiber 7, carbs 19, protein 4

55. Eggplant Salad

Preparation time: 10 minutes
Cooking time: 8 hours
Servings: 4

Ingredients:

- 24 ounces canned tomatoes, chopped
- 1 red onion, chopped
- 2 red bell peppers, chopped
- 1 big eggplant, roughly chopped
- 1 tablespoon smoked paprika
- 2 teaspoons cumin, ground
- Salt and black pepper to the taste
- Juice of 1 lemon

- 1 tablespoons parsley, chopped

Directions:
1. In your slow cooker, mix tomatoes with onion, bell peppers, eggplant, smoked paprika, cumin, salt, pepper and lemon juice, stir, cover and cook on Low for 8 hours
2. Add parsley, stir, divide into bowls and serve cold as a dinner salad.
3. Enjoy!

Nutrition Value: calories 251, fat 4, fiber 6, carbs 8, protein 3

56. Corn And Cabbage Soup
Preparation time: 10 minutes
Cooking time: 7 hours
Servings: 4

Ingredients:
- 1 small yellow onion, chopped
- 1 tablespoon olive oil
- 2 garlic cloves, minced
- 1 and ½ cups mushrooms, sliced
- 3 teaspoons ginger, grated
- A pinch of salt and black pepper
- 2 cups corn kernels
- 4 cups red cabbage, chopped
- 4 cups water
- 1 tablespoon nutritional yeast
- 2 teaspoons tomato paste
- 1 teaspoon sesame oil
- 1 teaspoon coconut aminos
- 1 teaspoon sriracha sauce

Directions:
1. In your slow cooker, mix olive oil with onion, garlic, mushrooms, ginger, salt, pepper, corn, cabbage, water, yeast and tomato paste, stir, cover and cook on Low for 7 hours.
2. Add sriracha sauce and aminos, stir, leave soup aside for a few minutes, ladle into bowls, drizzle sesame oil all over and serve.
3. Enjoy!

Nutrition Value: calories 300, fat 4, fiber 4, carbs 10, protein 4

57. Okra Soup
Preparation time: 10 minutes
Cooking time: 5 hours
Servings: 6

Ingredients:
- 1 green bell pepper, chopped
- 1 small yellow onion, chopped
- 3 cups veggie stock
- 3 garlic cloves, minced
- 16 ounces okra, sliced
- 2 cup corn
- 29 ounces canned tomatoes, crushed
- 1 and ½ teaspoon smoked paprika
- 1 teaspoon marjoram, dried
- 1 teaspoon thyme, dried
- 1 teaspoon oregano, dried
- Salt and black pepper to the taste

Directions:
1. In your slow cooker, mix bell pepper with onion, stock, garlic, okra, corn, tomatoes, smoked paprika, marjoram, thyme, oregano, salt and pepper, stir, cover and cook on High for 5 hours.
2. Ladle into bowls and serve.
3. Enjoy!

Nutrition Value: calories 243, fat 4, fiber 6, carbs 10, protein 3

58. Carrot Soup
Preparation time: 10 minutes
Cooking time: 5 hours
Servings: 6

Ingredients:
- 2 potatoes, cubed
- 3 pounds carrots, cubed
- 1 yellow onion, chopped
- 1-quart veggie stock
- Salt and black pepper to the taste
- 1 teaspoon thyme, dried
- 3 tablespoons coconut milk
- 2 teaspoons curry powder
- 3 tablespoons vegan cheese, crumbled
- A handful pistachios, chopped

Directions:
1. In your slow cooker, mix onion with potatoes, carrots, stock, salt, pepper, thyme and curry powder, stir, cover, cook on High for 1 hour and on Low for 4 hours.
2. Add coconut milk, stir, blend soup using an immersion blender, ladle soup into bowls, sprinkle vegan cheese and pistachios on top and serve.
3. Enjoy!

Nutrition Value: calories 241, fat 4, fiber 7, carbs 10, protein 4

59. Baby Carrots And Coconut Soup

Preparation time: 10 minutes
Cooking time: 7 hours
Servings: 6

Ingredients:

- 1 sweet potato, cubed
- 2 pounds baby carrots, peeled
- 2 teaspoons ginger paste
- 1 yellow onion, chopped
- 4 cups veggie stock
- 2 teaspoons curry powder
- Salt and black pepper to the taste
- 14 ounces coconut milk

Directions:

1. In your slow cooker, mix sweet potato with baby carrots, ginger paste, onion, stock, curry powder, salt and pepper, stir, cover and cook on High for 7 hours.
2. Add coconut milk, blend soup using an immersion blender, divide soup into bowls and serve.
3. Enjoy!

Nutrition Value: calories 100, fat 2, fiber 4, carbs 18, protein 3

60. Chinese Carrot Cream

Preparation time: 10 minutes
Cooking time: 5 hours
Servings: 6

Ingredients:

- 1 tablespoon coconut oil
- 3 garlic cloves, minced
- 1 yellow onion, chopped
- 1 pound carrots, chopped
- 2 cups veggie stock
- 2 cups water
- Salt and black pepper to the taste
- 1/3 cup peanut butter
- 2 teaspoons chili sauce

Directions:

1. In your slow cooker, mix oil with garlic, onion, carrots, stock, water, salt, pepper and chili sauce, stir, cover and cook on High for 4 hours and 30 minutes.
2. Add peanut butter, stir, cover, cook soup for 30 minutes more, blend using an immersion blender, divide soup into bowls and serve.
3. Enjoy!

Nutrition Value: calories 224, fat 14, fiber 6, carbs 18, protein 7

61. Seitan Stew

Preparation time: 10 minutes
Cooking time: 7 hours
Servings: 4

Ingredients:

- 1 pound seitan, chopped
- 2 tablespoons coconut aminos
- 1 yellow onion, chopped
- 5 cups veggie stock
- 2 tomatoes, chopped
- 3 garlic cloves, minced
- 3 potatoes, cubed
- 3 carrots, chopped
- 2 celery stalks, chopped
- Salt and black pepper to the taste

Directions:

1. In your slow cooker, mix seitan with aminos, onion, stock, tomatoes, garlic, potatoes, carrots, celery, salt and pepper, stir, cover and cook on Low for 7 hours.
2. Divide into bowls and serve.
3. Enjoy!

Nutrition Value: calories 300, fat 4, fiber 6, carbs 12, protein 3

62. Spicy Carrot Stew

Preparation time: 10 minutes
Cooking time: 3 hours
Servings: 6

Ingredients:

- 1 pound carrots, peeled and cut with a spiralizer
- 1 cup red onion, chopped
- 2 garlic cloves, minced
- 2 celery ribs, chopped
- 1 teaspoon coriander, ground
- 1 teaspoon cumin, ground
- ½ teaspoon turmeric, ground
- A pinch of cinnamon powder
- Salt and black pepper to the taste
- 1 cup water
- 4 cups veggie stock
- 1 cup lentils
- 15 ounces canned tomatoes, chopped
- 1 tablespoon tomato paste
- ¼ cup cilantro, chopped
- 1 tablespoon spicy red pepper sauce
- 1 tablespoon lemon juice

Directions:

1. In your slow cooker, mix carrots with onion, garlic, celery, coriander, cumin, turmeric, cinnamon, salt, pepper, water, stock, lentils, tomatoes, tomato paste and pepper sauce, stir, cover and cook on High for 3 hours.
2. Add lemon juice and cilantro, stir, divide into bowls and serve.
3. Enjoy!

Nutrition Value: calories 218, fat 4, fiber 4, carbs 8, protein 3

63. Tomato Soup

Preparation time: 10 minutes
Cooking time: 4 hours
Servings: 6

Ingredients:

- Zztjj[['po

Directions:

1. In your slow cooker, mix tomatoes with veggie stock, onion, tomato paste, basil, cumin, salt and pepper, stir, cover and cook on Low for 4 hours.
2. Add almond milk, blend soup using an immersion blender, ladle into bowls and serve.
3. Enjoy!

Nutrition Value: calories 212, fat 4, fiber 4, carbs 8, protein 5

64. Classic Tomato Soup

Preparation time: 10 minutes
Cooking time: 8 hours
Servings: 4

Ingredients:

- 1 tablespoon olive oil
- 1 teaspoon garlic, minced
- 1 red bell pepper, chopped
- 1 yellow onion, chopped
- 45 ounces canned tomatoes, chopped
- 1 cup veggie stock
- Salt and black pepper to the taste
- A pinch of red pepper flakes
- 1 tablespoon basil, chopped

Directions:

1. In your slow cooker, mix oil with onion, bell pepper, garlic, tomatoes, stock, salt and pepper, stir, cover and cook on Low for 8 hours.
2. Blend using an immersion blender, add pepper flakes and basil, stir, ladle into bowls and serve.
3. Enjoy!

Nutrition Value: calories 100, fat 2, fiber 4, carbs 8, protein 4

65. Collard Greens Mix

Preparation time: 10 minutes
Cooking time: 3 hours
Servings: 6

Ingredients:

- 1 yellow onion, chopped
- 10 cups collard greens, chopped
- 7 garlic cloves, minced
- 1 cup veggie stock
- 2 tablespoons apple cider vinegar
- 1 tablespoon smoked paprika
- 1 tablespoon chili powder
- A pinch of cayenne pepper
- 1 tablespoon coconut aminos

Directions:

1. In your slow cooker, mix onion with collard greens, garlic, stock, vinegar, paprika, chili powder, cayenne and aminos, stir, cover and cook on Low for 3 hours.
2. Divide between plates and serve.
3. Enjoy!

Nutrition Value: calories 172, fat 4, fiber 4, carbs 8, protein 4

66. Colored Collard Greens Dish

Preparation time: 10 minutes
Cooking time: 8 hours
Servings: 12

Ingredients:

- 28 ounces veggie stock
- 2 pounds collard greens, chopped
- 2 tablespoons stevia
- ½ cup yellow onion, chopped
- 2 tablespoons apple cider vinegar
- 1 teaspoon red pepper, crushed
- Salt and black pepper to the taste
- 15 ounces canned tomatoes, chopped
- 1 teaspoon smoked paprika
- 1 tablespoon cilantro, chopped

Directions:

1. In your slow cooker, mix collard greens with stock, stevia, onion, vinegar, red pepper, salt, pepper, tomatoes and paprika, stir, cover and cook on Low for 8 hours.
2. Add cilantro, stir, divide on plates and serve.
3. Enjoy!

Nutrition Value: calories 200, fat 3, fiber 5, carbs 8,

protein 3

67. Chinese Collard Greens Mix
Preparation time: 10 minutes
Cooking time: 3 hours
Servings: 4

Ingredients:
- 1 cup sweet onion, chopped
- 2 tablespoons olive oil
- 4 garlic cloves, minced
- 4 cups collard greens, chopped
- 1 tablespoon red miso paste
- ¼ cup parsley, chopped
- 1 cup water

Directions:
1. In your slow cooker, mix onion with oil, garlic, collard greens, water and miso paste, stir, cover, cook on High for 1 hour and on Low for 2 hours more.
2. Add parsley, stir, divide between plates and serve.
3. Enjoy!

Nutrition Value: calories 200, fat 2, fiber 3, carbs 6, protein 3

68. Fresh Collard Greens Mix
Preparation time: 10 minutes
Cooking time: 3 hours
Servings: 4

Ingredients:
- 8 cups collard greens, chopped
- 3 tablespoons olive oil
- 1 red onion, chopped
- 2 garlic cloves, minced
- 4 carrots, chopped
- 1 chipotle pepper, chopped
- 1 cup veggie stock
- A pinch of smoked sea salt

Directions:
1. In your slow cooker, mix collard greens with oil, onion, garlic, carrots, chipotle pepper, stock and salt, stir a bit, cover and cook on Low for 3 hours.
2. Divide between plates and serve.
3. Enjoy!

Nutrition Value: calories 234, fat 12, fiber 4, carbs 20, protein 5

69. Artichoke Soup
Preparation time: 10 minutes
Cooking time: 8 hours
Servings: 4

Ingredients:
- 2 celery stalks, chopped
- 1 carrot, chopped
- 1 yellow onion, chopped
- 3 garlic cloves, minced
- ½ teaspoon oregano, dried
- ½ teaspoon rosemary, dried
- ½ teaspoon fennel seeds
- ½ teaspoon thyme, dried
- A pinch of red pepper flakes
- ½ teaspoon garlic powder
- A pinch of salt and black pepper
- 40 ounces canned artichoke hearts, drained and chopped
- 5 and ½ cups veggie stock

Directions:
1. In your slow cooker, mix celery with carrot, onion, garlic, oregano, rosemary, fennel seeds, thyme, pepper flakes, garlic powder, salt, pepper, stock and artichokes, stir, cover and cook on Low for 8 hours.
2. Blend using an immersion blender, ladle into bowls and serve.
3. Enjoy!

Nutrition Value: calories 212, fat 3, fiber 5, carbs 6, protein 5

70. Intense Beet Soup
Preparation time: 10 minutes
Cooking time: 9 hours
Servings: 6

Ingredients:
- 4 beets, chopped
- 28 ounces canned tomatoes, chopped
- 2 potatoes, chopped
- 1 cup baby carrots, chopped
- 3 garlic cloves, minced
- 1 yellow onion, chopped
- Salt and black pepper to the taste
- 1 tablespoon parsley, chopped
- 1 and ½ teaspoons dill, dried
- 1 bay leaf
- 2 tablespoons stevia
- 6 tablespoons red vinegar
- 3 cups green cabbage
- 6 ounces tomato paste

Directions:

1. In your slow cooker, mix beets with tomatoes, potatoes, baby carrots, onion, salt, pepper, dill, bay leaf, stevia, vinegar, tomato paste and green cabbage, stir, cover and cook on Low for 8 hours.
2. Blend soup a bit using an immersion blender, add parsley, stir a bit, ladle into bowls and serve.
3. Enjoy!

Nutrition Value: calories 200, fat 3, fiber 6, carbs 5, protein 6

71. Brussels Sprouts Delight

Preparation time: 10 minutes
Cooking time: 3 hours
Servings: 4

Ingredients:

- 2 pounds Brussels sprouts, halved
- 1 tablespoon almonds, toasted and chopped
- 1 teaspoon red pepper flakes
- ¼ cup coconut aminos
- 2 tablespoons sriracha sauce
- 2 teaspoons garlic powder
- 1 teaspoon onion powder
- 1 tablespoon sweet paprika
- 2 tablespoons sesame oil
- 1 tablespoon balsamic vinegar
- A pinch of salt and black pepper

Directions:

1. In your slow cooker, mix Brussels sprouts with almonds, pepper flakes, aminos, sriracha sauce, garlic powder, onion powder, paprika, oil, vinegar salt and pepper, stir, cover and cook on Low for 3 hours.
2. Divide between plates and serve.
3. Enjoy!

Nutrition Value: calories 202, fat 4, fiber 3, carbs 13, protein 3

72. Mushroom Soup

Preparation time: 10 minutes
Cooking time: 5 hours
Servings: 6

Ingredients:

- 2 yellow onions, chopped
- ¼ cup barley
- 4 cups veggie stock
- 6 ounces brown mushrooms, halved
- A pinch of salt and black pepper
- 3 garlic cloves, minced
- 2 teaspoons thyme, chopped
- 12 ounces cabbage, shredded
- ½ teaspoon smoked paprika
- 4 cups water
- 1 tablespoon lemon juice

Directions:

1. In your slow cooker, mix onion with barley, stock, mushrooms, salt, pepper, garlic, thyme, cabbage, paprika, water and lemon juice, stir, cover and cook on High for 5 hours.
2. Divide soup into bowls and serve.
3. Enjoy!

Nutrition Value: calories 200, fat 5, fiber 7, carbs 10, protein 3

73. Beets And Capers Mix

Preparation time: 10 minutes
Cooking time: 6 hours
Servings: 4

Ingredients:

- 4 beets, peeled and sliced
- 1 cup veggie stock
- 2 tablespoons capers
- 2 tablespoons balsamic vinegar
- A bunch of parsley, chopped
- Salt and black pepper to the taste
- 1 tablespoon olive oil
- 1 garlic clove, chopped

Directions:

1. In your slow cooker, mix beets with stock, vinegar, parsley, capers, salt, pepper, oil and garlic, stir, cover and cook on High for 6 hours.
2. Divide between plates and serve right away.
3. Enjoy!

Nutrition Value: calories 101, fat 3, fiber 7, carbs 9, protein 2

74. Asparagus Soup

Preparation time: 10 minutes
Cooking time: 2 hours
Servings: 4

Ingredients:

- 2 pounds green asparagus, roughly chopped
- 5 veggie stock
- ½ cup coconut milk
- 3 tablespoons olive oil
- Salt and black pepper to the taste
- 1 yellow onion, chopped
- ¼ teaspoon lemon juice

Directions:
1. In your slow cooker, mix asparagus with stock, coconut milk, oil, salt, pepper, onion and lemon juice, stir, cover and cook on High for 2 hours.
2. Divide soup into bowls and serve.
3. Enjoy!

Nutrition Value: calories 130, fat 3, fiber 2, carbs 12, protein 3

75. Fennel Soup
Preparation time: 10 minutes
Cooking time: 4 hours
Servings: 4

Ingredients:
- 2 fennel bulbs, chopped
- 3 cups veggie stock
- 1 teaspoon cumin, ground
- 1 tablespoon olive oil
- Salt and black pepper to the taste
- 2 leeks, chopped

Directions:
1. In your slow cooker, mix fennel with stock, cumin, oil, leeks, salt and pepper, stir, cover and cook on High for 4 hours.
2. Ladle into bowls and serve hot.
3. Enjoy!

Nutrition Value: calories 132, fat 2, fiber 5, carbs 11, protein 3

76. Endives Soup
Preparation time: 10 minutes
Cooking time: 6 hours
Servings: 4

Ingredients:
- 2 tablespoons olive oil
- 2 scallions, chopped
- 3 endives, trimmed and chopped
- 6 cups veggie stock
- 3 garlic cloves chopped
- 1 tablespoon ginger, grated
- 1 teaspoon chili sauce
- A pinch of salt and black pepper
- ½ cup white rice

Directions:
- In your slow cooker, mix oil with scallions, endives, garlic, stock, ginger, chili sauce, salt, pepper and rice, stir, cover and cook on High for 6 hours.
- Ladle soup into bowls and serve.
- Enjoy!

Nutrition Value: calories 263., fat 4, fiber 7, carbs 17, protein 3

77. Special Minestrone Soup
Preparation time: 10 minutes
Cooking time: 4 hours
Servings: 8

Ingredients:
- 2 zucchinis, chopped
- 3 carrots, chopped
- 1 yellow onion, chopped
- A handful green beans
- 3 celery stalks, chopped
- 4 garlic cloves, minced
- 10 ounces canned garbanzo beans
- 1 pound lentils, cooked
- 4 cups veggie stock
- 28 ounces canned tomatoes, chopped
- 1 teaspoon curry powder
- ½ teaspoon garam masala
- ½ teaspoon cumin, ground
- A pinch of salt and black pepper

Directions:
1. In your slow cooker, mix zucchinis with carrots, onion, green beans, celery, garlic, garbanzo beans, lentils, stock, tomatoes, salt, pepper, cumin, curry powder and garam masala, stir, cover and cook on High for 4 hours.
2. Ladle soup into bowls and serve.
3. Enjoy!

Nutrition Value: calories 193, fat 12, fiber 7, carbs 34, protein 10

78. Green Chili Soup
Preparation time: 10 minutes
Cooking time: 6 hours
Servings: 6

Ingredients:
- 2 jalapeno chilies, chopped
- 1 cup yellow onion, chopped
- 1 tablespoon olive oil
- 4 poblano chilies, chopped
- 4 Anaheim chilies, chopped
- 3 cups corn
- 10 epazote leaves, shredded
- 6 cups water
- ½ bunch cilantro, chopped
- Salt and black pepper to the taste

Directions:

1. In your slow cooker, mix jalapenos with onion, oil, poblano chilies, Anaheim chilies, corn and water, stir, cover and cook on Low for 6 hours.
2. Add cilantro, epazote leaves, salt and pepper, stir, transfer to your blender, pulse well, divide into bowls and serve.
3. Enjoy!

Nutrition Value: calories 179, fat 5, fiber 5, carbs 33, protein 5

79. Caribbean Dish

Preparation time: 10 minutes
Cooking time: 4 hours and 40 minutes
Servings: 6

Ingredients:

- 2 tablespoons coconut oil
- 28 ounces canned black beans
- 2 yellow onions, chopped
- 4 garlic cloves, minced
- 1 green bell pepper, chopped
- 1 teaspoon thyme, dried
- 2 teaspoons chili flakes
- 1 tablespoon stevia
- 4 potatoes, cut into medium cubes
- A pinch of salt and cayenne pepper
- 28 ounces canned tomatoes, chopped
- 1 cup veggie stock
- 14 ounces coconut milk

Directions:

1. Heat up a pan with the oil over medium high heat, add onion, garlic, stevia, bell pepper, thyme, chili flakes, salt and cayenne, stir and cook for 3-4 minutes.
2. Add stock, stir, cook for 30 seconds more and transfer to your slow cooker.
3. Add beans, tomatoes and potatoes to your slow cooker as well, cover and cook on High for 4 hours.
4. Add coconut milk, stir, cover pot and cook on Low for 30 minutes more.
5. Divide mix between plates and serve.
6. Enjoy!

Nutrition Value: 475, fat 16, fiber 15, carbs 76, protein 14

80. Mediterranean Stew

Preparation time: 10 minutes
Cooking time: 7 hours
Servings: 10

Ingredients:

- 2 cups eggplant, cubed
- 1 butternut squash, peeled and cubed
- 2 cups zucchini, cubed
- 10 ounces tomato sauce
- 1 carrot, sliced
- 1 yellow onion, chopped
- ½ cup veggie stock
- 10 ounces okra
- 1/3 cup raisins
- 2 garlic cloves, minced
- ½ teaspoon turmeric powder
- ½ teaspoon cumin, ground
- ½ teaspoon red pepper flakes, crushed
- ¼ teaspoon sweet paprika
- ¼ teaspoon cinnamon powder

Directions:

1. In your slow cooker, mix eggplant with squash, zucchini, tomato sauce, carrot, onion, okra, garlic, stock, raisins, turmeric, cumin, pepper flakes, paprika and cinnamon, stir, cover and cook on Low for 7 hours.
2. Stir your stew one more time, divide into bowls and serve.
3. Enjoy!

Nutrition Value: calories 100, fat 3, fiber 4, carbs 24, protein 3

81. Chickpeas Delight

Preparation time: 10 minutes
Cooking time: 12 hours
Servings: 14

Ingredients:

- 6 cups chickpeas
- 11 cups water
- 1 yellow onion, chopped
- 1 tablespoon ginger, grated
- 20 garlic cloves, minced
- 8 Thai peppers, chopped
- 2 tablespoons cumin, ground
- 2 tablespoons coriander, ground
- 1 tablespoons red chili powder
- 2 tablespoons garam masala
- 2 tablespoons vegan tamarind paste
- Juice of ½ lemon

Directions:

1. In your slow cooker, mix chickpeas with water, stir, cover and cook on Low for 10 hours.
2. In your blender, mix onion with ginger, garlic, Thai peppers, cumin, coriander, chili powder, garam masala, tamarind paste and lemon juice

and pulse well.
3. Add this mix to slow cooker, toss, cover and cook on Low for 2 hours more.
4. Divide into bowls and serve.
5. Enjoy!

Nutrition Value: calories 355, fat 5, fiber 14, carbs 56, protein 17

82. Mexican Quinoa Dish

Preparation time: 10 minutes
Cooking time: 4 hours
Servings: 4

Ingredients:

- 15 ounces canned black beans, drained
- 30 ounces canned red enchilada sauce
- 15 ounces canned corn, drained
- 15 ounces canned tomatoes and green chilies, chopped
- 1 cup quinoa
- ½ cup water
- Salt and black pepper to the taste
- 1 cup vegan cheese, shredded

Directions:

1. In your slow cooker, mix black beans with corn, enchilada sauce, tomatoes and chilies, quinoa, water, salt and pepper and toss.
2. Sprinkle vegan cheese on top, cover and cook on High for 4 hours.
3. Divide into bowls and serve hot.
4. Enjoy!

Nutrition Value: calories 400, fat 3, fiber 14, carbs 32, protein 6

83. Sweet Potato Soup

Preparation time: 10 minutes
Cooking time: 5 hours and 20 minutes
Servings: 6

Ingredients:

- 5 cups veggie stock
- 3 sweet potatoes, peeled and chopped
- 2 celery stalks, chopped
- 1 cup yellow onion, chopped
- 1 cup almond milk
- 1 teaspoon tarragon, dried
- 2 garlic cloves, minced
- 2 cups baby spinach
- 8 tablespoons almonds, sliced
- A pinch of salt and black pepper

Directions:

1. In your slow cooker, mix stock with potatoes, celery, onion, almond milk, tarragon, garlic, salt and pepper, stir, cover and cook on High for 5 hours.
2. Blend soup using an immersion blender, add more salt and pepper if needed, also add spinach and almonds, toss, cover and leave aside for 20 minutes.
3. Divide soup into bowls and serve.
4. Enjoy!

Nutrition Value: calories 311, fat 5, fiber 4, carbs 12, protein 5

84. White Beans Stew

Preparation time: 10 minutes
Cooking time: 4 hours
Servings: 10

Ingredients:

- 2 pounds white beans
- 3 celery stalks, chopped
- 2 carrots, chopped
- 1 bay leaf
- 1 yellow onion, chopped
- 3 garlic cloves, minced
- 1 teaspoon rosemary, dried
- 1 teaspoon oregano, dried
- 1 teaspoon thyme, dried
- 10 cups water
- Salt and black pepper to the taste
- 28 ounces canned tomatoes, chopped
- 6 cups chard, chopped

Directions:

1. In your slow cooker, mix white beans with celery, carrots, bay leaf, onion, garlic, rosemary, oregano, thyme, water, salt, pepper, tomatoes and chard, toss, cover and cook on High for 4 hours.
2. Stir your stew one more time, divide into bowls and serve.
3. Enjoy!

Nutrition Value: calories 341, fat 8, fiber 12, carbs 20, protein 6

85. Spaghetti Squash Bowls

Preparation time: 10 minutes
Cooking time: 8 hours
Servings: 5

Ingredients:

- 1 spaghetti squash, halved
- 2 cups water

- 2 cups broccoli florets
- 1 tablespoon sesame seeds
- For the salad dressing:
- 1 and ½ tablespoon stevia
- 3 tablespoons wine vinegar
- 3 tablespoons olive oil
- 1 tablespoon coconut aminos
- 1 tablespoon ginger, grated
- 2 garlic cloves, minced
- 1 teaspoon sesame oil

Directions:
1. In your blender, mix stevia with vinegar, oil, aminos, ginger, garlic and sesame oil, pulse really well and leave aside for now.
2. In your slow cooker, mix spaghetti squash with water, cover and cook on Low for 8 hours.
3. Transfer squash to a cutting board, cool it down, scrape flesh and transfer to a bowl.
4. Add broccoli and sesame seeds and toss.
5. Add salad dressing, toss well and serve.
6. Enjoy!

Nutrition Value: calories 150, fat 4, fiber 6, carbs 26, protein 6

86. Italian Cauliflower Mix
Preparation time: 10 minutes
Cooking time: 3 hours and 30 minutes
Servings: 4

Ingredients:
- 1 cauliflower head, florets separated
- 2 teaspoons oregano, dried
- 1 cup red onion, chopped
- 2 garlic cloves, minced
- 1 teaspoon basil, dried
- 28 ounces canned tomatoes, chopped
- ½ cup veggie stock
- Salt and black pepper to the taste
- A pinch of red pepper flakes
- 6 zucchinis, cut with a spiralizer

Directions:
1. In your slow cooker, mix cauliflower with oregano, onion, garlic, basil, tomatoes, stock, pepper flakes, salt and pepper, stir, cover and cook on High for 3 hours and 30 minutes.
2. Divide zucchini noodles into bowls, divide cauliflower mix on top, toss a bit and serve.
3. Enjoy!

Nutrition Value: calories 251, fat 5, fiber 7, carbs 10, protein 4

87. Mushroom Delight
Preparation time: 10 minutes
Cooking time: 4 hours
Servings: 2

Ingredients:
- 1 pound mushrooms, halved
- 1 yellow onion, chopped
- 3 garlic cloves, minced
- 1 cup veggie stock
- 1 tablespoon coconut cream
- 2 teaspoons smoked paprika
- Salt and black pepper to the taste
- 4 tablespoons parsley, chopped

Directions:
1. In your slow cooker, mix mushrooms with garlic, onion, stock and paprika, stir, cover and cook on High for 4 hours.
2. Add parsley, coconut cream, salt and pepper, toss, divide into bowls and serve.
3. Enjoy!

Nutrition Value: calories 300, fat 6, fiber 12, carbs 16, protein 6

88. Quinoa And Veggie Mix
Preparation time: 10 minutes
Cooking time: 4 hours
Servings: 4

Ingredients:
- 3 cups veggie stock
- 1 and ½ cups quinoa
- 1 tablespoon olive oil
- 1 yellow onion, chopped
- 1 sweet red pepper, chopped
- 1 cup green beans, chopped
- 1 carrot, chopped
- 3 garlic cloves, minced
- 1 teaspoon basil, chopped
- Salt and black pepper to the taste

Directions:
1. In your slow cooker, mix stock with quinoa, oil, onion, red pepper, green beans, carrot, garlic, basil, salt and pepper, stir, cover and cook on Low for 4 hours.
2. Divide into bowls and serve.
3. Enjoy!

Nutrition Value: calories 312, fat 6, fiber 12, carbs 18, protein 5

89. Bulgur Chili

Preparation time: 10 minutes
Cooking time: 8 hours
Servings: 4

Ingredients:

- 2 cups white mushrooms, sliced
- ¾ cup bulgur, soaked in 1 cup hot water for 15 minutes and drained
- 2 cups yellow onion, chopped
- ½ cup red bell pepper, chopped
- 1 cup veggie stock
- 2 garlic cloves, minced
- 1 cup strong brewed coffee
- 14 ounces canned kidney beans, drained
- 14 ounces canned pinto beans, drained
- 2 tablespoons stevia
- 2 tablespoons chili powder
- 1 tablespoon cocoa powder
- 1 teaspoon oregano, dried
- 2 teaspoons cumin, ground
- 1 bay leaf
- Salt and black pepper to the taste

Directions:

1. In your slow cooker, mix mushrooms with bulgur, onion, bell pepper, stock, garlic, coffee, kidney and pinto beans, stevia, chili powder, cocoa, oregano, cumin, bay leaf, salt and pepper, stir gently, cover and cook on Low for 12 hours.
2. Discard bay leaf, divide chili into bowls and serve.
3. Enjoy!

Nutrition Value: calories 351, fat 4, fiber 6, carbs 20, protein 4

90. Cauliflower Chili

Preparation time: 10 minutes
Cooking time: 8 hours
Servings: 4

Ingredients:

- 30 ounces canned cannellini beans, drained
- 4 cups cauliflower florets
- 1 yellow onion, chopped
- 28 ounces canned tomatoes and juice
- 4 ounces canned roasted green chilies, chopped
- ½ cup hot sauce
- 1 tablespoon stevia
- 2 teaspoons cumin, ground
- 1 tablespoon chili powder
- A pinch of salt and cayenne pepper

Directions:

1. In your slow cooker, mix cannellini beans with cauliflower, onion, tomatoes and juice, roasted green chilies, hot sauce, stevia, cumin, chili powder, salt and cayenne pepper, stir, cover and cook on Low for 8 hours.
2. Divide into bowls and serve hot.
3. Enjoy!

Nutrition Value: calories 314, fat 6, fiber 6, carbs 29, protein 5

91. Quinoa Chili

Preparation time: 10 minutes
Cooking time: 6 hours
Servings: 6

Ingredients:

- 2 cups veggie stock
- ½ cup quinoa
- 30 ounces canned black beans, drained
- 28 ounces canned tomatoes, chopped
- 1 green bell pepper, chopped
- 1 yellow onion, chopped
- 2 sweet potatoes, cubed
- 1 tablespoon chili powder
- 2 tablespoons cocoa powder
- 2 teaspoons cumin, ground
- Salt and black pepper to the taste
- ¼ teaspoon smoked paprika

Directions:

1. In your slow cooker, mix stock with quinoa, black beans, tomatoes, bell pepper, onion, sweet potatoes, chili powder, cocoa, cumin, paprika, salt and pepper, stir, cover and cook on High for 6 hours.
2. Divide into bowls and serve hot.
3. Enjoy!

Nutrition Value: calories 342, fat 6, fiber 7, carbs 18, protein 4

92. Pumpkin Chili

Preparation time: 10 minutes
Cooking time: 5 hours
Servings: 6

Ingredients:

- 1 cup pumpkin puree
- 30 ounces canned kidney beans, drained
- 30 ounces canned roasted tomatoes, chopped
- 2 cups water
- 1 cup red lentils, dried
- 1 cup yellow onion, chopped

- 1 jalapeno pepper, chopped
- 1 tablespoon chili powder
- 1 tablespoon cocoa powder
- ½ teaspoon cinnamon powder
- 2 teaspoons cumin, ground
- A pinch of cloves, ground
- Salt and black pepper to the taste
- 2 tomatoes, chopped

Directions:
1. In your slow cooker, mix pumpkin puree with kidney beans, roasted tomatoes, water, lentils, onion, jalapeno, chili powder, cocoa, cinnamon, cumin, cloves, salt and pepper, stir, cover and cook on High for 5 hours.
2. Divide into bowls, top with chopped tomatoes and serve hot.
3. Enjoy!

Nutrition Value: calories 266, fat 6, fiber 4, carbs 12, protein 4

93. 3 Bean Chili

Preparation time: 10 minutes
Cooking time: 8 hours
Servings: 6

Ingredients:
- 15 ounces canned kidney beans, drained
- 30 ounces canned chili beans in sauce
- 15 ounces canned black beans, drained
- 2 green bell peppers, chopped
- 30 ounces canned tomatoes, crushed
- 2 tablespoons chili powder
- 2 yellow onions, chopped
- 2 garlic cloves, minced
- 1 teaspoon oregano, dried
- 1 tablespoon cumin, ground
- Salt and black pepper to the taste

Directions:
1. In your slow cooker, mix kidney beans with chili beans, black beans, bell peppers, tomatoes, chili powder, onion, garlic, oregano, cumin, salt and pepper, stir, cover and cook on Low for 8 hours.
2. Divide into bowls and serve.
3. Enjoy!

Nutrition Value: calories 314, fat 6, fiber 5, carbs 14, protein 4

94. Root Vegetable Chili

Preparation time: 10 minutes
Cooking time: 6 hours
Servings: 12

Ingredients:
- 2 cups turnips, cubed
- 2 cups rutabagas, cubed
- 2 cups sweet potatoes, cubed
- 2 cups parsnips, cubed
- 1 cup beets, cubed
- 1 cup carrots, cubed
- 1 and ½ cups yellow onion, chopped
- 8 ounces tempeh, rinsed and cubed
- 28 ounces canned tomatoes, chopped
- 1 cup veggie stock
- 15 ounces canned black beans, drained
- 15 ounces canned kidney beans, drained
- Salt and black pepper to the taste
- 1 teaspoon cumin, ground
- 1 teaspoon chili powder, ground
- A pinch of cayenne pepper
- ½ teaspoon nutmeg, ground
- ½ teaspoon sweet paprika
- ½ cup parsley, chopped

Directions:
1. In your slow cooker, mix turnips with rutabagas, sweet potatoes, parsnips, beets, carrots, onion, tempeh, tomatoes, stock, black and kidney beans, salt, pepper, cumin, chili powder, cayenne, nutmeg and paprika, stir, cover and cook on Low for 6 hours.
2. Add parsley, stir, divide into bowls and serve.
3. Enjoy!

Nutrition Value: calories 311, fat 6, fiber 6, carbs 16, protein 6

95. Brown Rice Soup

Preparation time: 10 minutes
Cooking time: 8 hours
Servings: 6

Ingredients:
- 70 ounces canned black beans, drained
- 1 cup yellow onion, chopped
- 1 tablespoon olive oil
- 2 carrots, chopped
- 1 jalapeno pepper, chopped
- 3 garlic cloves, minced
- 1 teaspoon cumin, ground
- 1 teaspoon chili powder
- 1 teaspoon oregano, dried
- Salt and black pepper to the taste

- 2 tablespoons tomato paste
- 4 cups veggie stock
- A splash of Tabasco sauce
- 2 cups brown rice, already cooked
- 1 tablespoon cilantro, chopped

Directions:
1. Drizzle the olive oil on the bottom of your slow cooker.
2. Add black beans, onion, carrots, jalapeno, garlic, cumin, chili, oregano, tomato paste, stock, Tabasco, salt, pepper and rice, stir, cover and cook on Low for 8 hours.
3. Add cilantro, stir, ladle into bowls and serve.
4. Enjoy!

Nutrition Value: calories 314, fat 5, fiber 8, carbs 18, protein 4

96. Butternut Squash Soup

Preparation time: 10 minutes
Cooking time: 8 hours
Servings: 6

Ingredients:
- 3 pounds butternut squash, peeled and cubed
- 1 yellow onion, chopped
- 4 cups veggie stock
- 14 ounces coconut milk
- Salt and black pepper to the taste
- 3 tablespoons red curry paste
- 1 tablespoon cilantro, chopped

Directions:
1. In your slow cooker, mix squash with onion, stock, milk, curry paste, salt and pepper, stir, cover and cook on Low for 8 hours
2. Blend using an immersion blender, ladle soup into bowls, sprinkle cilantro on top and serve.
3. Enjoy!

Nutrition Value: calories 237, fat 5, fiber 6, carbs 19, protein 6

97. Green Beans Soup

Preparation time: 10 minutes
Cooking time: 4 hours
Servings: 4

Ingredients:
- 1 pound green beans
- 1 yellow onion, chopped
- 4 carrots, chopped
- 4 garlic cloves, minced
- 1 tablespoon thyme, chopped
- 7 cups veggie stock
- Salt and black pepper to the taste

Directions:
1. In your slow cooker, mix green beans with onion, carrots, garlic, stock, salt and pepper, stir, cover and cook on High for 4 hours.
2. Add thyme, stir, ladle soup into bowls and serve.
3. Enjoy!

Nutrition Value: calories 231, fat 4, fiber 6, carbs 7, protein 5

98. Vegan Sandwich with Tofu & Lettuce Slaw

Preparation Time: 10 minutes + marinade time
Servings: 2

Ingredients
- ¼ pound firm tofu, sliced
- 2 low carb buns
- 1 tbsp olive oil
- Marinade
- 2 tbsp olive oil
- Salt and black pepper to taste
- 1 tsp allspice
- ½ tbsp xylitol
- 1 tsp thyme, chopped
- 1 habanero pepper, seeded and minced
- 2 green onions, thinly sliced
- 1 garlic clove
- Lettuce slaw
- ½ small iceberg lettuce, shredded
- ½ carrot, grated
- ½ red onion, grated
- 2 tsp liquid stevia
- 1 tbsp lemon juice
- Salt and black pepper
- 2 tbsp olive oil
- ½ tsp Dijon mustard
- Salt and black pepper to taste

Directions
1. Put the tofu slices in a bowl.
2. In a food processor, blend the marinade ingredients for a minute. Cover the tofu with this mixture and place in the fridge to marinate for 1 hour. In a large bowl, combine the lemon juice, stevia, olive oil, Dijon mustard, salt, and pepper. Stir in the lettuce, carrot, and onion; set aside.
3. Heat 1 teaspoon of oil in a skillet over medium heat and cook the tofu on both sides for 6 minutes in total. Remove to a plate. In the buns,

add the tofu and top with the slaw. Close the bread and serve.

Nutrition Value:
Calories: 687, Fat: 58.5g, Net Carbs: 10.5g, Protein: 21.3g

99. Southern Collard Greens
Preparation Time: 23 MINS
Servings: 5

Ingredients:
- 2 bunches collard greens
- 2 tbsp. olive oil
- 1 cut into thin rings small yellow onion
- 3 minced garlic cloves
- Pinch of red pepper flakes
- 1 cup water
- Salt, to taste

Directions:
1. Remove the tough stems of collard greens and then, cut into thin strands.
2. Place the oil in the Instant Pot and select "Sauté". Then add the onion and cook for about 4-5 minutes.
3. Add the garlic and red pepper flakes and cook for about 1 minute.
4. Select the "Cancel" and stir in collard greens and water.
5. Secure the lid and place the pressure valve to "Seal" position.
6. Select "Manual" and cook under "High Pressure" for about 3 minutes.
7. Select the "Cancel" and carefully do a Quick release.
8. Remove the lid and stir in salt.
9. Serve hot.

Nutrition Value:
Calories 106
Total Fat 6.9g
Net Carbs 2.38g
Protein 4.3g
Fiber 0.6g

100. Nicely Flavored Swiss Chard
Preparation Time: 13 MINS
Servings: 6

Ingredients:
- 2 ribs removed and chopped into bite-sized pieces large heads Swiss chard
- 2 tbsp. extra virgin olive oil
- ¼ tsp ground cumin
- 1/8 tsp crushed red pepper flakes
- 1/8 tsp cayenne pepper
- 1/3 cup water

Instructions:
1. In the pot of Instant Pot, add all ingredients and stir to combine.
2. Secure the lid and place the pressure valve to "Seal" position.
3. Select "Manual" and cook under "High Pressure" for about 3 minutes.
4. Select the "Cancel" and carefully do a Natural release.
5. Remove the lid and serve.

Nutrition Value:
Calories 50
Total Fat 4.8g
Net Carbs 0.31g
Protein 0.9g
Fiber 0.5g

101. American Style Kale
Preparation Time: 17 MINS
Servings: 4

Ingredients:
- 1 tbsp. olive oil
- 3 slivered garlic cloves
- 1 pound trimmed and chopped fresh kale
- ½ cup water
- Salt and freshly ground black pepper, to taste
- 1 tbsp. fresh lemon juice

Directions:
1. Place the oil in the Instant Pot and select "Sauté". Then add the garlic and cook for about 1 minute.
2. Add the kale and cook for about 1-2 minutes.
3. Select the "Cancel" and stir in water, salt and black pepper.
4. Secure the lid and place the pressure valve to "Seal" position.
5. Select "Manual" and cook under "High Pressure" for about 5 minutes.
6. Select the "Cancel" and carefully do a Quick release.
7. Remove the lid and stir in lemon juice.
8. Serve hot.

Nutrition Value:
Calories 90
Total Fat 12.7g
Net Carbs 3.17g
Protein 3.6g
Fiber 0.1g

102. Sweet & Sour Kale

Preparation Time: 17 MINS
Servings: 4

Ingredients:

- 1 tbsp. olive oil
- 1 thinly sliced small yellow onion
- 6 crushed garlic cloves
- 1 (10-ouncebag kale
- 1½ cups homemade chicken broth
- 2 tbsp. fresh lemon juice
- 1 tbsp. Erythritol
- 1 tsp crushed red pepper flakes
- Salt and freshly ground black pepper, to taste

Directions:

1. Place the oil in the Instant Pot and select "Sauté". Then add the onion and cook for about 3-4 minutes.
2. Add the garlic and cook for about 1 minute.
3. Select the "Cancel" and stir in remaining ingredients.
4. Secure the lid and place the pressure valve to "Seal" position.
5. Select "Manual" and cook under "High Pressure" for about 5 minutes.
6. Select the "Cancel" and carefully do a Quick release.
7. Remove the lid and serve.

Nutrition Value:

Calories 96
Total Fat 4.2g
Net Carbs 3.5g
Protein 4.5g
Fiber 1.7g

103. Super-Food Casserole

Preparation Time: 35 MINS
Servings: 8

Ingredients:

- 6 organic eggs
- ½ cup heavy cream
- Salt and freshly ground black pepper, to taste
- 1 cup shredded cheddar cheese
- 2½ cups trimmed and chopped fresh kale
- 1 chopped small yellow onion
- 1 tsp Herbs de Provence

Directions:

1. In a large bowl, add eggs, heavy cream, salt and black pepper and beat until well combined.
2. Add remaining ingredients and mix well.
3. Place the mixture into a baking dish evenly.
4. In the bottom of Instant Pot, arrange a steamer trivet and pour 1 cup of water.
5. Place the dish on top of the trivet.
6. Secure the lid and place the pressure valve to "Seal" position.
7. Select "Manual" and cook under "High Pressure" for about 20 minutes.
8. Select the "Cancel" and carefully do a Natural release.
9. Remove the lid and serve immediately.

Nutrition Value:

Calories 195
Total Fat 14.3g
Net Carbs 0.81g
Protein 11.4g
Fiber 0.9g

104. Traditional Indian Spinach

Preparation Time: 25 MINS
Servings: 4

Ingredients:

- 1 tbsp. olive oil
- 1 chopped small yellow onion
- 5 chopped garlic cloves
- 1 chopped green chili
- ½ tsp ground cumin
- ¼ tsp ground coriander
- 1 chopped tomato
- 10-ounce fresh spinach
- Salt and freshly ground black pepper, to taste
- 10-ounce cubed cottage cheese
- 2 tbsp. cream

Directions:

1. Place the oil in the Instant Pot and select "Sauté". Then add the onion, garlic, green chili and spices and cook for about 3-4 minutes.
2. Add the tomato and cook for about 2 minutes.
3. Select the "Cancel" and stir in spinach, salt and black pepper.
4. Secure the lid and place the pressure valve to "Seal" position.
5. Select "Manual" and cook under "High Pressure" for about 2 minutes.
6. Select the "Cancel" and carefully do a Natural release.
7. Remove the lid and with an immersion blender, puree the spinach mixture.
8. Select the "Sauté" and stir in cottage cheese.
9. Cook for about 2 minutes.
10. Select the "Cancel" and transfer spinach mixture

onto serving plates.
11. Top with cream and serve.

Nutrition Value:
Calories 130
Total Fat 5.6g
Net Carbs 2.22g
Protein 12.4g
Fiber 2.2g

105. Holiday Gathering Casserole
Preparation Time: 38 MINS
Servings: 8

Ingredients:
- 12 large organic eggs
- ½ cup unsweetened almond milk
- Salt and freshly ground black pepper, to taste
- 3 cups roughly chopped fresh baby spinach
- 1 cup seeded and chopped tomato
- 3 sliced large scallions
- 4 tomato slices
- ¼ cup shredded Parmesan cheese

Directions:
1. Lightly, grease a 1½ quart casserole dish that will fit in an Instant Pot. Keep aside.
2. In a large bowl, add eggs, milk, salt and pepper and beat until well combined.
3. In the bottom of prepared casserole dish, place spinach, chopped tomato, and scallions and stir to combine.
4. Top with egg mixture evenly and stir to combine.
5. Arrange tomatoes slices on top and sprinkle with Parmesan cheese.
6. In the bottom of Instant Pot, arrange a steamer trivet and pour 1 cup of water.
7. Fold a larger piece of foil in thirds to make a little carrier. Arrange the foil on top of steamer trivet.
8. Place the casserole dish over foil.
9. Secure the lid and place the pressure valve to "Seal" position.
10. Select "Manual" and cook under "High Pressure" for about 20 minutes.
11. Select the "Cancel" and carefully do a "Natural" release for about 10 minutes and then do a "Quick" release.
12. Remove the lid and serve warm.

Nutrition Value:
Calories 161
Total Fat 10.5g
Net Carbs 0.38g
Protein 14g
Fiber 0.8g

106. Simple Steamed Asparagus
Preparation Time: 12 MINS
Servings: 4

Ingredients:
- 1 pound trimmed fresh asparagus
- 4 tbsp. melted salted butter

Directions:
1. In the bottom of Instant Pot, arrange a steamer basket and pour 1 cup of water.
2. Place the asparagus into the steamer basket.
3. Secure the lid and place the pressure valve to "Seal" position.
4. Select the "Steam" and just use the default time of 2 minutes.
5. Select the "Cancel" and carefully do a "Quick" release.
6. Remove the lid and transfer the asparagus onto serving plates.
7. Drizzle with butter and serve.

Nutrition Value:
Calories 124
Total Fat 11.7g
Net Carbs 1.1g
Protein 2.6g
Fiber 2.4g

107. Buttered Asparagus
Preparation Time: 23 MINS
Servings: 4

Ingredients:
- 1 pound trimmed fresh asparagus
- 3 peeled whole garlic cloves
- 3 tbsp. softened butter
- 3 tbsp. grated Parmesan cheese

Directions:
1. Place asparagus and garlic in the center of a large piece of foil and top with butter.
2. Curve the edges of foil slightly to avoid the leakage of butter.
3. In the bottom of Instant Pot, arrange a steamer basket and pour 1 cup of water.
4. Place the asparagus into the steamer basket.
5. Secure the lid and place the pressure valve to "Seal" position.
6. Select the "Steam" and just use the default time of 8 minutes.
7. Select the "Cancel" and carefully do a "Quick" release.

8. Remove the lid and transfer asparagus onto serving plates.
9. Sprinkle with Parmesan and serve.

Nutrition Value:
Calories 108
Total Fat 9.1g
Net Carbs 1.3g
Protein 3.2g
Fiber 2.2g

108. Zesty Artichokes
Preparation Time: 35 MINS
Servings: 4

Ingredients:
- 4 (4-ounces artichokes
- 2 small lemons
- 2 cups homemade chicken broth
- 1 finely chopped celery stalk
- 1 tbsp. finely chopped tarragon leaves
- ¼ cup olive oil
- Salt, to taste

Directions:
1. Trim the stems of each artichoke so that they are 1-inch in length. Cut off 1-inch of the "petals" from the opposite end of the artichokes. Discard the stems and petal tips.
2. Zest the lemons and keep aside.
3. Cut 4 (¼-inch thin slices from the middle of one zested lemon, removing any seeds.
4. In the bottom of Instant Pot, arrange lemon slices and top each lemon slice with a trimmed artichoke, stem-side up.
5. Carefully, pour broth around the artichokes.
6. Secure the lid and place the pressure valve to "Seal" position.
7. Select "Manual" and cook under "High Pressure" for about 20 minutes.
8. Select the "Cancel" and carefully do a "Quick" release.
9. Meanwhile, for dipping sauce: peel the remaining lemon and cut the white pith.
10. in a food processor, add lemon zest, lemon fruit, celery, tarragon, olive oil and salt and pulse until smooth.
11. Remove the lid and serve artichokes with dipping sauce.

Nutrition Value:
Calories 185
Total Fat 13.5g
Net Carbs 3.4g
Protein 6.4g
Fiber 6.5g

109. Loveable Brussels Sprouts
Preparation Time: 21 MINS
Servings: 4

Ingredients:
- 2 tbsp. coconut oil
- ½ cup chopped yellow onion
- 2 tsp minced garlic
- 1 pound outer leaves removed Brussels sprout
- ½ cup water
- Salt and freshly ground black pepper, to taste

Directions:
1. Place 2 tsp of the coconut oil in the Instant Pot and select "Sauté". Then add the onion and garlic and cook for about 2-3 minutes.
2. Select the "Cancel" and stir in the broth.
3. Secure the lid and place the pressure valve to "Seal" position.
4. Select "Manual" and cook under "Low Pressure" for about 3 minutes.
5. Select the "Cancel" and carefully do a "Quick" release.
6. Remove the lid and drain excess liquid.
7. Serve immediately.

Nutrition Value:
Calories 115
Total Fat 7.2g
Net Carbs 3.02g
Protein 4.1g
Fiber 4.6g

110. Chinese Brussels Sprouts
Preparation Time: 35 MINS
Servings: 8

Ingredients:
- 2 pounds halved brussels sprouts
- ¼ cup soy sauce
- 2 tbsp. sriracha sauce
- 1 tbsp. fresh lime juice
- 2 tbsp. olive oil
- 1 tbsp. chopped almonds
- 1 tbsp. smoked paprika
- 1 tsp red pepper flakes
- 1 tsp garlic powder
- Salt and freshly ground black pepper, to taste

Directions:
1. In the pot of Instant Pot, add all ingredients and stir to combine.
2. Secure the lid and place the pressure valve to

"Seal" position.
3. Select "Manual" and cook under "High Pressure" for about 3 minutes.
4. Select the "Cancel" and carefully do a "Quick" release.
5. Remove the lid and serve.

Nutrition Value:
Calories 96
Total Fat 4.4g
Net Carbs 1.58g
Protein 4.8g
Fiber 4.8g

111. Garlicky Green Beans
Preparation Time: 20 MINS
Servings: 4

Ingredients:
- 1 pound fresh green beans
- 2 tbsp. butter
- 2 minced garlic cloves
- Salt and freshly ground black pepper, to taste
- 1½ cups water

Directions:
1. In the pot of Instant Pot, add all ingredients and stir to combine.
2. Secure the lid and place the pressure valve to "Seal" position.
3. Select "Manual" and cook under "High Pressure" for about 5 minutes.
4. Select the "Cancel" and carefully do a Quick release.
5. Remove the lid and serve hot.

Nutrition Value:
Calories 88
Total Fat 5.9g
Net Carbs 2.15g
Protein 2.2g
Fiber 3.9g

112. Southern Green Beans
Preparation Time: 35 MINS
Servings: 4

Ingredients:
- 1 pound frozen green beans
- 1 chopped small yellow onion
- 1 tsp minced garlic
- 1 tbsp. butter
- Salt and freshly ground black pepper, to taste
- 1 cup homemade chicken broth

Directions:

1. In the pot of Instant Pot, add all ingredients and stir to combine.
2. Secure the lid and place the pressure valve to "Seal" position.
3. Select "Manual" and cook under "High Pressure" for about 25 minutes.
4. Select the "Cancel" and carefully do a "Quick" release.
5. Remove the lid and serve.

Nutrition Value:
Calories 78
Total Fat 3.4g
Net Carbs 2.55g
Protein 3.5g
Fiber 4.3g

113. Holiday Dinner Table Casserole
Preparation Time: 35 MINS
Servings: 8

Ingredients:
For Casserole:
- 2 tbsp. butter
- 1 thinly sliced yellow onion
- Salt, to taste
- 8-ounce sliced button mushrooms
- 1¼ pounds trimmed and halved green beans
- 2 finely chopped garlic cloves
- 1 tsp Dijon mustard
- ½ cup homemade vegetable broth
- 5 tbsp. crème fraîche

For Crispy Onions:
- 1 sliced into thin rings medium yellow onion
- 2 tbsp. tapioca flour
- Salt, to taste
- Pinch of ground black pepper
- 3 tbsp. coconut oil

Directions:
1. For casserole: place the butter in the Instant Pot and select "Sauté". Then add the onion and cook for about 5 minutes.
2. Add the mushrooms and salt and cook for about 5 minutes.
3. Select the "Cancel" and stir in the green beans, garlic, mustard and broth.
4. Select "Manual" and cook under "High Pressure" for about 1 minute.
5. Select the "Cancel" and carefully do a "Quick" release.
6. Remove the lid and stir in the crème fraîche.
7. Meanwhile, for crispy onions: in a bowl, add onion rings, flour, salt and black pepper and

toss to coat well.
8. In a deep-frying pan, melt coconut oil over medium-high heat.
9. Add the onions rings and cook for about 3-4 minutes per side.
10. Remove from heat and transfer onion rings onto a plate.
11. Transfer the cooked green bean casserole into a serving dish and top with the crispy onions.
12. Serve immediately.

Nutrition Value:
Calories 124
Total Fat 8.7g
Net Carbs 1.35g
Protein 3g
Fiber 3.3g

114. Mexican Style Mushrooms
Preparation Time: 20 MINS
Servings: 4

Ingredients:
- 3 tbsp. olive oil
- 4 finely chopped garlic cloves
- 1 pound sliced white mushrooms
- 1 chipotle chile in adobo sauce
- ¼ tsp dried oregano
- ¼ tsp ground cumin
- ¼ tsp smoked paprika
- Salt, to taste
- 1 tbsp. apple cider vinegar
- 1 tbsp. fresh lime juice

Directions:
1. Place the oil in the Instant Pot and select "Sauté". Then add the mushrooms and garlic and cook for about 2-3 minutes.
2. Select the "Cancel" and stir in remaining ingredients.
3. Secure the lid and place the pressure valve to "Seal" position.
4. Select "Manual" and cook under "High Pressure" for about 2 minutes.
5. Select the "Cancel" and carefully do a Quick release.
6. Remove the lid and serve.

Nutrition Value:
Calories 121
Total Fat 10.9g
Net Carbs 1.25g
Protein 3.8g
Fiber 1.3g

115. Aromatic Mushrooms
Preparation Time: 19 MINS
Servings: 6

Ingredients:
- 1½ pounds cremini mushrooms
- 4 finely chopped garlic cloves
- ¼ tsp dried thyme
- ½ tsp dried oregano
- ½ tsp dried basil
- 2 bay leaves
- 1 cup homemade vegetable broth
- Salt and freshly ground black pepper, to taste
- ¼ cup half-and-half
- 2 tbsp. unsalted butter
- 2 tbsp. chopped fresh parsley leaves

Directions:
1. In the pot of Instant Pot, add all ingredients half-and-half, butter and parsley and stir to combine.

Secure the lid and place the pressure valve to "Seal" position.
Select "Manual" and cook under "High Pressure" for about 4 minutes.
Select the "Cancel" and carefully do a "Quick" release.
Remove the lid and stir in half-and-half and butter, and fresh parsley.
Serve warm.

Nutrition Value:
Calories 88
Total Fat 5.4g
Net Carbs 1.01g
Protein 4.2g
Fiber 0.8g

116. Thanksgiving Side Dish
Preparation Time: 28 MINS
Servings: 6

Ingredients:
- 1 pound trimmed fresh green beans
- 2 tbsp. olive oil
- ½ chopped yellow onion
- 1 minced garlic clove
- 10-ounce sliced fresh mushrooms
- ½ tbsp. fresh lemon juice
- Salt and freshly ground black pepper, to taste

Directions:
1. In the pot of Instant Pot, add green beans and enough water to cover.
2. Secure the lid and place the pressure valve to

"Seal" position.
3. Select "Manual" and cook under "High Pressure" for about 2 minutes.
4. Select the "Cancel" and carefully do a "Quick" release.
5. Remove the lid and drain the green beans.
6. Remove water from the pot and with paper towels, pat dry.
7. Place the oil in the Instant Pot and select "Sauté". Then add the onion and garlic and cook for about 3-4 minutes.
8. Add mushrooms and cook for about 5-6 minutes.
9. Stir in green beans, salt and black pepper and cook for about 1 minute.
10. Select the "Cancel" and serve.

Nutrition Value:
Calories 78
Total Fat 4.9g
Net Carbs 1.33g
Protein 3g
Fiber 3.3g

117. Authentic Sri Lankan Cabbage
Preparation Time: 25 MINS
Servings: 6

Ingredients:
- 1 tbsp. coconut oil
- 1 sliced chopped small yellow onion
- Salt, to taste
- 2 chopped garlic cloves
- ½ sliced long red chili
- 1 tbsp. mild curry powder
- 1 tbsp. ground turmeric
- 1 shredded medium head cabbage
- 1 peeled and sliced medium carrot
- ½ cup desiccated unsweetened coconut
- 2 tbsp. fresh lemon juice
- 1 tbsp. olive oil
- 1/3 cup water

Directions:
1. Place the coconut oil in the Instant Pot and select "Sauté". Then add the onion and salt and cook for about 3-4 minutes.
2. Add the garlic, chili and spices and cook for about 1 minute.
3. Select the "Cancel" and stir in remaining ingredients.
4. Secure the lid and place the pressure valve to "Seal" position.
5. Select "Manual" and cook under "High Pressure" for about 5 minutes.
6. Select the "Cancel" and carefully do a "Natural" release for about 5 minutes and then do a "Quick" release.
7. Remove the lid and serve.

Nutrition Value:
Calories 120
Total Fat 7.3g
Net Carbs 2.28g
Protein 2.7g
Fiber 5.6g

118. Bright Carrot Mash
Preparation Time: 19 MINS
Servings: 6

Ingredients:
- 1½ pounds peeled and roughly chopped carrots
- 1 tbsp. softened butter
- 1-2 drops liquid stevia
- Salt, to taste

Directions:
1. Arrange the trivet in the bottom of Instant Pot. Add 1 cup of water in Instant Pot.
2. Place carrot pieces on top of the trivet.
3. Secure the lid and place the pressure valve to "Seal" position.
4. Select "Manual" and cook under "High Pressure" for about 4 minutes.
5. Select the "Cancel" and carefully do a Quick release.
6. Remove the lid and transfer the carrots to a bowl.
7. Add remaining ingredients and with an immersion hand blender, blend until desired texture is achieved.
8. Serve immediately.

Nutrition Value:
Calories 63
Total Fat 1.9g
Net Carbs 1.86g
Protein 1g
Fiber 2.8g

119. Delish Carrots
Preparation Time: 35 MINS
Servings: 16

Ingredients:
- 2 tbsp. olive oil
- 1 chopped yellow onion
- 3 finely chopped garlic cloves
- 5 pounds halved medium baby carrots baby

Lunch

- ½ cup homemade vegetable broth
- 1 tsp Italian seasoning
- 1 tsp spike seasoning

Directions:
1. Place the oil in the Instant Pot and select "Sauté". Then add the onion and garlic and cook for about 4-5 minutes.
2. Add the carrots and cook for about 4-5 minutes.
3. Select the "Cancel" and stir in collard greens and water.
4. Secure the lid and place the pressure valve to "Seal" position.
5. Select "Manual" and cook under "High Pressure" for about 10 minutes.
6. Select the "Cancel" and carefully do a "Natural" release for about 10 minutes and then do a "Quick" release.
7. Remove the lid and serve.

Nutrition Value:
Calories 70
Total Fat 2.1g
Net Carbs 0.78g
Protein 1.2g
Fiber 4.3g

120. Glazed Carrots
Preparation Time: 19 MINS
Servings: 8

Ingredients:
- 2 pounds baby carrots
- 1/3 cup butter
- 2 tbsp. Erythritol
- 1/2 tsp ground cinnamon
- salt, to taste
- ½ cup water

Directions:
1. In the pot of Instant Pot, add all ingredients and stir to combine.
2. Secure the lid and place the pressure valve to "Seal" position.
3. Select "Manual" and cook under "High Pressure" for about 4 minutes.
4. Select the "Cancel" and carefully do a "Natural" release.
5. Remove the lid and serve.

Nutrition Value:
Calories 91
Total Fat 5.9g
Net Carbs 1.56g
Protein 0.8g
Fiber 3.4g

121. Sweet & Spicy Carrots
Preparation Time: 18 MINS
Servings: 4

Ingredients:
- 1 pound quartered lengthwise and halved carrots
- 1 tbsp. Erythritol
- 2 tbsp. butter
- 3 tsp ground mustard
- 1 tsp ground cumin
- ½ tsp cayenne pepper
- ¼ tsp red pepper flakes
- Salt and freshly ground black pepper, to taste
- 1/8 tsp ground cinnamon

Directions:
1. In the bottom of Instant Pot, arrange a steamer basket and pour 1 cup of water.
2. Place the carrots into the steamer basket.
3. Secure the lid and place the pressure valve to "Seal" position.
4. Select "Manual" and cook under "High Pressure" for about 1 minute.
5. Select the "Cancel" and carefully do a "Quick" release.
6. Remove the lid and transfer the carrots to a bowl.
7. Remove water from the pot and with paper towels, pat dry.
8. Select the "Sauté" mode for Power Pressure Cooker. In the pot of Pressure Cooker, melt butter and stir in the remaining ingredients.
9. Stir in the carrots and cook for about 1 minute.
10. Select the "Cancel" and serve warm with the sprinkling of cinnamon.

Nutrition Value:
Calories 112
Total Fat 6.6g
Net Carbs 3.50g
Protein 1.7g
Fiber 3.3g

122. Bell Pepper Gumbo
Preparation Time: 20 MINS
Servings: 3

Ingredients:
- tbsp. olive oil
- 4 minced garlic cloves
- ½ tsp cumin seeds
- 1 seeded and cut into long strips green bell pepper

- 1 seeded and cut into long strips red bell pepper
- 1 seeded and cut into long strips yellow bell pepper
- 1 seeded and cut into long strips bell pepper
- ½ tsp red chili powder
- ¼ tsp ground turmeric
- Salt and freshly ground black pepper, to taste
- ¼ cup water
- ½ tbsp. fresh lemon juice

Directions:
1. Place the oil in the Instant Pot and select "Sauté". Then add the garlic and cumin and cook for about 1 minute.
2. Select the "Cancel" and stir in remaining ingredients except for lemon juice.
3. Secure the lid and place the pressure valve to "Seal" position.
4. Select "Manual" and cook under "High Pressure" for about 2 minutes.
5. Select the "Cancel" and carefully do a "Quick" release.
6. Remove the lid and select "Sauté".
7. Stir in lemon juice and cook for about 1-2 minutes.
8. Select the "Cancel" and serve.

Nutrition Value:
Calories 101
Total Fat 5.3g
Net Carbs 4.6g
Protein 2g
Fiber 2.5g

123. Italian Bell Pepper Platter
Preparation Time: 20 MINS
Servings: 5

Ingredients:
- tbsp. olive oil
- 1 cut into thin strips yellow onion
- 5 seeded and cut into long strips green bell peppers
- very finely chopped medium ripe tomatoes
- chopped garlic cloves
- tbsp. fresh parsley
- Salt and freshly ground black pepper, to taste

Directions:
1. Place the oil in the Instant Pot and select "Sauté". Then add the onion and cook for about 3-4 minutes.
2. Add the bell peppers and garlic clove and cook for about 5 minutes.
3. Select the "Cancel" and stir in remaining ingredients.
4. Secure the lid and place the pressure valve to "Seal" position.
5. Select "Manual" and cook under "High Pressure" for about 5-6 minutes.
6. Select the "Cancel" and carefully do a "Quick" release.
7. Remove the lid and serve.

Nutrition Value:
Calories 82
Total Fat 3.2g
Net Carbs 2.7g
Protein 12.4g
Fiber 2.7g

DINNER

124. 2-Minutes Broccoli

Preparation Time: 12 MINS
Servings: 4

Ingredients:

- 4 cups broccoli florets
- Salt and freshly ground black pepper, to taste

Directions:

1. In the bottom of Instant Pot, arrange a steamer basket and pour 1 cup of water.
2. Place the broccoli into the steamer basket.
3. Secure the lid and place the pressure valve to "Seal" position.
4. Select "Manual" and cook under "High Pressure" for about 2 minutes.
5. Select the "Cancel" and carefully do a "Natural" release.
6. Remove the lid and transfer the broccoli to serving plates.
7. Sprinkle with salt and black pepper and serve.

Nutrition Value:

Calories 31
Total Fat 0.3g
Net Carbs 1.52g
Protein 2.6g
Fiber 2.4g

125. Brilliant Cheesy Broccoli

Preparation Time: 25 MINS
Servings: 2

Ingredients:

For Broccoli:

- 2 cups broccoli florets
- 1 tbsp. olive oil
- 2 tsp garlic powder
- ½ tbsp. smoked paprika
- Salt and freshly ground black pepper, to taste

For Cheese Sauce:

- 3 tbsp. butter
- 2 tbs. almond flour
- ½ cups unsweetened almond milk
- 1 cup shredded cheddar cheese
- 1 tsp garlic powder
- Salt, to taste

Directions:

1. For broccoli: in a bowl, add all ingredients and toss to coat well.
2. In the bottom of Instant Pot, arrange a steamer basket and pour 1 cup of water.
3. Place the broccoli into the steamer basket.
4. Secure the lid and place the pressure valve to "Seal" position.
5. Select "Manual" and cook under "Low Pressure" for about 10 minutes.
6. Select the "Cancel" and carefully do a "Natural" release.
7. Meanwhile, for cheese sauce: in a medium pan, melt butter over medium-high heat.
8. Add flour, beating continuously.
9. Slowly, add almond milk, beating continuously.
10. Cook for about 2-3 minutes or until thickened, stirring continuously.
11. Add cheese, garlic powder and salt and stir until smooth.
12. Remove the lid of Instant Pot and transfer broccoli ono serving plates.
13. To wit cheese sauce and serve.

Nutrition Value:

Calories 536
Total Fat 47.9g
Net Carbs 5g
Protein 19.3g
Fiber 4.3g

126. Easy-to-Prepare Broccoli

Preparation Time: 15 MINS
Servings: 4

Ingredients:

- 4 cups broccoli florets
- 6 minced garlic cloves
- 1 tbsp. butter
- 1 tbsp. fresh lime juice
- Salt, to taste

Directions:

1. In the bottom of Instant Pot, arrange a steamer basket and pour 1 cup of water.
2. Place the broccoli into the steamer basket.
3. Secure the lid and place the pressure valve to "Seal" position.
4. Select "Manual" and cook under "Low Pressure" for about 10 minutes.
5. Select the "Cancel" and carefully do a "Natural" release.
6. Remove the lid and transfer the broccoli to a plate.
7. Remove water from the pot and with paper

towels, pat dry.
8. Place the butter in the Instant Pot and select "Sauté". Then add the garlic and cook for about 30 seconds.
9. Add the broccoli and lime juice and cook for about 30 seconds.
10. Stir in salt and cook for about 1 minute.
11. Select the "Cancel" and serve.

Nutrition Value:
Calories 64
Total Fat 3.2g
Net Carbs 1.9g
Protein 2.9g
Fiber 2.5g

127. Luscious Broccoli Casserole
Preparation Time: 1 HOUR 4 MINS
Servings: 6

Ingredients:
- 2 tbsp. butter
- 1 chopped small yellow onion
- 4 minced garlic cloves
- 1 cup chopped broccoli florets
- 4 organic eggs
- ¼ cup unsweetened coconut milk
- Salt, to taste
- 1 tsp freshly grated lemon zest
- 1 tbsp. chopped fresh Italian parsley
- 1 tsp chopped fresh thyme
- 1½ cups shredded cheddar cheese

Directions:
1. Grease 1½ quart casserole dish that will fit in an Instant Pot. Keep aside.
2. Place the butter in the Instant Pot and select "Sauté". Then add the onion and garlic, and cook for about 7 minutes.
3. Add the broccoli and cook for about 4 minutes.
4. Select the "Cancel" and transfer the broccoli mixture to a large bowl.
5. In a large bowl, add remaining ingredients except for cheese and beat until well combined.
6. Add broccoli mixture and cheese and stir to combine.
7. Place the mixture into prepared casserole dish evenly.
8. With the glass lid, cover the casserole dish.
9. In the bottom of Instant Pot, arrange a steamer trivet and pour 1 cup of water.
10. Place the casserole dish on top of the trivet.
11. Secure the lid and place the pressure valve to "Seal" position.
12. Select "Manual" and cook under "High Pressure" for about 23 minutes.
13. Select the "Cancel" and carefully do a "Natural" release.
14. Remove the lid and serve warm.

Nutrition Value:
Calories 226
Total Fat 18.6g
Net Carbs 0.68g
Protein 11.7g
Fiber 1g

128. Better-Than-Real Mash
Preparation Time: 18 MINS
Servings: 8

Ingredients:
- ½ cup homemade chicken broth
- 1 chopped head cauliflower
- 2 tbsp. plain Greek yogurt
- Salt and ground black pepper, to taste
- 2 tsp melted butter
- 2 tbsp. chopped chives

Directions:
1. In the bottom of Instant Pot, arrange a steamer basket and pour broth.
2. Place the cauliflower into the steamer basket.
3. Secure the lid and place the pressure valve to "Seal" position.
4. Select "Manual" and cook under "High Pressure" for about 3 minutes.
5. Select the "Cancel" and carefully do a "Quick" release.
6. Remove the lid and transfer the cauliflower into a food processor.
7. Add yogurt, salt and black pepper and pulse until smooth.
8. Transfer the mashed cauliflower to a serving bowl.
9. Drizzle with melted ghee and serve with the garnishing of chives.

Nutrition Value:
Calories 40
Total Fat 1.2g
Net Carbs 0.75g
Protein 2.7g
Fiber 2.7g

129. Spicy Cauliflower
Preparation Time: 22 MINS
Servings: 4

Ingredients:

- 2 roughly chopped tomatoes
- ½ chopped small onion
- 1 green chile
- 1 tsp olive oil
- 1 tsp ground cumin
- ½ tsp ground turmeric
- ½ tsp paprika
- Salt and freshly ground black pepper, to taste
- 1 cut into small florets large head cauliflower
- ½ cup water
- 1 tbsp. chopped fresh cilantro

Directions:
1. In a food processor, add tomato, onion and green chile and pulse until smooth.
2. Place the oil in the Instant Pot and select "Sauté". Then add the pureed onion mixture and cook for about 2-3 minutes.
3. Add spices and cook for about 1 minute.
4. Select the "Cancel" and stir in cauliflower and water.
5. Secure the lid and place the pressure valve to "Seal" position.
6. Select "Manual" and cook under "Low Pressure" for about 2-3 minutes.
7. Select the "Cancel" and carefully do a Quick release.
8. Remove the lid and serve.

Nutrition Value:
Calories 74
Total Fat 1.7
Net Carbs 3.37g
Protein 4.5g
Fiber 5.8g

130. Veggie Mac and Cheese
Preparation Time: 23 MINS
Servings: 4

Ingredients:
- 2 cups grated into rice consistency cauliflower
- ½ cup shredded sharp cheddar cheese
- ½ cup half-and-half
- 2 tbsp. cream cheese
- Salt and freshly ground black pepper, to taste

Directions:
1. In a heatproof bowl that will fit in an Instant Pot, add all ingredients and stir to combine.
2. With a piece of foil, cover the bowl.
3. In the bottom of Instant Pot, arrange a steamer trivet and pour 1½ cups of water.
4. Place the casserole dish on top of the trivet.
5. Secure the lid and place the pressure valve to "Seal" position.
6. Select "Manual" and cook under "Low Pressure" for about 5 minutes.
7. Meanwhile, preheat the oven to broiler.
8. Select the "Cancel" and carefully do a "Natural" release for about 10 minutes and then do a "Quick" release.
9. Remove the lid transfer the bowl to a counter.
10. Remove the foil and broil for about 2-3 minutes.
11. Remove from oven and serve hot.

Nutrition Value:
Calories 126
Total Fat 10g
Net Carbs 1.07g
Protein 5.8g
Fiber 1.3g

131. Keto Soufflé
Preparation Time: 27 MINS
Servings: 6

Ingredients:
- 2 eggs
- 2-ounce softened cream cheese
- 1 cup sharp cheddar cheese
- ½ cup Asiago cheese
- ½ cup plain yogurt
- 2 tbsp. heavy cream
- 1 chopped head cauliflower
- ¼ cup minced fresh chives
- 2 tbsp. softened butter

Directions:
1. Grease 1¼ quart casserole dish that will fit in an Instant Pot. Keep aside.
2. In a food processor, add eggs, cream cheese, cheddar cheese, Asiago cheese, yogurt and heavy cream and pulse until smooth and frothy.
3. Add cauliflower and pulse until chunky.
4. Gently, fold in chives and butter.
5. Transfer the mixture to prepared casserole dish.
6. In the bottom of Instant Pot, arrange a steamer trivet and pour 1 cup of water.
7. Place the casserole dish on top of the trivet.
8. Secure the lid and place the pressure valve to "Seal" position.
9. Select "Manual" and cook under "High Pressure" for about 12 minutes.
10. Select the "Cancel" and carefully do a "Natural" release for about 10 minutes and then do a "Quick" release.
11. Remove the lid and serve.

Nutrition Value:
Calories 234
Total Fat 17.5g
Net Carbs 1.48g
Protein 11.7g
Fiber 3.1g

132. Indian Veggie Platter

Preparation Time: 22 MINS
Servings: 6

Ingredients:

- 4 dried red chilies
- 2 tbsp. shredded coconut
- 1 tsp coriander seeds
- 1 tsp cumin seeds
- ½ tsp mustard seeds
- ¼ tsp fenugreek seeds
- ½ tsp paprika
- 2 roughly chopped tomatoes
- ½ roughly chopped small yellow onion
- 5 chopped garlic cloves
- Salt, to taste
- 2 tbsp. butter
- 3 cups cauliflower
- 3 cups green beans
- 1 cup seeded and chopped bell pepper
- 2 cups water

Directions:

1. Heat a non-stick frying pan over medium heat and sauté red chilies, coconut and spices for about 1-2 minutes.
2. Remove from heat and keep aside to cool slightly.
3. In a spice grinder, add coconut mixture and grind into a coarse powder.
4. In a blender, add spice mixture, tomato, onion, garlic and salt and pulse until smooth.
5. Place the butter in the Instant Pot and select "Sauté". Then add the pureed tomato mixture and cook for about 4-5 minutes.
6. Select the "Cancel" and stir in veggies and water.
7. Secure the lid and place the pressure valve to "Seal" position.
8. Select "Manual" and cook under "Low Pressure" for about 14-15 minutes.
9. Select the "Cancel" and carefully do a Natural release.
10. Remove the lid and serve.

Nutrition Value:

Calories 93
Total Fat 4.9g
Net Carbs 1.95g
Protein 3.1g
Fiber 4.4g

133. French Veggie Combo

Preparation Time: 52 MINS
Servings: 8

Ingredients:

- 3 cups cubed into ¼-inch pieces eggplant
- Salt, to taste
- 4 tbsp. olive oil (divided)
- 1 chopped medium yellow onion
- 3 cups cubed into ¼-inch pieces zucchini
- 6 minced garlic cloves
- 2 seeded and cubed into ½-inch pieces bell peppers
- 2 tbsp. thinly sliced basil leaves (divided)
- ½ tsp red pepper flakes
- Freshly ground black pepper, to taste
- 2 cups cut into 1-inch pieces tomatoes
- 1 tbsp. chopped fresh parsley
- 1 tsp apple cider vinegar

Directions:

1. Arrange a colander in a sink.
2. Place eggplant pieces in the colander and sprinkle with some salt.
3. Keep aside to drain the moisture.
4. Place 2 tablespoons of the oil in the Instant Pot and select "Sauté". Then add the onion and cook for about 3-5 minutes.
5. Add the zucchini and garlic and cook for about 3-5 minutes.
6. Add the bell peppers and cook for about 3-5 minutes.
7. Add 1 tablespoon of basil leaves and stir to combine.
8. Select the "Cancel" and transfer the vegetable mixture to a bowl.
9. Place 2 tablespoons of the oil in the Instant Pot and select "Sauté". Then add the drained eggplant and cook for about 3-4 minutes.
10. Select the "Cancel" and stir in cooked veggie mixture red pepper flakes and black pepper.
11. Arrange tomato slices on top.
12. Secure the lid and place the pressure valve to "Seal" position.
13. Select "Manual" and cook under "High Pressure" for about 10 minutes.
14. Select the "Cancel" and carefully do a Quick release.

15. Remove the lid and select "Sauté".
16. Stir in vinegar and cook for about 6- 8 minutes.
17. Select the "Cancel" and serve hot with the garnishing of remaining basil.

Nutrition Value:
Calories 101
Total Fat 7.3g
Net Carbs 1.16g
Protein 1.8g
Fiber 2.9g

134. Provincial Ratatouille
Preparation Time: 26 MINS
Servings: 6

Ingredients:
- 1 sliced into thin circles large zucchini
- 1 sliced into thin circles medium eggplant
- 2 sliced into thin disks medium tomatoes
- 1 sliced into thin circles small yellow onion
- 1 tbsp. dried thyme (divided)
- Salt and freshly ground black pepper, to taste
- 2 finely chopped large garlic cloves
- 2 tbsp. olive oil
- 1 tbsp. apple cider vinegar
- 1 cup water

Directions:
1. In a bowl, add all vegetables and sprinkle with half of the thyme, salt and black pepper.
2. In the bottom of a foil lined round springform pan, spread some garlic.
3. Layer the vegetables into a tight snail-like circle over garlic, alternating between eggplant, zucchini, onion and tomato slices. (Keep the slices close together, overlapping slightly).
4. Sprinkle with the remaining garlic, thyme, salt and black pepper and drizzle with oil and vinegar.
5. In the bottom of Instant Pot, arrange a steamer trivet and pour 1 cup of water.
6. Place the pan on top of the trivet.
7. Secure the lid and place the pressure valve to "Seal" position.
8. Select "Manual" and cook under "Low Pressure" for about 6 minutes.
9. Select the "Cancel" and carefully do a "Natural" release for about 6 minutes and then do a "Quick" release.
10. Remove the lid and transfer the pan to a counter.
11. Carefully, transfer veggie mixture onto serving plates and serve.

Nutrition Value:
Calories 86
Total Fat 5.1g
Net Carbs 1.7g
Protein 2.1g
Fiber 4.4g

135. South-East Asian Curry
Preparation Time: 42 MINS
Servings: 4

Ingredients:
- 3 cups sliced fresh mushrooms
- ½ tsp minced garlic
- Salt, to taste
- ¼ tsp ground coriander
- ¼ tsp ground cumin
- ¼ tsp ground turmeric
- ¼ tsp red chili powder
- ½ cup unsweetened coconut milk
- ¼ cup plain Greek yogurt

Directions:
1. In a Pyrex dish that will fit in an Instant Pot, add all ingredients and stir to combine.
2. In the bottom of Instant Pot, arrange a steamer trivet and pour 1 cup of water.
3. Place the Pyrex dish on top of the trivet.
4. Secure the lid and place the pressure valve to "Seal" position.
5. Select "Manual" and cook under "High Pressure" for about 27 minutes.
6. Select the "Cancel" and carefully do a "Natural" release.
7. Remove the lid and serve.

Nutrition Value:
Calories 93
Total Fat 7.6g
Net Carbs 2.22g
Protein 3.3g
Fiber 1.3g

136. Summery Veggie Curry
Preparation Time: 29 MINS
Servings: 3

Ingredients:
For Spice Mixture:
- 1 tbsp. coriander seeds
- ½ tsp cumin seeds
- ½ tsp mustard seeds
- 2 tbsp. coconut shreds
- 2 tbsp. chopped peanuts

- 3 chopped garlic cloves
- 1 chopped hot green chile, chopped
- ½ tsp cayenne pepper
- ½ tsp ground turmeric
- Salt, to taste
- 1 tsp fresh lemon juice
- 1 cup plus 2 tsp water (divided)
- 6 baby eggplants

Directions:
1. Heat a non-stick frying pan over medium heat and sauté coriander, cumin and mustard seeds for about 2 minutes.
2. Add the coconut and peanuts and sauté for about 1-2 minutes.
3. Remove from heat and keep aside to cool slightly.
4. In a small food processor, add coconut mixture, garlic, chile, spices, lemon juice and 2 teaspoons of water and pulse until a coarse mixture is formed.
5. Carefully, make cross cuts on each eggplant, not all the way through.
6. Fill the spice mixture into the crosscut.
7. In the pot of Instant Pot, place the eggplants and with 1 cup of water and ¼ teaspoon of salt.
8. Secure the lid and place the pressure valve to "Seal" position.
9. Select "Manual" and cook under "High Pressure" for about 5 minutes.
10. Select the "Cancel" and carefully do a "Natural" release.
11. Remove the lid and serve.

Nutrition Value:
Calories 96
Total Fat 4.4g
Net Carbs 4.3g
Protein 4.1g
Fiber 5.1g

137. eritable Feast Curry

Preparation Time: 51 MINS
Servings: 8

Ingredients:
- 1 tbsp. coconut oil
- 1 finely chopped medium yellow onion
- 4 finely chopped garlic cloves
- 2 tbsp. curry powder
- 2½ cups cauliflower florets
- 2½ cups broccoli florets
- 3 tbsp. arrowroot starch
- Salt and freshly ground black pepper, to taste
- 2 cups water
- 1 (14-ouncecan unsweetened coconut milk
- 2 cups chopped fresh green beans

Directions:
1. Place the coconut oil in the Instant Pot and select "Sauté". Then add the onions for about 4-5 minutes.
2. Add the garlic and curry powder and cook for about 1 minute.
3. Select the "Cancel" and stir in remaining ingredients except for green beans.
4. Secure the lid and place the pressure valve to "Seal" position.
5. Select "Manual" and cook under "High Pressure" for about 20 minutes.
6. Select the "Cancel" and carefully do a "Natural" release.
7. Remove the lid and select "Sauté".
8. Stir in green beans and cook for about 5 minutes.
9. Select the "Cancel" and serve immediately.

Nutrition Value:
Calories 178
Total Fat 13.9g
Net Carbs 1.7g
Protein 3.5g
Fiber 4.5g

138. Italian Veggie Stew

Preparation Time: 51 MINS
Servings: 8

Ingredients:
- 2 tbsp. olive oil
- 1 minced celery stalk
- ½ minced medium yellow onion
- 2 minced garlic cloves
- 1 tsp Italian seasoning
- ½ tsp dried sage
- ½ tsp dried rosemary
- 10-ounce chopped Portobello mushrooms
- 10-ounce white button mushrooms
- 3¾ cups homemade vegetable broth
- 3 peeled and chopped medium carrots
- 3 cups chopped green beans
- 1 (15-ouncecan sugar-free diced tomatoes
- 1 (8-ouncecan sugar-free tomato sauce
- 1 tbsp. fresh lemon juice
- Salt and freshly ground black pepper, to taste
- 2 tbsp. arrowroot starch
- 3 tbsp. water

Directions:

1. Place the coconut oil in the Instant Pot and select "Sauté". Then add the celery, onion and garlic for about 4-5 minutes.
2. Add Italian seasoning and herbs and cook for about 1 minute.
3. Add mushrooms and cook for about 4-5 minutes.
4. Select the "Cancel" and stir in remaining ingredients except for arrowroot starch and water.
5. Secure the lid and place the pressure valve to "Seal" position.
6. Select "Manual" and cook under "High Pressure" for about 15 minutes.
7. Select the "Cancel" and carefully do a "Natural" release.
8. Meanwhile in a small bowl dissolve arrowroot starch in water.
9. Remove the lid and select "Sauté".
10. Stir in arrowroot starch mixture and cook for about 2-3 minutes.
11. Select the "Cancel" and serve hot.

Nutrition Value:
Calories 116
Total Fat 4.7g
Net Carbs 1.75g
Protein 6.6g
Fiber 4.1g

139. Spaghetti Squash
Preparation Time: 8-10 MIN
Servings: 5

Ingredients:
- 1 medium Spaghetti Squash (cca 4 lbs
- 1 cup Water

Directions:

1. With a knife cut the squash in half, across.
2. With a spoon remove seeds and placental tissue.
3. Place the steamer insert in the Instant Pot and then place squash halves in it.
4. Manually set the cooking time to 7 minutes at high pressure.
5. When done, quick release the pressure and carefully remove the squash from Instant Pot.
6. Using a fork scoop out the strands.
7. Serve with favorite low carb pasta sauce.

Nutrition Value:
Calories: 42
Total Fats: 0.4g
Net Carbs: 4g
Proteins: 1g

Fibers: 2.2g

140. Chili & Blue Cheese Stuffed Mushrooms
Preparation Time: 30 minutes
Servings: 2

Ingredients
- 1 tbsp olive oil
- 4 portobello mushrooms, stems removed
- 1 cup blue cheese, crumbled
- 2 sprigs fresh thyme, chopped
- ½ chili pepper chopped
- Salt and black pepper to taste
- 2 tbsp ground walnuts

Directions

1. Preheat the oven to 360 F.
2. Place the mushrooms on a lined baking sheet. In a bowl, add the blue cheese, chili pepper, and thyme and mix to combine. Fill the mushrooms with blue cheese mixture, top with walnuts, drizzle with olive oil and bake for 20 minutes. Serve with mixed leaf salad.

Nutrition Value:
Calories: 368, Fat:: 31.5g, Net Carbs:: 3.9g, Protein:: 18g

141 . Fresh Coconut Milk Shake with Blackberries
Preparation Time: 5 minutes
Servings: 2

Ingredients
- ½ cup water
- 1 ½ cups coconut milk
- 2 cups fresh blackberries
- ¼ tsp vanilla extract
- 1 tbsp vegan Protein: powder

Directions

1. In your a blender, combine all the ingredients and blend well until you attain a uniform and creamy consistency. Divide in glasses and serve!

Nutrition Value:
Calories: 253; Fat:: 22g, Net Carbs:: 5.6g, Protein:: 3.3g

142. Burritos Wraps with Avocado & Cauliflower
Preparation Time: 5 minutes
Servings: 2

Ingredients
- 1 tbsp butter
- ½ head cauliflower, cut into florets

- 2 zero carb flatbread
- 1 cup yogurt
- 1 cup tomato salsa
- 1 avocado, sliced
- 1 tbsp cilantro, chopped

Directions

1. Put the cauliflower in a food processor and pulse until it resembles rice. In a skillet, melt the butter and add the cauli rice. Sauté for 4-5 minutes until cooked through. Season with salt and black pepper. On flatbread, spread the yogurt all over and distribute the salsa on top. Top with cauli rice and scatter the avocado slices and cilantro on top. Fold and tuck the burritos and cut into two.

Nutrition Value:

Calories: 457, Fat: 31.3g, Net Carbs: 9.6g, Protein: 15.8g

143. Pizza Bianca with Mushrooms

Preparation Time: 17 minutes
Servings: 2

Ingredients

- 2 tbsp olive oil
- 4 eggs
- 2 tbsp water
- 1 jalapeño pepper, diced
- ¼ cup mozzarella cheese, shredded
- 2 chives, chopped
- 2 cups egg Alfredo sauce
- ½ tsp oregano
- ½ cup mushrooms, sliced

Directions

1. Preheat oven to 360 F.
2. In a bowl, whisk eggs, water, and oregano. Heat the olive oil in a large skillet. Pour in the egg mixture and cook until set, flipping once. Remove and spread the alfredo sauce and jalapeño pepper all over. Top with mozzarella cheese, mushrooms and chives. Bake for 5-10 minutes until the cheese melts.

Nutrition Value:

Calories: 312, Fat:: 23.5g, Net Carbs:: 2.4g, Protein:: 17.2g

144. Hot Pizza with Tomatoes, Cheese & Olives

Preparation Time: 30 minutes
Servings: 2

Ingredients

- 2 tbsp psyllium husk
- 1 cup cheddar cheese
- 2 tbsp cream cheese
- 2 tbsp pecorino cheese
- 1 tsp oregano
- ½ cup almond flour
- Topping
- 1 tomato, sliced
- 4 oz cheddar cheese, sliced
- ¼ cup tomato sauce
- 1 jalapeño pepper, sliced
- ½ cup black olives
- 2 tbsp basil, chopped

Directions

1. Preheat the oven to 375 F.
2. Microwave the cheddar cheese in an oven-proof bowl. In a separate bowl, combine cream cheese, pecorino cheese, psyllium husk, almond flour, and oregano. Add in the melted cheddar cheese and mix with your hands to combine.
3. Divide the dough in two. Roll out the two crusts in circles and place on a lined baking sheet. Bake for about 10 minutes.
4. Spread the tomato sauce over the crust and top with the cheddar cheese slices, jalapeño pepper, and tomato slices. Return to the oven and bake for another 10 minutes.
5. Garnish with black olives and basil.

Nutrition Value:

Calories: 576, Fat:: 42.3g, Net Carbs:: 7.5g, Protein:: 32.4g

145. Spicy Vegetarian Burgers with Fried Eggs

Preparation Time: 20 minutes
Servings: 2

Ingredients

- 1 garlic clove, minced
- 2 portobello mushrooms, chopped
- 1 cup cauli rice
- 1 tbsp peanut butter
- 1 tbsp basil, chopped
- 1 tbsp oregano
- Salt to taste
- 1 jalapeño pepper, minced
- ¼ red onion, sliced
- 2 eggs
- 2 low carb buns
- 2 tbsp mayonnaise
- 2 lettuce leaves

Directions

1. Sauté the mushrooms and cauli rice in warm peanut butter for 5 minutes. Remove to a bowl and add in garlic, oregano, basil, jalapeño pepper, and salt and mix well to obtain a dough. Make medium-sized burgers from the dough.
2. Cook the burgers in the same butter for 2 minutes per side and transfer to a serving plate. Reduce the heat and fry the eggs. Cut the low carb buns in half.
3. Add the lettuce leaves, burgers, eggs, red onion, and mayonnaise. Top with the other bun half.

Nutrition Value:
Calories: 456, Fat:: 37.5g, Net Carbs:: 9.3g, Protein:: 19g

146. Grilled Cauliflower Steaks with Haricots Vert

Preparation Time: 20 minutes
Servings: 2

Ingredients

- 2 tbsp olive oil
- 1 head cauliflower, sliced lengthwise into 'steaks'
- 2 tbsp chili sauce
- 1 tsp hot paprika
- 1 tsp oregano
- Salt and black pepper to taste
- 1 shallot, chopped
- 1 bunch haricots vert, trimmed
- 1 tbsp fresh lemon juice
- 1 tbsp cilantro, chopped

Directions

1. Preheat grill to medium heat. Steam the haricots vert in salted water over medium heat for 6 minutes. Drain, remove to a bowl and toss with lemon juice.
2. In a bowl, mix the olive oil, chili sauce, hot paprika, and oregano. Brush the cauliflower steaks with the mixture. Place them on the grill, close the lid and grill for 6 minutes.
3. Flip the cauliflower and cook further for 6 minutes. Remove the grilled caulis to a plate; sprinkle with salt, black pepper, shallots and cilantro. Serve with the steamed haricots vert.

Nutrition Value:
Calories: 234, Fat: 15.9g, Net Carbs: 8.4g, Protein: 5.2g

147. Tofu & Vegetable Stir-Fry

Preparation Time: 10 minutes + marinade time
Servings: 2

Ingredients

- 2 tbsp olive oil
- 1 ½ cups extra firm tofu, pressed and cubed
- 1 ½ tbsp flax seed meal
- Salt and black pepper, to taste
- 1 garlic clove, minced
- 1 tbsp soy sauce, sugar-free
- ½ head broccoli, break into florets
- 1 tsp onion powder
- 1 cup mushrooms, sliced
- 1 tbsp sesame seeds

Directions

1. In a bowl, add onion powder, tofu, salt, soy sauce, black pepper, flaxseed, and garlic. Toss the mixture to coat and allow to marinate for 20-30 minutes.
2. In a pan, warm oil over medium heat, add in broccoli, mushrooms and tofu mixture and stir-fry for 6-8 minutes. Serve sprinkled with sesame seeds.

Nutrition Value:
Calories: 423; Fat:: 31g, Net Carbs:: 7.3g, Protein:: 25.5g

148. Chili Lover's Frittata with Spinach & Cheese

Preparation Time: 17 minutes
Servings: 2

Ingredients

- 2 tbsp olive oil
- 1 cup spinach, chopped
- 2 red and yellow chilies, roasted and chopped
- 1 tbsp red wine vinegar
- 1 tbsp parsley, chopped
- 4 eggs
- ¼ cup Parmesan cheese, grated
- 2 tbsp goat cheese, crumbled
- ½ cup salad greens

Directions

1. In a bowl, mix the vinegar, half of the olive oil, and chilies. Coat the salad greens with the dressing.
2. In another bowl, whisk the eggs with salt, black pepper, parsley, spinach, and parmesan cheese.
3. Heat the remaining oil in the cast iron over medium heat and pour the egg mixture along with half of the goat cheese. Let cook for 3 minutes and when it is near done, sprinkle the remaining goat cheese on it, and transfer the cast iron to the oven.
4. Bake the frittata for 4 more minutes at 400 F. Garnish the frittata with salad greens and serve.

Nutrition Value:

Calories: 316, Fat: 28.3g, Net Carbs: 4.1g, Protein: 9.5g

149. Spicy Cauliflower Falafel

Preparation Time: 15 minutes
Servings: 2

Ingredients

- 4 tbsp olive oil
- 1 head cauliflower, cut into florets
- 1/3 cup silvered ground almonds
- ½ tsp ground cumin
- 1 tsp parsley, chopped
- Salt to taste
- 1 tsp chili pepper
- 3 tbsp coconut flour
- 2 eggs

Directions

1. Blitz the cauliflower in a food processor until a grain meal consistency is formed. Transfer to a bowl, add in the ground almonds, ground cumin, parsley, salt, chili pepper, and coconut flour, and mix until evenly combined.
2. Beat the eggs in a bowl and mix with the cauli mixture. Shape ¼ cup each into patties and set aside.
3. Warm olive oil in a frying pan over medium heat and fry the patties for 5 minutes on each side to be firm and browned. Remove onto a wire rack to cool, share into serving plates, and serve.

Nutrition Value:

Calories: 343, Fat: 31.2g, Net Carbs: 3.7g, Protein: 8.5g

150. Mediterranean Eggplant Squash Pasta

Preparation Time: 15 minutes
Servings: 2

Ingredients

- 2 tbsp butter
- 1 cup cherry tomatoes
- 2 tbsp parsley, chopped
- 1 eggplant, cubed
- ¼ cup Parmesan cheese
- 3 tbsp scallions, chopped
- 1 cup green beans
- 1 tsp lemon zest
- 10 oz butternut squash, spirals

Directions

1. In a saucepan over medium heat, add the butter to melt. Cook the spaghetti squash for 4-5 minutes and remove to a plate. In the same saucepan, cook eggplant for 5 minutes until tender.
2. Add the tomatoes and green beans, and cook for 5 more minutes. Stir in parsley, zest, and scallions, and remove the pan from heat. Stir in spaghetti squash and Parmesan cheese to serve.

Nutrition Value:

Calories: 388, Fat:: 17.8g, Net Carbs:: 9.6g, Protein:: 12g

151. Spiral Zucchini Noodles with Cheesy Sauce

Preparation Time: 20 minutes
Servings: 2

- ### Ingredients
- 2 tbsp olive oil
- 1 (28-ounce) can tomatoes, crushed
- 2 garlic cloves, minced
- 1 cup kale
- 1 onion, chopped
- 1 pound zucchinis, spiralized
- ¼ cup Parmesan cheese, shredded
- 10 kalamata olives, halved
- 2 tbsp basil, chopped
- Salt and black pepper to taste

Directions

1. Heat the olive oil in a pan over medium heat. Add zucchinis and cook for about 5 minutes. Transfer to a serving platter. In the same pan, sauté onion and garlic for 3 minutes.
2. Add in tomatoes, kale, salt, and pepper, reduce the heat and simmer for 8-10 minutes until thickened. Pour the sauce over zucchini noodles, scatter Parmesan cheese all over and top with olives and basil.

Nutrition Value:

Calories: 388, Fat:: 25.4g, Net Carbs:: 6.8g, Protein:: 15.5g

152. Cajun Flavored Stuffed Mushrooms

Preparation Time: 35 minutes
Servings: 2

Ingredients

- 2 tbsp coconut oil
- ½ head broccoli, cut into florets
- 1 pound cremini mushrooms, stems removed
- 1 onion, chopped
- ¼ cup almonds, chopped
- 1 garlic clove, minced
- 1 bell pepper, chopped
- 1 tsp cajun seasoning mix

- Salt and black pepper, to taste
- 1 cup Parmesan cheese, shredded

Directions

1. Blend the broccoli in a food processor until they become small rice-like granules.
2. Set oven to 360 F. Bake mushroom caps until tender for 8 to 12 minutes. In a skillet, melt the coconut oil; stir in bell pepper, garlic, and onion and sauté until fragrant. Place in black pepper, salt, and cajun seasoning mix. Fold in broccoli rice and almonds.
3. Equally separate the filling mixture among mushroom caps. Add a topping of Parmesan cheese and bake for 17 more minutes. Serve warm.

Nutrition Value:

Calories: 423; Fat:: 25.4g, Net Carbs:: 9.5g, Protein:: 21.7g

153. Keto Tortilla Wraps with Vegetables

Preparation Time: 10 minutes
Servings: 2

Ingredients

- 2 tsp olive oil
- 2 low carb tortillas
- 1 green onion, sliced
- 1 bell pepper, sliced
- ¼ tsp hot chilli powder
- 1 large avocado, sliced
- 1 cup cauli rice
- Salt and black pepper to taste
- ¼ cup sour cream
- 1 tbsp Mexican salsa
- 1 tbsp cilantro, chopped

Directions

1. Warm the olive oil in a skillet and sauté the green onion and bell pepper until they start to brown on the edges, for about 4 minutes; remove to a bowl. To the same pan, add in the cauli rice and stir-fry for 4-5 minutes. Combine with the onion and bell pepper mixture, season with salt, black pepper, and chili powder. Let cool for a few minutes.
2. Add in avocado, sour cream, and Mexican salsa and stir. Top with cilantro. Fold in the sides of each tortilla, and roll them in and over the filling to be enclosed. Wrap with foil, cut in halves, and serve.

Nutrition Value:

Calories: 373, Fat: 31.2g, Net Carbs: 8.6g, Protein: 7.6g

154. Roasted Cauliflower Gratin

Preparation Time: 21 minutes
Servings: 2-4

Ingredients

- 1/3 cup butter
- 2 tbsp melted butter
- 1 onion, chopped
- 2 heads cauliflower, cut into florets
- Salt and black pepper to taste
- ¼ cup almond milk
- ½ cup almond flour
- 1 ½ cup cheddar cheese, grated
- 1 tbsp ground almonds
- 1 tbsp parsley, chopped

Directions

1. Steam the cauliflower in salted water for 4-5 minutes. Drain and set aside.
2. Melt the 1/3 cup of butter in a saucepan over medium heat and sauté the onion for 3 minutes. Add the cauliflower, season with salt and black pepper and mix in almond milk. Simmer for 3 minutes.
3. Mix the remaining melted butter with almond flour. Stir into the cauliflower as well as half of the cheese. Sprinkle the top with the remaining cheese and ground almonds, and bake for 10 minutes until golden brown on the top. Serve sprinkled with parsley.

Nutrition Value:

Calories: 455, Fat: 38.3g, Net Carbs: 6.5g, Protein: 16.3g

155. Basil Spinach & Zucchini Lasagna

Preparation Time: 40 minutes
Servings: 2-4

Ingredients

- 2 zucchinis, sliced
- Salt and black pepper to taste
- 2 cups feta cheese
- 2 cups mozzarella cheese, shredded
- 3 cups tomato passata
- 1 cup spinach
- 1 tbsp basil, chopped

Directions

1. Mix the feta, mozzarella cheese, salt, and black pepper to evenly combine and spread ¼ cup of the mixture in the bottom of a greased baking dish. Layer 1/3 of the zucchini slices on top spread 1 cup of tomato sauce over, and scatter a 1/3 cup of spinach on top.

2. Repeat the layering process two more times to exhaust the ingredients while making sure to layer with the last ¼ cup of cheese mixture finally. Bake for 35 minutes until the cheese has a nice golden brown color. Remove the dish, sit for 5 minutes and serve sprinkled with basil.

Nutrition Value:

Calories: 411, Fat: 41.3g, Net Carbs: 3.2g, Protein: 6.5g

156. Broccoli & Asparagus Flan

Preparation Time: 65 minutes
Servings: 2-4

Ingredients

- A bunch of asparagus, stems trimmed
- 1 cup broccoli florets
- 1 cup water
- ½ cup whipping cream
- 1 cup almond milk
- 3 eggs
- 2 tbsp tarragon, chopped
- Salt and black pepper to taste
- A small pinch of nutmeg
- 2 tbsp Parmesan cheese, grated
- 3 cups water
- 2 tbsp butter, melted
- 1 tbsp butter, softened

Directions

1. Steam asparagus and broccoli in salted water over medium heat for 6 minutes. Drain and cut the tips of the asparagus and reserve for garnishing. Chop the remaining asparagus into small pieces.
2. In a blender, add the chopped asparagus, broccoli, whipping cream, almond milk, tarragon salt, nutmeg, black pepper, and Parmesan cheese and process until smooth. Pour the mixture through a sieve into a bowl and whisk the eggs into it.
3. Preheat the oven to 350 F. Grease ramekins with softened butter and share the asparagus mixture among the ramekins. Pour the melted butter over each one and top with 2-3 asparagus tips.
4. Pour the remaining water into a baking dish, place in the ramekins, and insert in the oven. Bake for 45 minutes or until their middle parts are no longer watery. Garnish the flan with the asparagus tips and serve.

Nutrition Value:

Calories: 298, Fat: 24,6g, Net Carbs: 4.5g, Protein: 17.5g

157. Grilled Vegetables & Tempeh Shish Kebab

Preparation Time: 26 minutes + marinade time
Servings: 2-4

Ingredients

- 2 tbsp olive oil
- 10 oz tempeh, cut into chunks
- 1 ½ cups water
- 1 red onion, cut into chunks
- 1 red bell pepper, cut chunks
- 1 yellow bell pepper, cut into chunks
- 1 cup zucchini, sliced
- 1 cup barbecue sauce, sugar-free
- 2 tbsp chives

Directions

1. In a pot over medium heat, pour the water. Bring to boil remove from heat and add the tempeh. Cover the pot and let tempeh steam for 5 minutes to remove its bitterness. Drain the tempeh after.
2. Pour the barbecue sauce in a bowl, add the tempeh to it, and coat with the sauce. Cover the bowl and marinate in the fridge for 2 hours. Preheat grill to medium heat. Thread the tempeh, yellow bell pepper, red bell pepper, zucchini, and onion.
3. Brush the grate of the grill with olive oil, place the skewers on it, and brush with barbecue sauce. Cook the skewers for 3 minutes on each side while rotating and brushing with more barbecue sauce.
4. Once ready, transfer the kabobs to a plate and serve sprinkled with chives.

Nutrition Value:

Calories: 228, Fat: 15g, Net Carbs: 3.6g, Protein: 13.2g

158. Grilled Tofu Kabobs with Arugula Salad

Preparation Time: 40 minutes + marinade time
Servings: 2-4

Ingredients

- 14 oz firm tofu, cut into strips
- 4 tsp sesame oil
- 1 lemon, juiced
- 5 tbsp soy sauce, sugar-free
- 3 tsp garlic powder
- 4 tbsp coconut flour
- ½ cup sesame seeds
- Arugula salad:
- 4 cups arugula, chopped
- 2 tsp extra virgin olive oil

- 2 tbsp pine nuts
- Salt and black pepper to season
- 1 tbsp balsamic vinegar

Directions

1. Stick the tofu strips on the skewers, height wise and place onto a plate.
2. In a bowl, mix sesame oil, lemon juice, soy sauce, garlic powder, and coconut flour. Pour the soy sauce mixture over the tofu, and turn in the sauce to be adequately coated. Cover the dish with cling film and marinate in the fridge for 2 hours.
3. Heat the griddle pan over high heat. Coat the tofu in the sesame seeds and grill in the griddle pan to be golden brown on both sides, about 12 minutes in total.
4. Arrange the arugula on a serving plate. Drizzle over olive oil and balsamic vinegar, and season with salt and black pepper. Sprinkle with pine nuts and place the tofu kabobs on top to serve.

Nutrition Value:

Calories: 411, Fat: 32.9g, Net Carbs: 7.1g, Protein: 21.6g

159. Sticky Tofu with Cucumber & Tomato Salad

Preparation Time: 40 minutes
Servings: 2-4

Ingredients

- 2 tbsp olive oil
- 12 ounces tofu
- 1 cup green onions, chopped
- 1 garlic clove, minced
- 2 tbsp vinegar
- 1 tbsp sriracha sauce

Salad

- 1 tbsp fresh lemon juice
- 2 tbsp extra virgin olive oil
- Sea salt and black pepper, to taste
- 1 tsp fresh dill weed
- 1 cup Greek yogurt
- 1 cucumber, sliced
- 2 tomatoes, sliced

Directions

1. Pat the tofu dry with kitchen paper and cut into slices. Put tofu slices, garlic, sriracha sauce, vinegar, and scallions in a bowl; allow to settle for approximately 30 minutes. Set oven to medium heat and add oil in a nonstick skillet to warm. Cook tofu for 5 minutes until golden brown.
2. In a salad plate, arrange tomatoes and cucumber slices, season with salt and black pepper, drizzle lemon juice and extra virgin olive oil and scatter dill all over. Top with the tofu and serve.

Nutrition Value:

Calories: 371; Fat:: 30.9g, Net Carbs:: 7.7g, Protein:: 17.3g

160. Stewed Vegetables

Preparation Time: 32 minutes
Servings: 2-4

Ingredients

- 2 tbsp butter
- 1 shallot, chopped
- 1 garlic clove, minced
- 1 tsp paprika
- 1 carrot, chopped
- 2 tomatoes, chopped
- 1 head cabbage, shredded
- 2 cups green beans, chopped
- 2 bell peppers, sliced
- Salt and black pepper to taste
- 2 tbsp parsley, chopped
- 1 cup vegetable broth

Directions

1. Melt butter in a saucepan over medium heat and sauté onion and garlic to be fragrant, 2 minutes.
2. Stir in bell peppers, carrot, cabbage, and green beans, paprika, salt, and pepper, add the vegetable broth and tomatoes, stir again, and cook the vegetables on low heat for 25 minutes to soften. Serve the stew sprinkled with parsley.

Nutrition Value:

Calories: 310, Fat: 26.4g, Net Carbs: 6g, Protein: 8g

161. Grilled Halloumi with Cauli-Rice & Almonds

Preparation Time: 5 minutes
Servings: 2-4

Ingredients

- 2 tbsp olive oil
- 4 oz halloumi, sliced
- 1 cauliflower head, grated
- ¼ cup oregano, chopped
- ¼ cup parsley, chopped
- ¼ cup mint, chopped
- ½ lemon juiced
- 2 tbsp almonds, chopped
- Salt and black pepper to taste

- 1 avocado, sliced to garnish

Directions
1. Heat a grill pan over medium heat. Drizzle the halloumi cheese with olive oil and add in the pan. Grill for 2 minutes on each side to be golden brown, set aside.
2. To make the cauli rice, add in the cauliflower and cook for 5-6 minutes until slightly cooked but crunchy. Stir in the cilantro, parsley, mint, lemon juice, salt and black pepper. Garnish the rice with avocado slices and almonds and serve with grilled halloumi.

Nutrition Value:
Calories: 255, Fat: 23g, Net Carbs: 3.3g, Protein: 7.6g

162. Portobello Bun Mushroom Burgers
Preparation Time: 15 minutes
Servings: 2-4

Ingredients
- 2 tbsp olive oil
- 4 portobello mushroom caps
- 1 clove garlic
- Salt and black pepper to taste
- ½ cup roasted red peppers, sliced
- 2 tomatoes, sliced
- 1 cup guacamole
- 1 zucchini, sliced
- ¼ cup feta cheese, crumbled
- 1 tbsp red wine vinegar
- 2 tbsp pitted kalamata olives, chopped
- ½ tsp dried oregano

Directions
1. Crush the garlic with salt in a bowl using the back of a spoon. Stir in 1 tablespoon of oil and brush the mushrooms and each inner side of the buns with the mixture.
2. Place the mushrooms in a preheated pan and grill them on both sides for 8 minutes until tender. Drizzle the zucchini with a little bit of olive oil, season with salt and pepper, and grill on both sides for 5-6 minutes.
3. In a bowl, mix the red peppers, olives, feta cheese, vinegar, oregano, and remaining oil; toss them. Assemble the burger: spread some guacamole on a slice of a mushroom bun, add 1-2 zucchini slices, a scoop of thevegetable mixture, a slice of tomato and another slice of mushroom bun.

Nutrition Value:
Calories: 221, Fat: 18.8g, Net Carbs: 4.3g, Protein: 4.5g

163. Soy Chorizo & Cabbage Bake
Preparation Time: 25 minutes
Servings: 2-4

Ingredients
- 1 pound soy chorizo, sliced
- 1 head green cabbage, cut into wedges
- 4 tbsp butter, melted
- 1 tsp garlic powder
- Salt and black pepper to taste
- 2 tbsp Parmesan cheese, grated
- 1 tbsp parsley, chopped

Directions
1. Preheat oven to 390 F, Grease a baking tray with cooking spray. Mix the butter, garlic, salt, and black pepper until evenly combined in a bowl.
2. Brush the mixture on all sides of the cabbage wedges. Place on the baking sheet, add in the soy chorizo and bake for 20 minutes to soften the cabbage. Sprinkle with Parmesan cheese and parsley.

Nutrition Value:
Calories: 268, Fat: 19.3g, Net Carbs: 4g, Protein: 17.5g

164. One-Pot Mushroom Stroganoff
Preparation Time: 15 minutes
Servings: 2-4

Ingredients
- 3 tbsp cashew butter
- 1 onion, chopped
- 4 cups baby bella mushrooms, cubed
- 2 cups vegetable broth
- ½ cup heavy cream
- ½ cup Parmesan cheese, grated
- 1 ½ tbsp dried Italian seasoning
- Salt and black pepper to taste

Directions
1. Melt the cashew butter in a saucepan over medium heat, sauté the onion for 3 minutes until soft.
2. Stir in the mushrooms and cook until tender, for about 3 minutes. Add the vegetable broth, mix, and bring to boil for 4 minutes until the liquid reduces slightly.
3. Pour in the heavy cream and Parmesan cheese. Stir to melt the cheese. Also, mix in the Italian seasoning. Season with salt and pepper, simmer for 40 seconds and turn the heat off. Ladle stroganoff over a bed of spaghetti squash and serve.

Nutrition Value:
Calories: 255, Fat: 21g, Net Carbs: 5.4g, Protein: 7.8g

165. Vegetable Stew
Preparation Time: 25 minutes
Servings: 2-4

Ingredients
- 2 tbsp olive oil
- 1 turnip, chopped
- 1 onion, chopped
- 2 garlic cloves, pressed
- ½ cup celery, chopped
- 1 carrot, chopped
- 1 cup wild mushrooms, sliced
- 2 tbsp dry white wine
- 2 tbsp rosemary, chopped
- 1 thyme sprig, chopped
- 4 cups vegetable stock
- ½ tsp chili pepper
- 1 tsp smoked paprika
- 2 tomatoes, chopped
- 1 tbsp flax seed meal

Directions
1. Cook onion, carrot, celery, mushrooms, paprika, chili pepper, and garlic in warm oil over medium heat for 5-6 minutes until tender; set the vegetables aside.
2. Stir in wine to deglaze the stockpot's bottom. Place in thyme and rosemary. Pour in tomatoes, vegetable stock, reserved vegetables and turnip and allow to boil.
3. On low heat, allow the mixture to simmer for 15 minutes while covered. Stir in flax seed meal to thicken the stew. Plate into individual bowls and serve.

Nutrition Value:
Calories: 164; Fat:: 11.3g, Net Carbs:: 8.2g, Protein:: 3.3g

166. Sautéed Tofu with Pistachios
Preparation Time: 15 minutes
Servings: 2-4

Ingredients
- 2 tbsp olive oil
- 8 oz firm tofu, cubed
- 1 tbsp tomato paste
- 1 tbsp balsamic vinegar
- 1 tsp garlic powder
- 1 tsp onion powder
- Salt and black pepper to taste
- 1 cup pistachios, chopped

Directions
1. Heat the oil in a skillet over medium heat and cook the tofu for 3 minutes while stirring to brown.
2. Mix the tomato paste, garlic powder, onion powder, and vinegar; add to the tofu. Stir, season with salt and black pepper, and cook for another 4 minutes.
3. Add the pistachios. Stir and cook on low heat for 3 minutes to be fragrant.

Nutrition Value:
Calories: 335, Fat: 27g, Net Carbs: 6.3g, Protein: 16.5g

167. Zucchini Spaghetti with Avocado & Capers
Preparation Time: 15 minutes
Servings: 2-4

Ingredients
- 2 tbsp olive oil
- 4 zucchinis, julienned or spiralized
- ½ cup pesto
- 2 avocados, sliced
- ¼ cup capers
- ¼ cup basil, chopped
- ¼ cup sun-dried tomatoes, chopped

Directions
1. Cook zucchini spaghetti in half of the warm olive oil over medium heat for 4 minutes.
2. Transfer to a plate. Stir in pesto, basil, salt, tomatoes, and capers. Top with avocado slices.

Nutrition Value:
Calories: 449, Fat: 42g, Net Carbs:: 8.4g, Protein:: 6.3g

168. Mushroom & Cheese Cauliflower Risotto
Preparation Time: 15 minutes
Servings: 2-4

Ingredients
- 3 tbsp olive oil
- 1 onion, chopped
- ¼ cup vegetable broth
- 1/3 cup Parmesan cheese
- 4 tbsp heavy cream
- 3 tbsp chives, chopped
- 2 pounds mushrooms, sliced
- 1 large head cauliflower, break into florets
- 2 tbsp parsley, chopped

Directions

1. In a food processor, pulse the cauliflower florets until you attain a rice-like consistency.
2. Heat 2 tbsp oil in a saucepan. Add the mushrooms and cook over medium heat for about 3 minutes. set aside. Heat the remaining oil and cook the onion for 2 minutes.
3. Stir in the cauliflower and broth, and cook until the liquid is absorbed, about 7-8 minutes. Stir in the heavy cream and Parmesan cheese, Top with chives and parsley to serve.

Nutrition Value:

Calories: 255, Fat:: 21g, Net Carbs:: 5.3g, Protein:: 10.3g

169. Avocado Boats

Preparation Time: 10 minutes
Servings: 2-4

Ingredients

- 2 avocados, halved and stoned
- 1 tomato, chopped
- 1 cucumber, chopped
- ¼ cup walnuts, ground
- 2 carrots, chopped
- 1 garlic clove
- 1 tsp lemon juice
- 1 tbsp soy sauce
- Salt and black pepper, to taste

Directions

1. To make the filling, in a mixing bowl, mix soy sauce, tomato, carrots, avocado pulp, cucumber, lemon juice, walnuts, and garlic.
2. Add black pepper and salt. Plate the mixture into the avocado halves. Scatter walnuts over to serve.

Nutrition Value:

Calories: 272; Fat:: 25g, Net Carbs:: 6.1g, Protein:: 4g

170. Basil Tofu with Cashew Nuts

Preparation Time: 13 minutes
Servings: 2-4

Ingredients

- 3 tsp olive oil
- 1 cup extra firm tofu, cubed
- ¼ cup cashew nuts
- 1 ½ tbsp coconut aminos
- 3 tbsp vegetable broth
- 1 garlic clove, minced
- 1 tsp cayenne pepper
- ½ tsp turmeric powder
- Salt and black pepper, to taste
- 2 tsp sunflower seeds
- 10 basil leaves, torn
- 1 tbsp balsamic vinegar

Directions

1. Warm olive oil in a frying pan over medium heat. Add in tofu and fry until golden, turning once, for about 6 minutes. Pour in the cashew nuts and cook for 2 minutes. Stir in the remaining ingredients except for the balsamic vinegar and basil, set heat to medium-low and cook for 5 more minutes.
2. Drizzle with the balsamic vinegar, season to taste, sprinkle with basil and serve.

Nutrition Value:

Calories: 245; Fat:: 19.6g, Net Carbs:: 5.5g, Protein:: 12.3g

171. Stuffed Mushrooms

Preparation Time: 30 minutes
Servings: 2-4

Ingredients

- 2 tbsp olive oil
- ¼ tsp chilli flakes
- 1 cup gorgonzola cheese, crumbled
- 1 onion, chopped
- 1 garlic clove, minced
- 1 pound mushrooms, stems removed
- Salt and black pepper, to taste
- ¼ cup walnuts, toasted and chopped
- 2 tbsp parsley, chopped

Directions

1. Put to a pan over medium heat and warm the olive oil. Sauté garlic and onion, until soft, for about 5 minutes. Sprinkle with black pepper and salt, and remove to a bowl.
2. Add in walnuts and gorgonzola cheese and stir until heated through. Divide the filling among the mushroom caps and set on a greased baking sheet.
3. Bake in the oven for 30 minutes at 360 F and remove to a wire rack to cool slightly. Add fresh parsley and serve.

Nutrition Value:

Calories: 139; Fat:: 11.2g, Net Carbs:: 7.4g, Protein:: 4.8g

172. Steamed Bok Choy with Thyme & Garlic

Preparation Time: 25 minutes
Servings: 2-4

Ingredients

- 2 pounds Bok choy, sliced

- 2 tbsp coconut oil
- 2 tbsp soy sauce, sugar-free
- 1 tsp garlic, minced
- ½ tsp thyme, chopped
- ½ tsp red pepper flakes, crushed
- Salt and black pepper, to the taste

Directions

1. In a pot, steam bok choy in salted water over medium heat, for 6 minutes; drain and set aside. Place a pan over medium heat and warm the coconut oil. Add in garlic and cook until soft.
2. Stir in the bok choy, red pepper, soy sauce, black pepper, salt, and thyme and cook until everything is heated through, for about 1-2 minutes.

Nutrition Value:

Calories: 132; Fat:: 9.5g, Net Carbs:: 3.5g, Protein:: 4.9g

173. Stir-Fried Brussels Sprouts with Tofu & Leeks

Preparation Time: 20 minutes
Servings: 2-4

Ingredients

2 tbsp olive oil
2 garlic cloves, minced
1 leek, sliced
10 ounces tofu, crumbled
2 tbsp water
2 tbsp soy sauce, sugar-free
1 tbsp tomato puree
½ pound Brussels sprouts, halved
½ red chilli, seeded and sliced
Salt and black pepper, to taste
Lime wedges to serve

Directions

1. In a saucepan over medium heat, warm the oil. Add the leek and garlic and cook until tender, about 2-3 minutes. Place in the soy sauce, water, red chilli and tofu.
2. Cook for 5 minutes until the tofu starts to brown. Add in brussels sprouts, season with black pepper and salt, and cook for 10 minutes while stirring frequently. Garnish with lime wedges to serve.

Nutrition Value:

Calories: 183; Fat:: 12.5g, Net Carbs:: 7.7g, Protein:: 13.2g

174. Colorful Peppers Stuffed with Mushrooms & "Rice"

Preparation Time: 40 minutes
Servings: 2-4

Ingredients

- 2 tbsp olive oil
- 1 head cauliflower, grated
- 2 pounds mixed bell peppers, tops removed
- 1 cup mushrooms, sliced
- 1 onion, chopped
- 1 cup celery, chopped
- 1 garlic clove, minced
- 1 tsp dried oregano
- 1 tsp chili powder
- 2 tomatoes, pureed
- Sea salt and pepper, to taste
- 2 tbsp parsley, chopped

Directions

1. Preheat oven to 360 F and lightly oil a casserole dish.
2. Warm the olive oil over medium heat in a pan. Add in garlic, celery, and onion and sauté until soft and translucent. Stir in chili powder, tomatoes, mushrooms, oregano, parsley, and cauliflower rice. Cook for 6 minutes until the cauliflower rice becomes tender. Season with salt and black pepper.
3. Split the cauliflower mixture among the bell peppers. Set in the casserole dish and bake for 30 minutes until the skin of the peppers starts to brown. Serve with full-Fat: Greek yogurt.

Nutrition Value:

Calories:: 233; Fat: 8g, Net Carbs: 8.4g, Protein: 7.6g,

175. Fennel & Celeriac with Chili Tomato Sauce

Preparation Time: 20 minutes
Servings: 2-4

Ingredients

- 2 tbsp olive oil
- 1 garlic clove, crushed
- ½ celeriac, sliced
- ½ fennel bulb, sliced
- ¼ cup vegetable stock
- Sea salt and black pepper, to taste

Sauce

- 2 tomatoes, halved
- 2 tbsp olive oil
- ½ cup onions, chopped
- 2 cloves garlic, minced
- 1 chili, minced
- 1 bunch fresh basil, chopped

- 1 tbsp fresh cilantro, chopped
- Salt and black pepper, to taste

Directions

1. Set a pan over medium-high heat and warm olive oil. Add in garlic and sauté for 1 minute. Stir in celeriac and fennel slices, stock and cook until softened. Sprinkle with black pepper and salt.
2. Brush olive oil to the tomato halves. Microwave for 15 minutes; get rid of any excess liquid. Remove the cooked tomatoes to a food processor; add the rest of the ingredients for the sauce and puree to obtain the desired consistency. Serve the celeriac and fennel topped with tomato sauce.

Nutrition Value:

Calories: 145; Fat:: 15g, Net Carbs:: 5.3g, Protein:: 2.1g

176. Steamed Asparagus with Feta

Preparation Time: 30 minutes
Servings: 2-4

Ingredients

- 1 pound asparagus, cut off stems
- 2 tbsp olive oil
- 1 cup feta cheese, crumbled
- 2 garlic cloves, minced
- 1 tsp cajun spice mix
- 1 tsp mustard
- 1 bell pepper, chopped
- ¼ cup vegetable broth
- Salt and black pepper, to taste

Directions

1. Steam asparagus in salted water in a pot over medium heat until tender for 10 minutes; then drain.
2. Heat olive oil in a pan over medium heat and place in garlic; cook for 30 seconds until soft. Stir in the rest of the ingredients, including reserved asparagus, and cook for an additional 4 minutes. Serve topped with feta cheese in a platter.

Nutrition Value:

Calories: 211; Fat:: 16.5g, Net Carbs:: 2.8g, Protein:: 8.8g

177. Roasted Pumpkin with Almonds & Cheddar

Preparation Time: 45 minutes
Servings: 2-4

Ingredients

- 2 tbsp olive oil
- 1 large pumpkin, peeled and sliced
- ½ cup almonds, ground
- ½ cup cheddar cheese, grated
- 2 tbsp thyme, chopped

Directions

1. Preheat the oven to 360 F.
2. Arrange the pumpkin slices on a baking dish, drizzle with olive oil, and bake for 35 minutes. Mix the almonds and cheese, and when the pumpkin is ready, remove it from the oven, and sprinkle the cheese mixture all over. Bake for 5 more minutes. Sprinkle with thyme to serve.

Nutrition Value:

Calories: 154, Fat: 8.6g, Net Carbs: 5.1g, Protein: 4.5g

178. Smoked Vegetable Bake with Parmesan

Preparation Time: 35 minutes
Servings: 2-4

Ingredients

- 2 tbsp olive oil
- 1 onion, chopped
- 1 celery, chopped
- 2 carrots, sliced
- ½ pound artichokes, halved
- 1 cup vegetable broth
- 1 tsp turmeric
- Salt and black pepper, to taste
- ½ tsp liquid smoke
- 1 cup Parmesan cheese, shredded
- 2 tbsp chives, chopped

Directions

1. Preheat oven to 360 F and grease a baking dish with olive oil. Place in the artichokes, onion, and celery. Combine vegetable broth with turmeric, black pepper, liquid smoke, and salt.
2. Spread this mixture over the vegetables and bake for about 25 minutes. Sprinkle with Parmesan cheese and return in the oven to bake for another 5 minutes until the cheese melts. Decorate with fresh chives and serve.

Nutrition Value:

Calories: 231; Fat:: 15.5g, Net Carbs:: 9.3g, Protein:: 11g

179. Sauteed Spinach with Spicy Tofu

Preparation Time: 25 minutes
Servings: 2-4

Ingredients

- 2 tbsp olive oil

- 14 ounces block tofu, pressed and cubed
- 1 celery stalk, chopped
- 1 bunch scallions, chopped
- 1 tsp cayenne pepper
- 1 tsp garlic powder
- 2 tbsp Worcestershire sauce
- Salt and black pepper, to taste
- 1 pound spinach, chopped
- ½ tsp turmeric powder
- ¼ tsp dried basil

Directions

1. In a large skillet over medium heat, warm 1 tablespoon of olive oil. Stir in tofu cubes and cook for 8 minutes. Place in scallions and celery; cook for 5 minutes until soft. Stir in cayenne, Worcestershire sauce, black pepper, salt, and garlic; cook for 3 more minutes; set aside.
2. In the same pan, warm the remaining 1 tablespoon of oil. Add in spinach and the remaining seasonings and cook for 4 minutes. Mix in tofu mixture and serve warm.

Nutrition Value:
Calories: 205; Fat:: 12.5g, Net Carbs:: 7.8g, Protein:: 7.7g

180. Traditional Greek Eggplant Casserole

Preparation Time: 50 minutes
Servings: 2-4

Ingredients

- 2 large eggplants, cut into strips
- ½ cup celery, chopped
- ½ cup carrots, chopped
- 1 white onion, chopped
- 1 egg
- 1 tomato, chopped
- 1 tsp olive oil
- 2 cups grated Parmesan, divided into 2
- 1 cup feta cheese, crumbled
- 2 cloves garlic, minced
- 1 tsp Greek seasoning
- Salt and black pepper to taste
- Sauce:
- 1 cup heavy cream
- 2 tbsp butter, melted
- ½ cup mozzarella cheese, grated
- 1 tsp Greek seasoning
- 2 tbsp almond flour

Directions

1. Preheat the oven to 350 F. Heat olive oil in a skillet over medium heat and sauté the onion, garlic, tomato, celery, and carrots for 5 minutes; set aside to cool.
2. Mix the egg, 1 cup of parmesan cheese, feta cheese, and salt in a bowl; set aside.
3. Pour the heavy cream in a pot and bring to heat over a medium fire while continually stirring. Stir in the remaining parmesan cheese, and 1 teaspoon of Greek seasoning; set aside.
4. Spread a small amount of the cream sauce at the bottom of the baking dish and place the eggplant strips in a single layer on top of the sauce. Spread a layer of feta cheese on the eggplants, sprinkle some veggies on it, and repeat the layering process from the sauce until all the ingredients are exhausted.
5. In a small bowl, evenly mix the melted butter, almond flour, and 1 teaspoon of Greek seasoning. Spread the top of the mousaka layers with this mixture and sprinkle with mozzarella cheese. Cover the dish with foil and place it in the oven to bake for 25 minutes. Remove the foil and bake for 5 minutes until the cheese is slightly burned. Slice the mousaka and serve warm.

Nutrition Value:
Calories: 612, Fat: 33.5g, Net Carbs: 13.5g, Protein: 36.6g

Poppy Seed Coleslaw

Preparation Time: 3 hours 15 minutes
Servings: 2-4

Ingredients

Dressing

- 2 tbsp olive oil
- 1 cup poppy seeds
- 2 cups water
- 2 tbsp green onions, chopped
- 1 garlic clove, minced
- 1 lime, freshly squeezed
- Salt and black pepper, to taste
- ¼ tsp dill, minced
- 1 tbsp yellow mustard

Salad

- ½ head white cabbage, shredded
- 1 carrot, shredded
- 1 shallot, sliced
- 2 tbsp Kalamata olives, pitted

Directions

1. In a food processor, place olive oil, water, green onion, mustard, dill, lime juice, salt, and black pepper to taste. Pulse until well incorporated.

Add in poppy seeds and mix well.
2. Place cabbage, carrot, and onion in a bowl and mix to combine. Transfer to a salad plate, pour the dressing over and top with kalamata olives to serve.

Nutrition Value:

Calories: 235; Fat:: 17.3g, Net Carbs:: 6.4g, Protein:: 8.1g

182. Tofu & Hazelnut Loaded Zucchini

Preparation Time: 50 minutes
Servings: 2-4

Ingredients

- 2 tbsp olive oil
- 12 ounces firm tofu, drained and crumbled
- 2 garlic cloves, pressed
- ½ cup onions, chopped
- 2 cups crushed tomatoes
- ¼ tsp dried oregano
- Salt and black pepper to taste
- ¼ tsp chili pepper
- 2 zucchinis, cut into halves, scoop out the insides
- ¼ cup hazelnuts, chopped
- 2 tbsp cilantro, chopped

Directions

1. Sauté onion, garlic, and tofu in olive oil for 5 minutes until softened. Place in scooped zucchini flesh, 1 cup of tomatoes, oregano, and chili pepper. Season with salt, and pepper and cook for 6 minutes.
2. Preheat oven to 390 F. Pour the remaining tomatoes in a baking dish. Spoon the tofu mixture into the zucchini shells. Arrange the zucchini boats in the baking dish. Bake for about 30 minutes. Sprinkle with hazelnuts and continue baking for 5 to 6 more minutes. Scatter with cilantro to serve.

Nutrition Value:

Calories: 234; Fat:: 18.3g, Net Carbs:: 5.9g, Protein:: 12.5g

183. Parsnip & Carrot Strips with Walnut Sauce

Preparation Time: 15 minutes
Servings: 2-4

Ingredients

- 2 tbsp olive oil
- 2 carrots, cut into strips
- 2 parsnips, cut into strips
- ½ cup water
- Salt and black pepper to taste
- 1 tsp rosemary, chopped
- Walnut sauce
- ½ cup walnuts
- 3 tbsp nutritional yeast
- Salt and black pepper, to taste
- ¼ tsp onion powder
- ½ tsp garlic powder
- ¼ cup olive oil

Directions

1. Set a pan over medium heat and warm oil; cook the parsnips and carrots for 1 minute as you stir. Add in water and cook for an additional 6 minutes. Sprinkle with rosemary, salt, and pepper; transfer to a serving platter.
2. Place all sauce ingredients in a food processor and pulse until you attain the required consistency. Pour the sauce over the vegetables and serve.

Nutrition Value:

Calories: 338; Fat:: 28.6g, Net Carbs:: 9.7g, Protein:: 6.5g

184. Cauliflower & Celery Bisque

Preparation Time: 30 minutes
Servings: 2-4

Ingredients

- 2 tbsp olive oil
- 1 onion, finely chopped
- 1 garlic clove, minced
- 1 head cauliflower, cut into florets
- ½ cup celery, chopped
- 4 cups vegetable broth
- ½ cup heavy cream
- Salt and black pepper to taste
- 1 tbsp parsley, chopped

Directions

1. Set a large pot over medium heat and warm the olive oil. Add celery, garlic and onion and sauté until translucent, about 5 minutes. Place in vegetable broth, and cauliflower.
2. Bring to a boil, reduce the heat and simmer for 15-20 minutes. Transfer the soup to an immersion blender and blend to achieve the required consistency; top with parsley to serve.

Nutrition Value:

Calories: 187; Fat:: 13.5g, Net Carbs:: 5.6g, Protein:: 4.1g

185. Balsamic Roasted Vegetables with Feta & Almonds

Preparation Time: 45 minutes
Servings: 2-4

Ingredients

- 4 tbsp olive oil
- 1 red bell pepper, sliced
- 1 green bell pepper, sliced
- 1 orange bell pepper, sliced
- ½ head broccoli, cut into florets
- 2 zucchinis, sliced
- 8 white pearl onions, peeled
- 2 garlic cloves, halved
- 2 thyme sprigs, chopped
- 1 tsp dried sage, crushed
- 2 tbsp balsamic vinegar
- Sea salt and cayenne pepper, to taste
- 1 cup feta cheese, crumbled
- ½ cup almonds, toasted and chopped

Directions

1. Preheat oven to 375 F. Mix all vegetables with olive oil, seasonings, and balsamic vinegar; shake well. Spread the vegetables out in a baking dish and roast in the oven for 40 minutes or until tender, flipping once halfway through.
2. Remove from the oven to a serving plate. Scatter the feta cheese and almonds all over and serve.

Nutrition Value:

Calories: 276; Fat:: 23.3g, Net Carbs:: 7.9g, Protein:: 8.1g

186. Cauliflower-Kale Dip

Preparation Time: 10 minutes
Servings: 2-4

Ingredients

- ¼ cup olive oil
- 1 pound cauliflower, cut into florets
- 2 cups kale
- Salt and black pepper, to taste
- 1 garlic clove, minced
- 1 tbsp sesame paste
- 1 tbsp fresh lime juice
- ½ tsp garam masala

Directions

1. In a large pot filled with salted water over medium heat, steam cauliflower until tender for 5 minutes. Add in the kale and continue to cook for another 2-3 minutes.
2. Drain, transfer to a blender and pulse until smooth. Place in garam masala, oil, black paper, fresh lime juice, garlic, salt and sesame paste.

Blend the mixture until well combined. Decorate with some additional olive oil and serve.

Nutrition Value:

Calories: 185; Fat:: 16.5g, Net Carbs:: 3.9g, Protein:: 3.5g

187. Tofu & Vegetable Casserole

Preparation Time: 45 minutes
Servings: 2-4

Ingredients

- 10 oz tofu, pressed and cubed
- 2 tsp olive oil
- 1 cup leeks, chopped
- 1 garlic clove, minced
- ½ cup celery, chopped
- ½ cup carrot, chopped
- 1 ½ pounds Brussels sprouts, shredded
- 1 habanero pepper, chopped
- 2 ½ cups mushrooms, sliced
- 1 ½ cups vegetable stock
- 2 tomatoes, chopped
- 2 thyme sprigs, chopped
- 1 rosemary sprig, chopped
- 2 bay leaves
- Salt and ground black pepper to taste

Directions

1. Set a pot over medium heat and warm oil. Add in garlic and leeks and sauté until soft and translucent, about 3 minutes. Add in tofu and cook for another 4 minutes. Add the habanero pepper, celery, mushrooms, and carrots. Cook as you stir for 5 minutes. Stir in the rest of the ingredients.
2. Simmer for 25 to 35 minutes or until cooked through. Remove and discard the bay leaves.

Nutrition Value:

Calories: 328; Fat:: 18.5g, Net Carbs:: 9.7g, Protein:: 21g

188. Cauliflower-Based Waffles with Zucchini & Cheese

Preparation Time: 45 minutes
Servings: 2

Ingredients

- 2 green onions
- 1 tbsp olive oil
- 2 eggs
- 1/3 cup Parmesan cheese
- 1 cup zucchini, shredded and squeezed
- 1 cup mozzarella cheese, grated

- ½ head cauliflower
- 1 tsp garlic powder
- 1 tbsp sesame seeds
- 2 tsp thyme, chopped

Directions

1. Chop the cauliflower into florets, toss the pieces a the food processor and pulse until rice is formed. Remove to a clean kitchen towel and press to eliminate excess moisture. Return to the food processor and add zucchini, spring onions, and thyme; pulse until smooth and transfer to a bowl.
2. Stir in the rest of the ingredients and mix to combine. Leave to rest for 10 minutes. Heat waffle iron and spread in the mixture, evenly. Cook until golden brown, for about 5 minutes.

Nutrition Value:

Calories: 336, Fat:: 21g, Net Carbs:: 7.2g, Protein:: 32.6g

189. Pumpkin & Bell Pepper Noodles with Avocado Sauce

Preparation Time: 15 minutes
Servings: 2-4

Ingredients

- ½ pound pumpkin, spiralized
- ½ pound bell peppers, spiralized
- 2 tbsp olive oil
- 2 avocados, chopped
- 1 lemon, juiced and zested
- 2 tbsp sesame oil
- 2 tbsp cilantro, chopped
- 1 onion, chopped
- 1 jalapeño pepper, deveined and minced
- Salt and black pepper, to taste
- 2 tbsp pumpkin seeds

Directions

1. Toast the pumpkin seeds in a dry nonstick skillet, stirring frequently for a minute until golden; set aside. Add in oil and sauté bell peppers and pumpkin for 8 minutes. Remove to a serving platter.
2. Combine avocados, sesame oil, onion, jalapeño pepper, lemon juice, and lemon zest in a food processor and pulse to obtain a creamy mixture. Adjust the seasoning and pour over the vegetable noodles, top with the pumpkin seeds and serve.

Nutrition Value:

Calories: 673; Fat:: 59g, Net Carbs:: 9.8g, Protein:: 22.9g

190. Curried Cauliflower & Mushrooms Traybake

Preparation Time: 30 minutes
Servings: 2-4

Ingredients

- 1 head cauliflower, cut into florets
- 1 cup mushrooms, halved
- 4 garlic cloves, minced
- 1 red onion, sliced
- 2 tomatoes, chopped
- ¼ cup coconut oil, melted
- 1 tsp chili paprika paste
- ½ tsp curry powder
- Salt and black pepper, to taste

Directions

1. Set oven to 380 F and grease a baking dish with the coconut oil.
2. In a large bowl, toss the cauliflower and mushrooms, garlic, onion, tomatoes, chili paprika paste, curry, black pepper, and salt. Spread out on the baking dish and roast for 20-25 minutes, turning once. Place in a plate and drizzle over the cooking juices to serve.

Nutrition Value:

Calories: 171; Fat:: 15.7g, Net Carbs:: 6.9g, Protein:: 3.5g

191. Tasty Tofu & Swiss Chard Dip

Preparation Time: 10 minutes
Servings: 2-4

Ingredients

- 2 tbsp mayonnaise
- 2 cups Swiss chard
- ½ cup tofu, pressed, drained, crumbled
- ¼ cup almond milk
- 1 tsp nutritional yeast
- 1 garlic clove, minced
- 2 tbsp olive oil
- Salt and pepper to taste
- ½ tsp paprika
- ½ tsp mint leaves, chopped

Directions

1. Fill a pot with salted water and boil Swiss chard over medium heat for 5-6 minutes, until wilted.
2. Puree the remaining ingredients, except for the mayonnaise, in a food processor. Season with salt and pepper. Stir in the Swiss chard and mayonnaise to get a homogeneous mixture.

Nutrition Value:

Calories: 136; Fat:: 11g, Net Carbs:: 6.3g, Protein:: 3.1g

192. One-Pot Ratatouille with Pecans

Preparation Time: 47 minutes
Servings: 2-4

Ingredients

- 2 tbsp olive oil
- 1 eggplant, sliced
- 1 zucchini, sliced
- 1 red onion, sliced
- 14 oz canned tomatoes
- 1 red bell peppers, sliced
- 1 yellow bell pepper, sliced
- 1 cloves garlic, sliced
- ¼ cup basil leaves, chop half
- 2 sprigs thyme
- 1 tbsp balsamic vinegar
- ½ lemon, zested
- ¼ cup pecans, chopped
- Salt and black pepper to taste

Directions

1. Place a casserole pot over medium heat and warm the olive oil. Sauté the eggplants, zucchinis, and bell peppers for 5 minutes. Spoon the veggies into a large bowl.
2. In the same pan, sauté garlic, onion, and thyme leaves for 5 minutes and return the cooked veggies to the pan along with the canned tomatoes, balsamic vinegar, chopped basil, salt, and pepper to taste. Stir and cover the pot, and cook the ingredients on low heat for 30 minutes.
3. Stir in the remaining basil leaves, lemon zest, and adjust the seasoning to serve.

Nutrition Value:

Calories: 188, Fat: 13g, Net Carbs: 8.3g, Protein: 4.5g

193. Baked Parsnip Chips with Yogurt Dip

Preparation Time: 20 minutes
Servings: 2-4

Ingredients

- 3 tbsp olive oil
- 1/3 cup natural yogurt
- 1 tsp lime juice
- 1 tbsp parsley, chopped
- Salt and black pepper, to taste
- 1 garlic clove, minced
- 2 cups parsnips, sliced

Directions

1. Preheat the oven to 300 F. Set parsnip slices on a baking sheet; toss with garlic powder, 1 tbsp of olive oil, and salt. Bake for 15 minutes, tossing once halfway through, until slices are crisp and slightly browned.
2. In a bowl, mix yogurt, lime juice, black pepper, 2 tbsp of olive oil, garlic, and salt until well combined. Serve the chips with yogurt dip.

Nutrition Value:

Calories: 176; Fat:: 12.7g, Net Carbs:: 8.7g, Protein:: 1.9g

194. Roasted Cauliflower with Bell Peppers & Onion

Preparation Time: 40 minutes
Servings: 2-4

Ingredients

- 1 pound cauliflower, cut into florets
- 2 bell peppers, halved
- ¼ cup olive oil
- 2 onions, quartered
- Salt and black pepper, to taste
- ½ tsp cayenne pepper
- 1 tsp curry powder

Directions

1. Preheat oven to 425 F. Line a large baking sheet with parchment paper and spread out the cauliflower, onion, and bell peppers. Sprinkle olive oil, curry powder, black pepper, salt and cayenne pepper and toss to combine well.
2. Roast for 35 minutes as you toss in intervals until they start to brown.

Nutrition Value:

Calories: 186; Fat:: 15.1g, Net Carbs:: 8.2g, Protein:: 3.9g

195. Oven-Roasted Asparagus with Romesco Sauce

Preparation Time: 15 minutes
Servings: 2-4

Ingredients

- 1 pound asparagus spears, trimmed
- 2 tbsp olive oil
- Salt and black pepper, to taste
- ½ tsp paprika
- Romesco sauce
- 2 red bell peppers, roasted
- 2 tsp olive oil
- 2 tbsp almond flour
- ½ cup scallions, chopped
- 1 garlic clove, minced
- 1 tbsp lemon juice
- ½ tsp chili pepper

- Salt and black pepper, to taste
- 2 tbsp rosemary, chopped

Directions
1. In a food processor, pulse together the bell peppers, salt, black pepper, garlic, lemon juice, scallions, almond flour, 2 tsp of olive oil and chili pepper. Mix evenly and set aside.
2. Preheat oven to 390 F and line a baking sheet with parchment paper. Add asparagus spears to the baking sheet. Toss with 2 tbsp of olive oil, paprika, black pepper, and salt. Bake until cooked through for 9 minutes. Transfer to a serving plate, pour the sauce over and garnish with rosemary to serve.

Nutrition Value:
Calories: 145; Fat:: 11g, Net Carbs:: 5.9g, Protein:: 4.1g

196. Parmesan Brussels Sprouts with Onion
Preparation Time: 45 minutes
Servings: 2-4

Ingredients
- 1 ½ pounds brussels sprouts, halved
- 2 large red onions, sliced
- 2 tbsp olive oil
- Salt and black pepper, to taste
- 1 tbsp fresh chives, chopped
- 2 tbsp Parmesan cheese, shredded

Directions
1. Set oven to 400 F and spread sprout halves and onion slices on a baking sheet. Season with black pepper and drizzle with olive oil; toss to coat.
2. Roast in the oven for 30 minutes, until the vegetables become soft. Sprinkle with Parmesan cheese and bake for 5-10 more minutes until the cheese melts. Serve scattered with chives.

Nutrition Value:
Calories:: 179; Fat: 9g, Net Carbs: 8.6g, Protein: 7.5g

197. Chocolate Nut Granola
Preparation Time: 1 hour
Servings: 2-4

Ingredients
- ¼ cup cocoa powder
- 1/3 tbsp coconut oil, melted
- ¼ cup almond flakes
- ¼ cup almond milk
- ¼ tbsp xylitol
- 1/8 tsp salt
- 1/3 tsp lime zest
- ¼ tsp ground cinnamon
- ¼ cup pecans, chopped
- ¼ cup almonds, slivered
- 1 tbsp pumpkin seeds
- 2 tbsp sunflower seeds
- 2 tbsp flax seed

Directions
1. Preheat oven to 300 F and line a baking dish with parchment paper. Set aside.
2. Mix almond flakes, cocoa powder, ground cinnamon, almonds, xylitol, pumpkin seeds, sunflower seeds, flax seed, and salt in a bowl.
3. In a separate bowl, whisk coconut oil, almond milk and lemon zest until combined. Pour over the other mixture and stir to coat.
4. Lay the mixture in an even layer onto the baking dish Bake for 50 minutes, making sure that you shake gently in intervals of 15 minutes. Let cool completely before serving.

Nutrition Value:
Calories: 273; Fat:: 26.2g, Net Carbs:: 8.9g, Protein:: 4.6g

198. Mozzarella & Bell Pepper Avocado Cups
Preparation Time: 10 minutes
Servings: 2-4

Ingredients
- 2 avocados
- ½ cup fresh mozzarella, chopped
- 2 tbsp olive oil
- 2 cups green bell peppers, chopped
- 1 onion, chopped
- ½ tsp garlic puree
- Salt and black pepper, to taste
- ½ tomato, chopped
- 2 tbsp basil, chopped

Directions
1. Halve the avocados and scoop out 2 teaspoons of flesh; set aside.
2. Sauté olive oil, garlic, onion, and bell peppers in a skillet over medium heat for 5 minutes until tender. Remove to a bowl and leave to cool. Mix in the reserved avocado, tomato, salt, mozzarella, and black pepper. Fill the avocado halves with the mixture and serve sprinkled with basil.

Nutrition Value:
Calories: 273; Fat:: 22.5g, Net Carbs:: 6.9g, Protein:: 8.3g

199. Green Mac and Cheese

Calories: 165; Fat:: 14.7g, Net Carbs:: 3.2g, Protein:: 6.2g

Preparation Time: 15 minutes
Servings: 2-4

Ingredients

- 4 zucchinis, spiralized
- 2 tbsp butter, melted
- Salt and black pepper, to taste
- 1 cup heavy cream
- 1 cup cream cheese
- 1 tsp garlic paste
- ½ tsp onion flakes

Directions

1. Shake zucchinis with melted butter, salt and pepper. Cook in a saucepan over medium heat for 5-6 minutes. Remove to a serving plate.
2. In the same pan, pour the heavy cream, garlic paste, and cream cheese and heat through, stirring frequently. Reduce heat to low and simmer for 2-3 minutes until thickened. Adjust the seasoning.
3. Coat the zucchinis in the cheese sauce and serve immediately in serving bowls.

Nutrition Value:
Calories: 686; Fat:: 72g, Net Carbs:: 3.9g, Protein:: 10g

200. Roasted Tomatoes with Vegan Cheese Crust

Preparation Time: 15 minutes
Servings: 2-4

Ingredients

- 3 tomatoes, sliced
- 2 tbsp olive oil
- ½ cup pepitas seeds
- 1 tbsp nutritional yeast
- Salt and black pepper, to taste
- 1 tsp garlic puree
- 2 tbsp parsley. chopped

Directions

1. Preheat oven to 380 F and grease a baking pan with olive oil. Drizzle olive oil over the tomatoes.
2. In a food processor, add pepitas seeds, nutritional yeast, garlic puree, salt and pepper, and pulse until the desired consistency is attained. Press the mixture firmly onto each slice of tomato. Set the tomato slices on the prepared baking pan and bake for 10 minutes. Serve sprinkled with parsley.

Nutrition Value:

SIDES

201. Mashed Cauliflower
Preparation Time: 10 minutes
Cooking time: 15 minutes
Servings: 4

Ingredients:
- 2 teaspoon minced garlic
- 10 oz cauliflower
- 1 teaspoon lemon juice
- 3 tablespoon almond milk
- 1 teaspoon salt
- ½ teaspoon chili flakes
- 2 cups of water

Directions:
1. Pour water in the saucepan and add cauliflower.
2. Close the lid and boil it for 15 minutes or until the vegetable is soft.
3. Then strain the cauliflower and transfer it in the blender.
4. Add minced garlic, almond milk, lemon juice, salt, and chili flakes.
5. Blend the vegetable until smooth and soft.
6. Transfer the cooked mashed cauliflower in the serving bowls.

Nutrition Value: calories 46, fat 2.8, fiber 2.1, carbs 4.9, protein 1.8

202. Fragrant Cauliflower Steaks
Preparation Time: 10 minutes
Cooking time: 10 minutes
Servings: 6

Ingredients:
- 2-pound cauliflower head
- 1 teaspoon Taco seasoning
- 1 teaspoon ground thyme
- 1 tablespoon butter
- 4 oz Parmesan, grated

Directions:
1. Preheat the grill to 365F.
2. Meanwhile, slice the cauliflower head into steaks.
3. Rub every cauliflower steak with Taco seasoning and ground thyme.
4. Place the steaks on the grill and grill for 2 minutes from each side.
5. After this, rub the cauliflower with butter and cook for 1 minute more from each side.
6. Then sprinkle the cauliflower steaks with grated cheese and cook for 3 minutes only on one side.

Nutrition Value: calories 118, fat 6.1, fiber 3.8, carbs 9.1, protein 9.1

203. Fried Cheese
Preparation Time: 10 minutes
Cooking time: 5 minutes
Servings: 6

Ingredients:
- 1-pound goat cheese log
- 1/3 cup almond flour
- 1 egg, whisked
- 1 teaspoon chili pepper
- ½ teaspoon garlic powder
- 1 tablespoon olive oil

Directions:
1. Cut the goat cheese into medium pieces.
2. Then mix up together almond flour, chili pepper, and garlic powder. Stir it.
3. Dip the goat cheese pieces in the whisked egg.
4. Then coat them in the almond flour mixture.
5. Preheat the skillet and pour olive oil inside.
6. When the olive oil is hot, place the goat cheese inside and cook for 30 seconds from each side.
7. Serve the cooked side dish hot.

Nutrition Value: calories 362, fat 28.4, fiber 0.2, carbs 2.3, protein 24.4

204. Cabbage Salad
Preparation Time: 8 minutes
Cooking time: 5 minutes
Servings: 2

Ingredients:
- 8 oz white cabbage, shredded
- ½ avocado, peeled
- 2 tablespoons lemon juice
- 1 teaspoon avocado oil
- ¼ cup spinach, chopped
- 3 tablespoon water

Directions:
1. Place avocado, lemon juice, spinach, avocado oil, and water in the blender.
2. Blend the mixture until smooth.
3. Place the cabbage in the salad bowl.
4. Pour the green mixture over the cabbage.

5. Mix up the salad well and let it marinate for at least 5 minutes.

Nutrition Value: calories 156, fat 12.4, fiber 6.4, carbs 11.4, protein 2.6

205. Hummus

Preparation Time: 10 minutes
Cooking time: 15 minutes
Servings: 6

Ingredients:
- 2-pound cauliflower head
- 1 teaspoon salt
- 1 teaspoon garlic powder
- 1 teaspoon chili flakes
- 3 tablespoon olive oil
- 1 tablespoon tahini paste
- 1 cup of water

Directions:
1. Boil cauliflower head in 1 cup of water for 15 minutes or until tender.
2. Meanwhile, mix up together salt, garlic powder, chili flakes, olive oil, and tahini paste.
3. Strain the cauliflower. Leave 5 tablespoons of cauliflower water.
4. Blend the vegetable until you get a mashed mixture.
5. Add 5 tablespoons of remaining cauliflower water and tahini paste mixture.
6. Blend the hummus for 2 minutes more.
7. Transfer it in the bowl.

Nutrition Value: calories 114, fat 8.5, fiber 4.1, carbs 8.9, protein 3.5

206. Roasted Halloumi

Preparation Time: 8 minutes
Cooking time: 5 minutes
Servings: 3

Ingredients:
- 10 oz halloumi cheese
- 1 tablespoon olive oil
- 1 teaspoon ground black pepper
- ½ teaspoon dried oregano
- ¼ teaspoon dried cilantro

Directions:
1. Preheat grill to 375F.
2. Meanwhile, mix up together olive oil, ground black pepper, dried oregano, and dried cilantro.
3. Brush the cheese with the olive oil mixture from each side.
4. Place Halloumi cheese on the grill and cook it for 2.5 minutes from each side.

Nutrition Value: calories 387, fat 32.9, fiber 0.3, carbs 3, protein 20.5

207. Roasted Cabbage

Preparation Time: 10 minutes
Cooking time: 15 minutes
Servings: 3

Ingredients:
- 11 oz white cabbage
- 1 tablespoon olive oil
- 1 teaspoon white pepper
- 1 teaspoon onion powder

Directions:
1. Cut the white cabbage into wedges.
2. Rub the vegetable with white pepper and onion powder.
3. Then sprinkle with olive oil.
4. Preheat the oven to 375F.
5. Place the cabbage wedges in the tray and transfer in the preheated oven.
6. Cook the side dish for 15 minutes or until the edges of the cabbage are light brown.

Nutrition Value: calories 71, fat 4.8, fiber 2.8, carbs 7.1, protein 1.5

208. Deviled Eggs

Preparation Time: 10 minutes
Cooking time: 6 minutes
Servings: 3

Ingredients:
- 3 eggs
- 1 tablespoon mustard
- 1 teaspoon chives, chopped
- ¾ teaspoon turmeric

Directions:
1. Boil the eggs for 6 minutes.
2. Meanwhile, mix p together chives, turmeric, and mustard.
3. When the eggs are cooked, chill them in icy water and peel.
4. Cut the eggs into halves.
5. Remove the egg yolks and add them in the mustard mixture.
6. Mash it until smooth.
7. Fill the egg whites with the egg yolk mixture.

Nutrition Value: calories 82, fat 5.5, fiber 0.7, carbs 2, protein 6.5

209. Fried Broccoli

Preparation Time: 7 minutes

Cooking time: 13 minutes
Servings: 4

Ingredients:
- 2 cups broccoli florets
- 1 teaspoon onion powder
- 2 tablespoon coconut oil
- 1 teaspoon almond flakes
- 1 teaspoon salt

Directions:
1. Preheat the oven to 365F.
2. Place the broccoli florets in the tray.
3. Add coconut oil, almond flakes, salt, and onion powder.
4. Mix up the broccoli well.
5. Transfer the tray in the oven and cook for 10 minutes.
6. Then stir the broccoli and cook it for 2-3 minutes more.

Nutrition Value: calories 86, fat 7.8, fiber 1.4, carbs 3.7, protein 1.7

210. Brussel Sprouts with Nuts
Preparation Time: 10 minutes
Cooking time: 30 minutes
Servings: 4

Ingredients:
- 2 cups Brussel sprouts
- 3 oz pecans, chopped
- 3 tablespoon coconut oil
- 1 teaspoon salt
- 1 teaspoon garlic powder
- 1 teaspoon cayenne pepper

Directions:
1. Cut Brussel sprouts into halves and place in the tray.
2. Mix up together coconut oil, salt, garlic powder, and cayenne pepper.
3. Put the mixture over Brussel sprouts.
4. Add pecans.
5. Preheat the oven to 360F.
6. Put the tray with Brussel sprouts in the oven and cook for 30 minutes or until sprouts are tender.

Nutrition Value: calories 259, fat 25.6, fiber 4.1, carbs 7.8, protein 4

211. Zucchini Pasta
Preparation Time: 10 minutes
Cooking time: 5 minutes
Servings: 4

Ingredients:
- 2 zucchini, trimmed
- 1 tablespoon olive oil
- ¼ cup almond milk
- ½ teaspoon salt
- ½ teaspoon ground black pepper
- ¼ cup spinach
- ½ avocado, peeled

Directions:
1. Make the noodles from zucchini with the help of spiralizer.
2. Preheat the olive oil in the skillet and add zucchini noodles.
3. Sprinkle "noodles" with almond milk, salt, and ground black pepper.
4. Cook the mixture for 3 minutes over the medium-high heat.
5. Meanwhile, blend together spinach and avocado.
6. Add the avocado mixture in the zucchini noodles and stir until homogenous.
7. Cook the meal for 2 minutes more.

Nutrition Value: calories 133, fat 12.2, fiber 3.2, carbs 6.5, protein 2.1

212. Shirataki Noodles
Preparation Time: 10 minutes
Cooking time: 5 minutes
Servings: 3

Ingredients:
- 10 oz shirataki noodles
- 1 cup of coconut milk
- 1 tablespoon lemon juice
- ¾ teaspoon ground ginger
- ¼ teaspoon cayenne pepper
- ½ teaspoon salt

Directions:
1. In the saucepan combine together coconut milk. Lemon juice, ground ginger, cayenne pepper, and salt.
2. Stir it, close the lid and cook over the high heat until it starts to boil.
3. After this, add shirataki noodles, stir gently, and close the lid.
4. Cook the noodles for 15 minutes.
5. Strain the cooked noodles.

Nutrition Value: calories 207, fat 19.2, fiber 11.9, carbs 4.9, protein 2.6

213. Low Carb Baked Vegetables
Preparation Time: 10 minutes

Cooking time: 25 minutes
Servings: 4

Ingredients:

- 2 green peppers
- 1 cup white mushrooms
- 1 white onion, peeled
- 1 eggplant
- 1 teaspoon cayenne pepper
- 1 tablespoon almond butter
- ½ teaspoon salt

Directions:

1. Chop the green peppers and mushrooms roughly.
2. Then peel the eggplant and chop it too.
3. Combine together all the ingredients in the mixing bowl.
4. Add salt and cayenne pepper. Stir well.
5. Then cut the onion into 4 parts and separate into the petals. Add it into the vegetable mix.
6. Preheat the oven to 365F.
7. Line the baking tray with baking paper.
8. Put all the vegetables on the tray and flatten them.
9. Add almond butter and put in the oven.
10. Bake the vegetables for 25 minutes or until they are tender.

Nutrition Value: calories 81, fat 2.7, fiber 6.3, carbs 13.6, protein 3.4

214. Rutabaga Swirls

Preparation Time: 5 minutes
Cooking time: 5 minutes
Servings: 4

Ingredients:

- 8 oz rutabaga, peeled
- 1 tablespoon almond butter
- ½ teaspoon cayenne pepper
- ¾ teaspoon salt

Directions:

1. Cut rutabaga into very thin strips.
2. Sprinkle the strips with cayenne pepper and salt. Stir well.
3. Preheat the skillet and add almond butter. Melt it.
4. Add rutabaga strips and roast them for 5 minutes over the medium-high heat. Stir the strips constantly.
5. When the rutabaga swirls are light brown: they are cooked.

Nutrition Value: calories 46, fat 2.4, fiber 1.9, carbs 5.5, protein 1.6

215. Fettuccine

Preparation Time: 10 minutes
Cooking time: 4 minutes
Servings: 1

Ingredients:

- 1 zucchini
- ¾ teaspoon salt
- ¾ teaspoon ground paprika
- 2 tablespoon almond milk

Directions:

1. Wash and trim zucchini.
2. Then cut it into halves and remove the seeds.
3. With the help of potato peeler slice the zucchini on fettuccine noodles.
4. Transfer the noodles in the pan, add salt, ground paprika, and almond milk.
5. Simmer fettuccine over the medium heat for 4 minutes.
6. Then sprinkle the cooked meal with ground paprika and stir gently.

Nutrition Value: calories 105, fat 7.7, fiber 3.4, carbs 9.1, protein 3.3

216. French Fries

Preparation Time: 8 minutes
Cooking time: 15 minutes
Servings: 5

Ingredients:

- 3 cups Jicama fries
- 1 teaspoon onion powder
- 1 teaspoon garlic powder
- 1 teaspoon turmeric
- 1 teaspoon smoked paprika
- ½ teaspoon salt
- 3 tablespoons avocado oil

Directions:

1. Place Jicama fries into the mixing bowl.
2. Add onion powder, garlic powder, turmeric, and smoked paprika.
3. Then add salt and shake the mixture until homogenous.
4. Preheat the oven to 365F.
5. Make the layer of Jicama fries in the tray and sprinkle avocado oil. Use 2 trays if needed.
6. Place the tray in the oven and bake fries for 15 minutes or until light brown.

Nutrition Value: calories 45, fat 1.2, fiber 4.2, carbs 8.1, protein 0.9

217. Broccoli Fritters
Preparation Time: 10 minutes
Cooking time: 5 minutes
Servings: 4

Ingredients:
- 2 tablespoon flax meal
- ½ teaspoon salt
- 1 cup broccoli
- 1 egg, beaten
- 1 teaspoon ground black pepper
- ½ cup almond flour
- 1 tablespoon olive oil
- 3 oz tofu, crumbled

Directions:
1. Blend broccoli until smooth.
2. Then add salt, flax meal, beaten egg, ground black pepper, and tofu.
3. Blend the mixture till you get the homogenous texture.
4. Make the medium fritters from the broccoli mixture.
5. Coat every fritter in almond flour.
6. Preheat olive oil in the skillet.
7. Roast broccoli fritters for 2 minutes from each side or till light brown.

Nutrition Value: calories 105, fat 8.6, fiber 2.3, carbs 4, protein 5.3

218. Spinach in Cream
Preparation Time: 8 minutes
Cooking time: 15 minutes
Servings: 4

Ingredients:
- 3 cups spinach
- 1 cup heavy cream
- 1 teaspoon salt
- ½ teaspoon minced garlic
- 4 oz Provolone cheese

Directions:
1. Chop spinach and put in a saucepan.
2. Add salt and minced garlic.
3. Pour heavy cream in spinach, stir gently, close the lid and simmer for 10 minutes. Stir it from time to time.
4. Meanwhile, shred cheese.
5. Add shredded cheese in the saucepan and stir until homogenous.
6. Remove the saucepan from the heat and leave it to rest for 5 minutes.

Nutrition Value: calories 209, fat 18.7, fiber 0.5, carbs 2.4, protein 8.5

219. Dill Radish
Preparation Time: 10 minutes
Cooking time: 15 minutes
Servings: 4

Ingredients:
- 2 cups radish
- 1 tablespoon coconut oil
- 1 teaspoon salt
- ¼ cup of coconut milk
- 2 tablespoon dried dill

Directions:
1. Wash and trim radish.
2. Then cut them into halves and sprinkle with salt, coconut milk, coconut oil, and dried dill.
3. Mix up the radish carefully.
4. Place the radish in the tray in one layer.
5. Preheat the oven to 350F and put the tray inside.
6. Cook radish for 15 minutes or until the edges of the radish starts to be light brown.

Nutrition Value: calories 77, fat 7.1, fiber 1.5, carbs 3.7, protein 1

220. Curry Rice
Preparation Time: 5 minutes
Cooking time: 15 minutes
Servings: 2

Ingredients:
- 1 tablespoon curry paste
- ½ pound cauliflower, riced
- 1 teaspoon salt
- 1 tablespoon almond butter
- 1 cup of water

Directions:
1. Pour water in the saucepan.
2. Add all the remaining ingredients and close the lid.
3. Cook rice for 15 minutes.
4. Then strain the rice and transfer in the serving bowls.

Nutrition Value: calories 128, fat 9, fiber 3.6, carbs 9.6, protein 4.3

221. Garlic Artichokes
Preparation Time: 5 minutes
Cooking time: 15 minutes
Servings: 2

Ingredients:
- 1 teaspoon minced garlic
- 2 artichokes, trimmed
- ½ teaspoon salt
- 1 tablespoon canola oil

Directions:
1. Rub the artichokes with minced garlic, salt, and canola oil.
2. Place the vegetables in the pan.
3. Transfer the pan in preheated to the 350F oven.
4. Cook the side dish for 15 minutes. Cooked artichokes should be tender but not soft.

Nutrition Value: calories 124, fat 7.2, fiber 6.9, carbs 14, protein 4.3

222. Turnip Slaw

Preparation Time: 15 minutes
Cooking time: 5 minutes
Servings: 4

Ingredients:
- 11 oz turnip, peeled
- ½ carrot, peeled
- 1 tablespoon lemon juice
- 1 tablespoon fresh dill, chopped
- 1 tablespoon keto mayonnaise
- ¼ teaspoon ground black pepper

Directions:
1. Grate turnip into rough pieces or cut into thin strips.
2. Then grate the carrot.
3. Mix up together all the vegetables.
4. Add lemon juice, chopped dill, mayonnaise, and ground black pepper.
5. Stir the salad and leave for 10 minutes to marinate.

Nutrition Value: calories 28, fat 0.1, fiber 1.8, carbs 6.4, protein 1

223. Sauteed Cabbage

Preparation Time: 10 minutes
Cooking time: 35 minutes
Servings: 5

Ingredients:
- 1-pound cabbage, shredded
- 1 teaspoon salt
- 1 teaspoon smoked paprika
- ½ onion, diced
- 1 teaspoon tomato paste
- 1 cup almond milk
- 1 tablespoon macadamia nuts, crushed

Directions:
1. Pour almond milk in the saucepan and bring it to boil.
2. Add salt, smoked paprika, shredded cabbage, tomato paste, and diced onion.
3. Stir until the cabbage gets the light red color.
4. Close the lid and cook cabbage for 10 minutes over the medium heat.
5. Then add macadamia nuts, stir, and cook for 25 minutes more over the low heat.

Nutrition Value: calories 152, fat 12.9, fiber 3.9, carbs 9.6, protein 2.6

224. Spiced Rutabaga

Preparation Time: 10 minutes
Cooking time: 10 minutes
Servings: 3

Ingredients:
- 1 teaspoon cayenne pepper
- ½ teaspoon salt
- 1 teaspoon dried rosemary
- 1 teaspoon dried oregano
- 1 teaspoon dried dill
- 12 oz rutabaga, peeled
- 2 tablespoons sesame oil

Directions:
1. Cut rutabaga into halves.
2. Sprinkle halves with dried rosemary, salt, cayenne pepper, dill, and oregano.
3. Put the edges on the preheated to 360F grill and sprinkle with sesame oil.
4. Grill rutabaga for 10 minutes. Flip rutabaga halves from time to time.

Nutrition Value: calories 128, fat 9.4, fiber 3.6, carbs 10.7, protein 1.5

225. Swiss Chard

Preparation Time: 8 minutes
Cooking time: 15 minutes
Servings: 2

Ingredients:
- 2 cups swiss chard
- 1 tablespoon olive oil
- 1 teaspoon salt
- ½ teaspoon ground black pepper

Directions:
1. Chop swiss chard and transfer in the saucepan.
2. Add salt, olive oil, and ground black pepper.
3. Stir gently, close the lid, and saute vegetables for

15 minutes over the medium heat. Stir the vegetable time to time while cooking.

Nutrition Value: calories 68, fat 7.1, fiber 0.7, carbs 1.7, protein 0.7

226. Broccoli Cream

Preparation time: 10 minutes
Cooking time: 20 minutes
Servings: 4

Ingredients:

- 1 pound broccoli florets
- 4 cups vegetable stock
- 2 shallots, chopped
- 1 teaspoon chili powder
- A pinch of salt and black pepper
- 2 garlic cloves, minced
- 2 tablespoons olive oil, chopped
- 1 tablespoon dill, chopped

Directions:

1. Heat up a pot with the oil over medium high heat, add the shallots and the garlic and sauté for 2 minutes.
2. Add the broccoli and the other ingredients, bring to a simmer and cook over medium heat for 18 minutes.
3. Blend the mix using an immersion blender, divide the cream into bowls and serve.

Nutrition Value: calories 111, fat 8, fiber 3.3, carbs 10.2, protein 3.7

227. Cauliflower and Tomatoes Mix

Preparation time: 10 minutes
Cooking time: 30 minutes
Servings: 4

Ingredients:

- 1 pound cauliflower florets
- ½ pound cherry tomatoes, halved
- 2 tablespoons avocado oil
- 2 shallots, chopped
- 2 garlic cloves, minced
- A pinch of salt and black pepper
- 1 cup vegetable stock
- 1 tablespoon coriander, chopped
- ½ teaspoon allspice, ground

Directions:

1. Heat up a pan with the oil over medium heat, add the shallots and the garlic and sauté for 2 minutes.
2. Add the cauliflower and the other ingredients, toss, bring to a simmer and cook over medium heat for 28 minutes more.
3. Divide everything between plates and serve.

Nutrition Value: calories 57, fat 1.7, fiber 3.9, carbs 10.7, protein 3.1

228. Shallots and Kale Soup

Preparation time: 10 minutes
Cooking time: 20 minutes
Servings: 4

Ingredients:

- 4 cups chicken stock
- 1 pound kale, torn
- 2 shallots, chopped
- A pinch of salt and black pepper
- 1 tablespoon olive oil
- 2 teaspoons coconut aminos
- 1 tablespoon cilantro, chopped

Directions:

1. Heat up a pot with the oil over medium heat, add the shallots and sauté for 5 minutes.
2. Add the kale, stock and the other ingredients, bring to a simmer and cook over medium heat for 15 minutes more.
3. Divide the soup into bowls and serve.

Nutrition Value: calories 98, fat 4.1, fiber 1.7, carbs 13.1, protein 4.1

229. Hot Kale Pan

Preparation time: 10 minutes
Cooking time: 23 minutes
Servings: 4

Ingredients:

- 1 red onion, chopped
- 1 pound kale, roughly torn
- 1 cup baby bella mushrooms, halved
- A pinch of salt and black pepper
- 1 tablespoon olive oil
- 3 garlic cloves, minced
- ½ teaspoon hot paprika
- ½ tablespoon red pepper flakes, crushed
- 1 tablespoon dill, chopped
- 3 tablespoons coconut aminos

Directions:

1. Heat up a pan with the oil over medium heat, add the onion and the garlic and sauté for 5 minutes.
2. Add the mushrooms, and sauté them for 3 minutes more.
3. Add the kale and the other ingredients, toss,

cook over medium heat for 15 minutes more, divide into bowls and serve.

Nutrition Value: calories 100, fat 3, fiber 1, carbs 2, protein 6

230. Baked Broccoli
Preparation time: 10 minutes
Cooking time: 20 minutes
Servings: 4

Ingredients:
- 2 garlic cloves, minced
- 2 tablespoons olive oil
- 1 pound broccoli florets
- ½ teaspoon nutmeg, ground
- ½ teaspoons rosemary, dried
- A pinch of salt and black pepper

Directions:
1. In a roasting pan, combine the broccoli with the garlic and the other ingredients, toss and bake at 400 degrees F for 20 minutes.
2. Divide the mix between plates and serve.

Nutrition Value: calories 150, fat 4.1, fiber 1, carbs 3.2, protein 2

231. Leeks Cream
Preparation time: 10 minutes
Cooking time: 30 minutes
Servings: 4

Ingredients:
- 4 leeks, sliced
- 4 cups vegetable stock
- 1 tablespoon olive oil
- 2 shallots, chopped
- 1 tablespoon rosemary, chopped
- A pinch of salt and black pepper
- 1 cup heavy cream
- 1 tablespoon chives, chopped

Directions:
1. Heat up a pot with the oil over medium high heat, add the shallots and the leeks and sauté for 5 minutes.
2. Add the stock and the other ingredients except the chives, bring to a simmer and cook over medium heat for 25 minutes stirring from time to time.
3. Blend the soup using an immersion blender, ladle it into bowls, sprinkle the chives on top and serve.

Nutrition Value: calories 150, fat 3, fiber 1, carbs 2, protein 6

232. Fennel Soup
Preparation time: 10 minutes
Cooking time: 25 minutes
Servings: 4

Ingredients:
- 2 fennel bulb, sliced
- 2 tablespoons olive oil
- 2 shallots, chopped
- 3 garlic cloves, minced
- 4 cups chicken stock
- A pinch of salt and black pepper
- 1 cup heavy cream
- 1 tablespoon dill, chopped

Directions:
1. Heat up a pot with the oil over medium heat, add the shallots and the garlic and sauté for 5 minutes.
2. Add the fennel and the other ingredients, bring to a simmer, cook over medium heat for 20 minutes more, blend using an immersion blender, divide into bowls and serve.

Nutrition Value: calories 140, fat 2, fiber 1, carbs 5, protein 10

233. Cauliflower and Green Beans
Preparation time: 10 minutes
Cooking time: 30 minutes
Servings: 4

Ingredients:
- 1 pound cauliflower florets
- 1 red onion, chopped
- 1 tablespoon olive oil
- 2 garlic cloves minced
- 1 cup tomato passata
- A pinch of salt and black pepper
- ½ pound green beans, trimmed and halved
- 1 tablespoon cilantro, chopped

Directions:
1. Heat up a pot with the oil over medium high heat, add the onion and the garlic and sauté for 5 minutes.
2. Add the cauliflower and the other ingredients, toss and cook everything for 25 minutes more.
3. Divide everything between plates and serve.

Nutrition Value: calories 93, fat 3.7, fiber 5.9, carbs 13.7, protein 4.1

234. Bok Choy Soup
Preparation time: 10 minutes
Cooking time: 25 minutes

Servings: 4

Ingredients:

- 2 tablespoons coconut oil, melted
- 1 pound bok choy, torn
- 2 shallots, chopped
- 4 cups chicken stock
- 1 cup heavy cream
- 1 tablespoon cilantro, chopped
- A pinch of salt and black pepper
- ½ teaspoon nutmeg, ground

Directions:

1. Heat up a pot with the oil over medium heat, add the shallots and sauté for 5 minutes.
2. Add the bok choy and the other ingredients, bring to a simmer and cook over medium heat for 20 minutes.
3. Blend the soup using an immersion blender, divide into bowls and serve.

Nutrition Value: calories 192, fat 18.8, fiber 1.2, carbs 5.1, protein 3.2

235. Cabbage Sauté

Preparation time: 10 minutes
Cooking time: 20 minutes
Servings: 4

Ingredients:

- 2 garlic cloves, minced
- 2 shallots, chopped
- 1 tablespoon olive oil
- 1 green cabbage head, shredded
- 1 cup tomatoes, cubed
- 1 teaspoon lime juice
- A pinch of salt and black pepper
- 1 tablespoon cilantro, chopped

Directions:

1. Heat up a pan with the oil over medium high heat, add the shallots and the garlic and sauté for 5 minutes.
2. Add the cabbage and the other ingredients, toss and cook over medium heat for 15 minutes more.
3. Divide everything between plates and serve.

Nutrition Value: calories 89, fat 3.8, fiber 5.1, carbs 13.5, protein 2.9

236. Mustard Greens Sauté

Preparation time: 10 minutes
Cooking time: 20 minutes
Servings: 4

Ingredients:

- 1 tablespoon olive oil
- 1 pound mustard greens, roughly chopped
- 2 garlic cloves, minced
- 2 spring onions, chopped
- A pinch of salt and black pepper
- ½ cup chicken stock
- 1 tablespoon balsamic vinegar
- 1 tablespoon cilantro, chopped

Directions:

1. Heat up a pan with the oil over medium heat, add the garlic and the spring onions, stir and sauté for 5 minutes.
2. Add the mustard greens and the other ingredients, bring to a simmer and cook over medium heat for 15 minutes more.
3. Divide everything between plates and serve.

Nutrition Value: calories 150, fat 12, fiber 2, carbs 4, protein 8

237. Bok Choy and Tomatoes

This is just fantastic!
Preparation time: 10 minutes
Cooking time: 20 minutes
Servings: 4

Ingredients:

- 1 pound bok choy
- 2 shallots, chopped
- 1 tablespoon olive oil
- 2 cups tomatoes, cubed
- 1 tablespoon balsamic vinegar
- ½ cup vegetable stock
- A pinch of salt and black pepper
- 1 teaspoon rosemary, dried
- 1 teaspoon fennel powder
- 1 tablespoon chives, chopped

Directions:

1. Heat up a pan with the oil over medium heat, add the shallots and sauté for 3 minutes.
2. Add the bok choy and the other ingredients, bring to a simmer and cook over heat for 17 minutes.
3. Divide the mix between plates and serve.

Nutrition Value: calories 120, fat 8, fiber 1, carbs 3, protein 7

238. Sesame Savoy Cabbage

Preparation time: 5 minutes
Cooking time: 20 minutes
Servings: 4

Ingredients:

- 2 garlic cloves, minced
- 2 spring onions, chopped
- 1 Savoy cabbage, shredded
- 1 tablespoon olive oil
- ½ cup tomato passata
- 1 tablespoon sesame seeds

Directions:

1. Heat up a pan with the oil over medium heat, add the spring onions and the garlic and sauté for 5 minutes.
2. Add the cabbage and the rest of the ingredients, toss, cook over medium heat for 15 minutes more, divide between plates and serve.

Nutrition Value: calories 120, fat 3, fiber 1, carbs 3, protein 6

239. Chili Collard Greens

This will really make everyone love your cooking!
Preparation time: 10 minutes
Cooking time: 20 minutes
Servings: 4

Ingredients:

- 1 tablespoon chili powder
- 1 bunch collard greens, roughly chopped
- 1 tablespoon olive oil
- ½ cup chicken stock
- 2 shallots, chopped
- 1 teaspoon hot paprika
- ½ teaspoon cumin, ground
- A pinch of salt and black pepper
- 1 tablespoon lime juice

Directions:

1. Heat up a pan with the oil over medium high heat, add the shallots and sauté for 5 minutes.
2. Add the collard greens and the other ingredients, toss and cook over medium heat for 15 minutes more.
3. Divide everything between plates and serve.

Nutrition Value: calories 245, fat 20, fiber 1, carbs 5, protein 12

240. Artichokes Soup

Preparation time: 10 minutes
Cooking time: 35 minutes
Servings: 6

Ingredients:

- 1 tablespoon olive oil
- 2 shallots, chopped
- 10 ounces canned artichokes, drained and quartered
- 4 cups chicken stock
- 1 teaspoon smoked paprika
- 1 teaspoon cumin, ground
- A pinch of red pepper flakes
- 3 celery stalks, chopped
- 2 tomatoes, cubed
- 2 tablespoons lime juice
- A pinch of salt and black pepper

Directions:

1. Heat up a pot with the oil over medium high heat, add the shallots and sauté for 5 minutes.
2. Add the artichokes and the other ingredients, bring to a simmer and cook over medium heat for 30 minutes more.
3. Ladle the soup into bowls and serve.

Nutrition Value: calories 150, fat 3, fiber 2, carbs 4, protein 8

241. Ginger and Bok Choy Soup

Preparation time: 10 minutes
Cooking time: 25 minutes
Servings: 4

Ingredients:

- 4 cups bok choy, roughly chopped
- 2 spring onions, chopped
- 1 quart vegetable stock
- A pinch of salt and black pepper
- 2 teaspoons ginger, grated

Directions:

1. Put the stock into a pot, bring to a simmer over medium heat, add the bok choy and the other ingredients, bring to a simmer and cook for 25 minutes.
2. Blend the soup using an immersion blender, divide into bowls and serve.

Nutrition Value: calories 140, fat 2, fiber 1, carbs 3, protein 7

242. Spinach Soup

Preparation time: 10 minutes
Cooking time: 15 minutes
Servings: 4

Ingredients:

- 1 tablespoon olive oil
- ½ teaspoon coriander, ground
- 2 shallots, chopped
- 2 garlic cloves, minced

- 1 tablespoon ginger, grated
- 1 pound spinach leaves, torn
- 4 cups chicken stock
- A pinch of salt and black pepper
- 1 tablespoon cilantro, chopped

Directions:
1. Heat up a pot with the oil over medium high heat, add the shallots and the garlic and sauté for 2 minutes.
2. Add the ginger, spinach and the other ingredients, bring to a simmer and cook over medium heat for 13 minutes more.
3. Ladle the soup into bowls and serve.

Nutrition Value: calories 143, fat 6, fiber 3, carbs 7, protein 7

243. Asparagus Soup

Preparation time: 10 minutes
Cooking time: 20 minutes
Servings: 4

Ingredients:

- 1 asparagus bunch, trimmed and halved
- 1 tablespoon olive oil
- 2 shallots, chopped
- 1 teaspoon lime juice
- 4 cups chicken stock
- 1 cup heavy cream
- A pinch of salt and black pepper
- 1 tablespoon oregano, chopped

Directions:
1. Heat up a pot with the oil over medium heat, add the shallots and sauté for 2 minutes.
2. Add the asparagus and the other ingredients except the cream and the oregano, bring to a simmer and cook over medium heat for 18 minutes more.
3. Add the cream, blend the soup using an immersion blender, divide into bowls and serve with the oregano sprinkled on top.

Nutrition Value: calories 130, fat 1, fiber 1, carbs 2, protein 3

244. Baked Endives

Preparation time: 10 minutes
Cooking time: 20 minutes
Servings: 4

Ingredients:

- ¼ cup parmesan, grated
- 2 endives, trimmed and halved lengthwise
- 1 tablespoon olive oil
- 2 garlic cloves, minced
- A pinch of salt and black pepper
- ½ teaspoon sweet paprika

Directions:
1. Arrange the endives on a lined baking sheet, add the oil and the other ingredients, toss, introduce in the oven at 400 degrees F and bake for 20 minutes.
2. Divide between plates and serve.

Nutrition Value: calories 120, fat 2, fiber 2, carbs 5, protein 8

245. Baked Asparagus

Preparation time: 10 minutes
Cooking time: 15 minutes
Servings: 4

Ingredients:

- 1 tablespoon avocado oil
- 2 bunches of asparagus, trimmed
- 2 tablespoons lime juice
- ½ cup parmesan, grated
- A pinch of salt and black pepper

Directions:
1. Arrange the asparagus on a lined baking sheet, add the oil and the other ingredients, toss and bake at 400 degrees F for 15 minutes.
2. Divide between plates and serve.

Nutrition Value: calories 160, fat 7, fiber 2, carbs 6, protein 10

246. Asparagus and Tomatoes

Preparation time: 10 minutes
Cooking time: 20 minutes
Servings: 4

Ingredients:

- ¼ cup shallots, chopped
- 2 tablespoons olive oil
- 4 asparagus spears, trimmed and halved
- 1 pound cherry tomatoes, halved
- A pinch of salt and black pepper
- 1 cup cheddar cheese, grated

Directions:
1. In a roasting pan, combine the asparagus with the shallots and the other ingredients, toss and bake at 400 degrees F for 20 minutes.
2. Divide the mix between plates and serve.

Nutrition Value: calories 200, fat 12, fiber 2, carbs 5, protein 14

247. Endives and Mustard Sauce

Preparation time: 10 minutes
Cooking time: 20 minutes
Servings: 4

Ingredients:

- 2 endives, trimmed and halved lengthwise
- 2 tablespoons olive oil
- 2 shallots, chopped
- A pinch of salt and black pepper
- 2 tablespoons parmesan, grated
- 2 tablespoons mustard
- ¼ cup heavy cream

Directions:

1. Heat up a pan with the oil over medium heat, add the shallots and sauté for 2 minutes.
2. Add the endives and the other ingredients except the parmesan, toss, and cook over medium heat for 15 minutes more.
3. Add the parmesan, toss, cook everything for 3 minutes more, divide between plates and serve.

Nutrition Value: calories 256, fat 23, fiber 2, carbs 5, protein 13

248. Mexican Peppers Mix

Preparation time: 10 minutes
Cooking time: 16 minutes
Servings: 4

Ingredients:

- 4 bell peppers, cut into medium chunks
- ½ cup tomato juice
- 2 tablespoons jarred jalapenos, chopped
- 1 cup tomatoes, chopped
- ¼ cup yellow onion, chopped
- ¼ cup green peppers, chopped
- 2 cups tomato sauce
- Salt and black pepper to the taste
- 2 teaspoons onion powder
- ½ teaspoon red pepper, crushed
- 1 teaspoon chili powder
- ½ teaspoons garlic powder
- 1 teaspoon cumin, ground

Directions:

1. In a pan that fits your air fryer, mix tomato juice, jalapenos, tomatoes, onion, green peppers, salt, pepper, onion powder, red pepper, chili powder, garlic powder, oregano and cumin, stir well, introduce in your air fryer and cook at 350 degrees F for 6 minutes
2. Add bell peppers and cook at 320 degrees F for 10 minutes more.
3. Divide peppers mix between plates and serve them as a side dish.
4. Enjoy!

Nutrition Value: calories 180, fat 4, fiber 3, carbs 7, protein 14

249. Garlic Eggplants

Preparation time: 10 minutes
Cooking time: 10 minutes
Servings: 4

Ingredients:

- 2 tablespoons olive oil
- 2 garlic cloves, minced
- 3 eggplants, halved and sliced
- 1 red chili pepper, chopped
- 1 green onion stalk, chopped
- 1 tablespoon ginger, grated
- 1 tablespoon coconut aminos
- 1 tablespoon balsamic vinegar

Directions:

1. Heat up a pan that fits your air fryer with the oil over medium-high heat, add eggplant slices and cook for 2 minutes.
2. Add chili pepper, garlic, green onions, ginger, coconut aminos and vinegar, introduce in your air fryer and cook at 320 degrees F for 7 minutes.
3. Divide between plates and serve as a side dish.
4. Enjoy!

Nutrition Value: calories 130, fat 2, fiber 4, carbs 7, protein 9

250. Broccoli and Mushrooms Mix

Preparation time: 30 minutes
Cooking time: 8 minutes
Servings: 2

Ingredients:

- 10 ounces mushrooms, halved
- 1 broccoli head, florets separated
- 1 garlic clove, minced
- 1 tablespoon balsamic vinegar
- 1 yellow onion, chopped
- 1 tablespoon olive oil
- Salt and black pepper
- 1 teaspoon basil, dried
- 1 avocado, peeled, pitted and roughly cubed
- A pinch of red pepper flakes

Directions:

1. In a bowl, mix mushrooms with broccoli, onion, garlic and avocado.
2. In another bowl, mix vinegar, oil, salt, pepper and basil and whisk well.
3. Pour this over veggies, toss to coat, leave aside for 30 minutes, transfer to your air fryer's basket and cook at 350 degrees F for 8 minutes,
4. Divide between plates and serve with pepper flakes on top as a side dish.
5. Enjoy!

Nutrition Value: calories 182, fat 3, fiber 3, carbs 5, protein 8

251. Green Beans Side Salad

Preparation time: 10 minutes
Cooking time: 15 minutes
Servings: 4

Ingredients:
- 1-pint cherry tomatoes
- 1 pound green beans
- 2 tablespoons olive oil
- Salt and black pepper to the taste

Directions:
1. In a bowl, mix cherry tomatoes with green beans, olive oil, salt and pepper, toss, transfer to a pan that fits your air fryer and cook at 400 degrees F for 15 minutes.
2. Divide between plates and serve as a side dish.
3. Enjoy!

Nutrition Value: calories 142, fat 6, fiber 5, carbs 8, protein 9

252. Red Potatoes and Green Beans

Preparation time: 10 minutes
Cooking time: 15 minutes
Servings: 4

Ingredients:
- 1 pound red potatoes, cut into wedges
- 1 pound green beans
- 2 garlic cloves, minced
- 2 tablespoons olive oil
- Salt and black pepper to the taste
- ½ teaspoon oregano, dried

Directions:
1. In a pan that fits your air fryer, combine potatoes with green beans, garlic, oil, salt, pepper and oregano, toss, introduce in your air fryer and cook at 380 degrees F for 15 minutes.
2. Divide between plates and serve as a side dish.
3. Enjoy!

Nutrition Value: calories 201, fat 6, fiber 4, carbs 8, protein 5

253. Baby Potatoes Salad

Preparation time: 10 minutes
Cooking time: 20 minutes
Servings: 4

Ingredients:
- 1 and ½ pounds baby potatoes, halved
- 2 garlic cloves, chopped
- 2 red onions, chopped
- 9 ounces cherry tomatoes
- 3 tablespoons olive oil
- 1 and ½ tablespoons balsamic vinegar
- 2 thyme springs, chopped
- Salt and black pepper to the taste

Directions:
1. In your food processor, mix garlic with onions, oil, vinegar, thyme, salt and pepper and pulse really well.
2. In a bowl, mix potatoes with tomatoes and balsamic mix, toss, transfer to your air fryer and cook at 380 degrees F for 20 minutes.
3. Divide between plates and serve cold as a side dish.
4. Enjoy!

Nutrition Value: calories 201, fat 6, fiber 3, carbs 14, protein 6

254. Arabic Plums Mix

Preparation time: 10 minutes
Cooking time: 12 minutes
Servings: 4

Ingredients:
- 3 tablespoons stevia
- 3 ounces almonds, peeled and chopped
- 12 ounces plumps, pitted
- 2 tablespoons veggie stock
- 2 yellow onions, chopped
- 2 garlic cloves, minced
- Salt and black pepper to the tastes
- 1 teaspoon cumin powder
- 1 teaspoon turmeric powder
- 1 teaspoon ginger powder
- 1 teaspoon cinnamon powder
- 3 tablespoons olive oil

Directions:
1. In a pan that fits your air fryer, combine almonds with plums, stevia, stock, onions, garlic, salt, pepper, cumin, turmeric, ginger,

cinnamon and oil, toss, introduce in your air fryer and cook at 350 degrees F for 12 minutes.
2. Divide plums mix between plates and serve as a side dish
3. Enjoy!

Nutrition Value: calories 152, fat 3, fiber 6, carbs 12, protein 4

255. Lemony Baby Potatoes

Preparation time: 10 minutes
Cooking time: 25 minutes
Servings: 6

Ingredients:

- 2 tablespoons olive oil
- 2 springs rosemary, chopped
- 2 tablespoons parsley, chopped
- 2 tablespoons oregano, chopped
- Salt and black pepper to the taste
- 1 tablespoon lemon rind, grated
- 3 garlic cloves, minced
- 2 tablespoons lemon juice
- 2 pounds baby potatoes

Directions:

1. In a bowl, mix baby potatoes with oil, rosemary, parsley, oregano, salt, pepper, lemon rind, garlic and lemon juice, toss, transfer potatoes to your air fryer's basket and cook at 356 degrees F for 25 minutes.
2. Divide potatoes between plates and serve as a side dish.
3. Enjoy!

Nutrition Value: calories 204, fat 4, fiber 5, carbs 17, protein 6

256. White Mushrooms Mix

Preparation time: 10 minutes
Cooking time: 15 minutes
Servings: 2

Ingredients:

- Salt and black pepper to the taste
- 7 ounces snow peas
- 8 ounces white mushrooms, halved
- 1 yellow onion, cut into rings
- 2 tablespoons coconut aminos
- 1 teaspoon olive oil

Directions:

1. In a bowl, snow peas with mushrooms, onion, aminos, oil, salt and pepper, toss well, transfer to a pan that fits your air fryer, introduce in the fryer and cook at 350 degrees F for 15 minutes.
2. Divide between plates and serve as a side dish
3. Enjoy!

Nutrition Value: calories 175, fat 4, fiber 2, carbs 12, protein 7

257. Gold Potatoes and Bell Pepper Mix

Preparation time: 10 minutes
Cooking time: 25 minutes
Servings: 4

Ingredients:

- 4 gold potatoes, cubed
- 1 yellow onion, chopped
- 2 teaspoons olive oil
- 1 green bell pepper, chopped
- Salt and black pepper to the taste
- ½ teaspoon thyme, dried

Directions:

1. Heat up your air fryer at 350 degrees F, add oil, heat it up, add onion, bell pepper, salt and pepper, stir and cook for 5 minutes.
2. Add potatoes and thyme, stir, cover and cook at 360 degrees F for 20 minutes.
3. Divide between plates and serve as a side dish.
4. Enjoy!

Nutrition Value: calories 201, fat 4, fiber 4, carbs 12, protein 7

258. Delicious Potato Mix

Preparation time: 10 minutes
Cooking time: 25 minutes
Servings: 6

Ingredients:

- 6 ounces jarred roasted red bell peppers, chopped
- 3 garlic cloves, minced
- 2 tablespoons parsley, chopped
- Salt and black pepper to the taste
- 2 tablespoons chives, chopped
- 4 potatoes, peeled and cut into wedges
- Cooking spray

Directions:

1. In a pan that fits your air fryer, combine roasted bell peppers with garlic, parsley, salt, pepper, chives, potato wedges and the oil, toss, transfer to your air fryer and cook at 350 degrees F for 25 minutes.
2. Divide between plates and serve as a side dish.
3. Enjoy!

Nutrition Value: calories 212, fat 6, fiber 4, carbs 11,

protein 5

259. Chinese Long Beans Mix

Preparation time: 10 minutes
Cooking time: 10 minutes
Servings: 3

Ingredients:

- ½ teaspoon coconut aminos
- 1 tablespoon olive oil
- A pinch of salt and black pepper
- 4 garlic cloves, minced
- 4 long beans, trimmed and sliced

Directions:

1. In a pan that fits your air fryer, combine long beans with oil, aminos, salt, pepper and garlic, toss, introduce in your air fryer and cook at 350 degrees F for 10 minutes.
2. Divide between plates and serve as a side dish.
3. Enjoy!

Nutrition Value: calories 170, fat 3, fiber 3, carbs 7, protein 3

260. Easy Portobello Mushrooms

Preparation time: 10 minutes
Cooking time: 12 minutes
Servings: 4

Ingredients:

- 4 big Portobello mushroom caps
- 1 tablespoon olive oil
- 1 cup spinach, torn
- 1/3 cup vegan breadcrumbs
- ¼ teaspoon rosemary, chopped

Directions:

1. Rub mushrooms caps with the oil, place them in your air fryer's basket and cook them at 350 degrees F for 2 minutes.
2. Meanwhile, in a bowl, mix spinach, rosemary and breadcrumbs and stir well.
3. Stuff mushrooms with this mix, place them in your air fryer's basket again and cook at 350 degrees F for 10 minutes.
4. Divide them between plates and serve as a side dish.
5. Enjoy!

Nutrition Value: calories 152, fat 4, fiber 7, carbs 9, protein 5

261. Summer Squash Mix

Preparation time: 10 minutes
Cooking time: 10
Servings: 4

Ingredients:

- 3 ounces coconut cream
- ½ teaspoon oregano, dried
- Salt and black pepper
- 1 big yellow summer squash, peeled and cubed
- 1/3 cup carrot, cubed
- 2 tablespoons olive oil

Directions:

1. In a pan that fits your air fryer, combine squash with carrot, oil, oregano, salt, pepper and coconut cream, toss, transfer to your air fryer and cook at 400 degrees F for 10 minutes.
2. Divide between plates and serve as a side dish.
3. Enjoy!

Nutrition Value: calories 170, fat 4, fiber 7, carbs 8, protein 6

262. Corn Side Salad

Preparation time: 10 minutes
Cooking time: 10 minutes
Servings: 4

Ingredients:

- 3 cups corn
- A drizzle of olive oil
- Salt and black pepper to the taste
- 1 teaspoon sweet paprika
- 1 tablespoon stevia
- ½ teaspoon garlic powder
- ½ iceberg lettuce head, cut into medium strips
- ½ romaine lettuce head, cut into medium strips
- 1 cup canned black beans, drained
- 3 tablespoons cilantro, chopped
- 4 green onions, chopped
- 12 cherry tomatoes, sliced

Directions:

1. Put the corn in a pan that fits your air fryer, drizzle the oil, add salt, pepper, paprika, stevia and garlic powder, introduce in your air fryer and cook at 350 degrees F for 10 minutes.
2. Transfer corn to a salad bowl, add lettuce, black beans, tomatoes, green onions and cilantro, toss, divide between plates and serve as a side salad.
3. Enjoy!

Nutrition Value: calories 162, fat 6, fiber 4, carbs 7, protein 6

263. Colored Veggie Mix

Preparation time: 10 minutes
Cooking time: 12 minutes
Servings: 6

Sides

Ingredients:
- 1 zucchini, sliced in half and roughly chopped
- 1 orange bell pepper, roughly chopped
- 1 green bell pepper, roughly chopped
- 1 red onion, roughly chopped
- 4 ounces brown mushrooms, halved
- Salt and black pepper to the taste
- 1 teaspoon Italian seasoning
- 1 cup cherry tomatoes, halved
- ½ cup kalamata olives, pitted and halved
- ¼ cup olive oil
- 3 tablespoons balsamic vinegar
- 2 tablespoons basil, chopped

Directions:
1. In a bowl, mix zucchini with mushrooms, orange bell pepper, green bell pepper, red onion, salt, pepper, Italian seasoning and oil, toss well, transfer to preheated air fryer at 380 degrees F and cook them for 12 minutes.
2. In a large bowl, combine mixed veggies with tomatoes, olives, vinegar and basil, toss, divide between plates and serve cold as a side dish.
3. Enjoy!

Nutrition Value: calories 180, fat 5, fiber 8, carbs 10, protein 6

264. Leeks Medley

Preparation time: 10 minutes
Cooking time: 12 minutes
Servings: 4

Ingredients:
- 6 leeks, roughly chopped
- 1 tablespoon cumin, ground
- 1 tablespoon mint, chopped
- 1 tablespoon parsley, chopped
- 1 teaspoon garlic, minced
- A drizzle of olive oil
- Salt and black pepper to the taste

Directions:
1. In a pan that fits your air fryer, combine leeks with cumin, mint, parsley, garlic, salt, pepper and the oil, toss, introduce in your air fryer and cook at 350 degrees F for 12 minutes.
2. Divide leeks medley between plates and serve as a side dish.
3. Enjoy!

Nutrition Value: calories 131, fat 7, fiber 3, carbs 10, protein 6

265. Corn and Tomatoes

Preparation time: 10 minutes
Cooking time: 13 minutes
Servings: 4

Ingredients:
- 2 cups corn
- 4 tomatoes, roughly chopped
- 1 tablespoon olive oil
- Salt and black pepper to the taste
- 1 tablespoon oregano, chopped
- 1 tablespoon parsley, chopped
- 2 tablespoons soft tofu, pressed and crumbled

Directions:
1. In a pan that fits your air fryer, combine corn with tomatoes, oil, salt, pepper, oregano and parsley, toss, introduce the pan in your air fryer and cook at 320 degrees F for 10 minutes.
2. Add tofu, toss, introduce in the fryer for 3 minutes more, divide between plates and serve as a side dish.
3. Enjoy!

Nutrition Value: calories 171, fat 7, fiber 8, carbs 9, protein 6

266. Broccoli, Tomatoes and Carrots

Preparation time: 10 minutes
Cooking time: 14 minutes
Servings: 2

Ingredients:
- 1 broccoli head, florets separated and steamed
- 1 tomato, chopped
- 3 carrots, chopped and steamed
- 2 ounces soft tofu, crumbled
- 1 teaspoon parsley, chopped
- 1 teaspoon thyme, chopped
- Salt and black pepper to the taste

Directions:
1. In a pan that fits your air fryer, combine broccoli with tomato, carrots, thyme, parsley, salt and pepper, toss, introduce the fryer and cook at 350 degrees F for 10 minutes.
2. Add tofu, toss, introduce in the fryer for 4 minutes more, divide between plates and serve as a side dish.
3. Enjoy!

Nutrition Value: calories 174, fat 4, fiber 7, carbs 12, protein 3

267. Oregano Bell Peppers

Preparation time: 10 minutes
Cooking time: 15 minutes

Servings: 4

Ingredients:

- 1 tablespoon olive oil
- 1 sweet onion, chopped
- 1 red bell pepper, chopped
- 1 orange bell pepper, chopped
- 1 green bell pepper, chopped
- Salt and black pepper to the taste
- ½ cup cashew cheese, shredded
- 1 tablespoon oregano, chopped

Directions:

1. In a pan that fits your air fryer, combine onion with red bell pepper, green bell pepper, orange bell pepper, salt, pepper, oregano and oil, toss, introduce in the fryer and cook at 320 degrees F for 10 minutes.
2. Add cashew cheese, toss, introduce in the fryer for 4 minutes more, divide between plates and serve as a side dish.
3. Enjoy!

Nutrition Value: calories 172, fat 4, fiber 6, carbs 8, protein 7

268. Yellow Lentils Mix

Preparation time: 10 minutes
Cooking time: 15 minutes
Servings: 2

Ingredients:

- 1 cup yellow lentils, soaked in water for 1 hour and drained
- 1 hot chili pepper, chopped
- 1-inch ginger piece, grated
- ½ teaspoon turmeric powder
- 1 teaspoon garam masala
- Salt and black pepper to the taste
- 2 teaspoons olive oil
- ½ cup cilantro, chopped
- 1 and ½ cup spinach, chopped
- 4 garlic cloves, minced
- ¾ cup red onion, chopped

Directions:

1. In a pan that fits your air fryer, mix lentils with chili pepper, ginger, turmeric, garam masala, salt, pepper, olive oil, cilantro, spinach, onion and garlic, toss, introduce in your air fryer and cook at 400 degrees F for 15 minutes.
2. Divide lentils mix between plates and serve as a side dish.
3. Enjoy!

Nutrition Value: calories 202, fat 2, fiber 8, carbs 12, protein 4

269. Creamy Zucchini and Sweet Potatoes

Preparation time: 10 minutes
Cooking time: 16 minutes
Servings: 8

Ingredients:

- 1 cup veggie stock
- 2 tablespoons olive oil
- 2 sweet potatoes, peeled and cut into medium wedges
- 8 zucchinis, cut into medium wedges
- 2 yellow onions, chopped
- 1 cup coconut milk
- Salt and black pepper to the taste
- 1 tablespoon coconut aminos
- ¼ teaspoon thyme, dried
- ¼ teaspoon rosemary, dried
- 4 tablespoons dill, chopped
- ½ teaspoon basil, chopped

Directions:

1. Heat up a pan that fits your air fryer with the oil over medium heat, add onion, stir and cook for 2 minutes.
2. Add zucchinis, thyme, rosemary, basil, potato, salt, pepper, stock, milk, aminos and dill, stir, introduce in your air fryer, cook at 360 degrees F for 14 minutes, divide between plates and serve as a side dish.
3. Enjoy!

Nutrition Value: calories 133, fat 3, fiber 4, carbs 10, protein 5

270. Baked Brussels Sprouts

Preparation time: 10 minutes
Cooking time: 20 minutes
Servings: 4

Ingredients:

- 1 pound Brussels sprouts, trimmed and halved
- 1 tablespoon avocado oil
- 2 garlic cloves, minced
- A pinch of salt and black pepper
- ¼ cup cilantro, chopped

Directions:

1. In a roasting pan, combine the sprouts with the oil and the other ingredients, toss and bake at 400 degrees F for 20 minutes.
2. Divide everything between plates and serve.

Nutrition Value: calories 100, fat 3, fiber 1, carbs 2, protein 6

271. Roasted Tomatoes

Preparation time: 10 minutes
Cooking time: 25 minutes
Servings: 4

Ingredients:

- 1 pound tomatoes, halved
- A pinch of salt and black pepper
- 2 tablespoons olive oil
- 1 teaspoon rosemary, dried
- 1 teaspoon basil, dried
- 1 tablespoon chives, chopped

Directions:

1. In a roasting pan combine the tomatoes with the oil and the other ingredients, toss gently and bake at 390 degrees F for 25 minutes.
2. Divide the mix between plates and serve.

Nutrition Value: calories 122, fat 12, fiber 1, carbs 3, protein 14

272. Brussels Sprouts and Green Beans

Preparation time: 10 minutes
Cooking time: 20 minutes
Servings: 4

Ingredients:

- 1 tablespoon avocado oil
- 1 pound Brussels sprouts, trimmed and halved
- ½ pound green beans, trimmed and halved
- ½ teaspoon garlic powder
- A pinch of salt and black pepper
- 1 tablespoon lime juice

Directions:

1. In a roasting pan, combine the sprouts with the green beans and the other ingredients, toss, introduce in the oven at 375 degrees F and bake for 20 minutes.
2. Divide between plates and serve.

Nutrition Value: calories 80, fat 5, fiber 2, carbs 5, protein 7

273. Crispy Radishes

Preparation time: 10 minutes
Cooking time: 20 minutes
Servings: 4

Ingredients:

- Cooking spray
- 15 radishes, sliced
- Salt and black pepper to the taste
- 1 tablespoon chives, chopped

Directions:

1. Arrange radish slices on a lined baking sheet and spray them with cooking oil.
2. Season with salt and pepper and sprinkle chives, introduce in the oven at 375 degrees F and bake for 10 minutes.
3. Flip them and bake for 10 minutes more.
4. Serve them cold.
5. Enjoy!

Nutrition Value: calories 30, fat 1, fiber 0.4, carbs 1, protein 0.1

274. Creamy Radishes

Preparation time: 10 minutes
Cooking time: 25 minutes
Servings: 1

Ingredients:

- 7 ounces radishes, cut in halves
- 2 tablespoons sour cream
- 2 bacon slices
- 1 tablespoon green onion, chopped
- 1 tablespoon cheddar cheese, grated
- Hot sauce to the taste
- Salt and black pepper to the taste

Directions:

1. Put radishes into a pot, add water to cover, bring to a boil over medium heat, cook them for 10 minutes and drain.
2. Heat up a pan over medium high heat, add bacon, cook until it's crispy, transfer to paper towels, drain grease, crumble and leave aside.
3. Return pan to medium heat, add radishes, stir and sauté them for 7 minutes.
4. Add onion, salt, pepper, hot sauce and sour cream, stir and cook for 7 minutes more.
5. Transfer to a plate, top with crumbled bacon and cheddar cheese and serve.
6. Enjoy!

Nutrition Value: calories 340, fat 23, fiber 3, carbs 6, protein 15

275. Radish Soup

Preparation time: 10 minutes
Cooking time: 20 minutes
Servings: 4

Ingredients:

- 2 bunches radishes, cut in quarters
- Salt and black pepper to the taste

- 6 cups chicken stock
- 2 stalks celery, chopped
- 3 tablespoons coconut oil
- 6 garlic cloves, minced
- 1 yellow onion, chopped

Directions:
1. Heat up a pot with the oil over medium heat, add onion, celery and garlic, stir and cook for 5 minutes.
2. Add radishes, stock, salt and pepper, stir, bring to a boil, cover and simmer for 15 minutes.
3. Divide into soup bowls and serve.
4. Enjoy!

Nutrition Value: calories 120, fat 2, fiber 1, carbs 3, protein 10

276. Tasty Avocado Salad

Preparation time: 10 minutes
Cooking time: 0 minutes
Servings: 4

Ingredients:
- 2 avocados, pitted and mashed
- Salt and black pepper to the taste
- ¼ teaspoon lemon stevia
- 1 tablespoon white vinegar
- 14 ounces coleslaw mix
- Juice from 2 limes
- ¼ cup red onion, chopped
- ¼ cup cilantro, chopped
- 2 tablespoons olive oil

Directions:
1. Put coleslaw mix in a salad bowl.
2. Add avocado mash and onions and toss to coat.
3. In a bowl, mix lime juice with salt, pepper, oil, vinegar and stevia and stir well.
4. Add this over salad, toss to coat, sprinkle cilantro and serve.
5. Enjoy!

Nutrition Value: calories 100, fat 10, fiber 2, carbs 5, protein 8

277. Avocado And Egg Salad

Preparation time: 10 minutes
Cooking time: 7 minutes
Servings: 4

Ingredients:
- 4 cups mixed lettuce leaves, torn
- 4 eggs
- 1 avocado, pitted and sliced
- ¼ cup mayonnaise
- 2 teaspoons mustard
- 2 garlic cloves, minced
- 1 tablespoon chives, chopped
- Salt and black pepper to the taste

Directions:
1. Put water in a pot, add some salt, add eggs, bring to a boil over medium high heat, boil for 7 minutes, drain, cool, peel and chop them.
2. In a salad bowl, mix lettuce with eggs and avocado.
3. Add chives and garlic, some salt and pepper and toss to coat.
4. In a bowl, mix mustard with mayo, salt and pepper and stir well.
5. Add this over salad, toss well and serve right away.
6. Enjoy!

Nutrition Value: calories 234, fat 12, fiber 4, carbs 7, protein 12

278. Avocado And Cucumber Salad

Preparation time: 10 minutes
Cooking time: 0 minutes
Servings: 4

Ingredients:
- 1 small red onion, sliced
- 1 cucumber, sliced
- 2 avocados, pitted, peeled and chopped
- 1 pound cherry tomatoes, halved
- 2 tablespoons olive oil
- ¼ cup cilantro, chopped
- 2 tablespoons lemon juice
- Salt and black pepper to the taste

Directions:
1. In a large salad bowl, mix tomatoes with cucumber, onion and avocado and stir.
2. Add oil, salt, pepper and lemon juice and toss to coat well.
3. Serve cold with cilantro on top.
4. Enjoy!

Nutrition Value: calories 140, fat 4, fiber 2, carbs 4, protein 5

279. Delicious Avocado Soup

Preparation time: 10 minutes
Cooking time: 10 minutes
Servings: 4

Ingredients:
- 2 avocados, pitted, peeled and chopped

- 3 cups chicken stock
- 2 scallions, chopped
- Salt and black pepper to the taste
- 2 tablespoons ghee
- 2/3 cup heavy cream

Directions:

1. Heat up a pot with the ghee over medium heat, add scallions, stir and cook for 2 minutes.
2. Add 2 and ½ cups stock, stir and simmer for 3 minutes.
3. In your blender, mix avocados with the rest of the stock, salt, pepper and heavy cream and pulse well.
4. Add this to the pot, stir well, cook for 2 minutes and season with more salt and pepper.
5. Stir well, ladle into soup bowls and serve.
6. Enjoy!

Nutrition Value: calories 332, fat 23, fiber 4, carbs 6, protein 6

280. Delicious Avocado And Bacon Soup

Preparation time: 10 minutes
Cooking time: 10 minutes
Servings: 4

Ingredients:

- 2 avocados, pitted and cut in halves
- 4 cups chicken stock
- 1/3 cup cilantro, chopped
- Juice from ½ lime
- 1 teaspoon garlic powder
- ½ pound bacon, cooked and chopped
- Salt and black pepper to the taste

Directions:

1. Put stock in a pot and bring to a boil over medium high heat.
2. In your blender, mix avocados with garlic powder, cilantro, lime juice, salt and pepper and blend well.
3. Add this over stock and blend using an immersion blender.
4. Add bacon, more salt and pepper the taste, stir, cook for 3 minutes, ladle into soup bowls and serve.
5. Enjoy!

Nutrition Value: calories 300, fat 23, fiber 5, carbs 6, protein 17

281. Thai Avocado Soup

Preparation time: 10 minutes
Cooking time: 10 minutes
Servings: 4

Ingredients:

- 1 cup coconut milk
- 2 teaspoons Thai green curry paste
- 1 avocado, pitted, peeled and chopped
- 1 tablespoon cilantro, chopped
- Salt and black pepper to the taste
- 2 cups veggie stock
- Lime wedges for serving

Directions:

1. In your blender, mix avocado with salt, pepper, curry paste and coconut milk and pulse well.
2. Transfer this to a pot and heat up over medium heat.
3. Add stock, stir, bring to a simmer and cook for 5 minutes.
4. Add cilantro, more salt and pepper, stir, cook for 1 minute more, ladle into soup bowls and serve with lime wedges on the side.
5. Enjoy!

Nutrition Value: calories 240, fat 4, fiber 2, carbs 6, protein 12

282. Simple Arugula Salad

Preparation time: 10 minutes
Cooking time: 0 minutes
Servings: 4

Ingredients:

- 1 white onion, chopped
- 1 tablespoon vinegar
- 1 cup hot water
- 1 bunch baby arugula
- ¼ cup walnuts, chopped
- 2 tablespoons cilantro, chopped
- 2 garlic cloves, minced
- 2 tablespoons olive oil
- Salt and black pepper to the taste
- 1 tablespoon lemon juice

Directions:

1. In a bowl, mix water with vinegar, add onion, leave aside for 5 minutes, drain well and press.
2. In a salad bowl, mix arugula with walnuts and onion and stir.
3. Add garlic, salt, pepper, lemon juice, cilantro and oil, toss well and serve.
4. Enjoy!

Nutrition Value: calories 200, fat 2, fiber 1, carbs 5, protein 7

283. Arugula Soup

Preparation time: 10 minutes
Cooking time: 13 minutes
Servings: 6

Ingredients:

- 1 yellow onion, chopped
- 1 tablespoon olive oil
- 2 garlic cloves, minced
- ½ cup coconut milk
- 10 ounces baby arugula
- ¼ cup mixed mint, tarragon and parsley
- 2 tablespoons chives, chopped
- 4 tablespoons coconut milk yogurt
- 6 cups chicken stock
- Salt and black pepper to the taste

Directions:

1. Heat up a pot with the oil over medium high heat, add onion and garlic, stir and cook for 5 minutes.
2. Add stock and milk, stir and bring to a simmer.
3. Add arugula, tarragon, parsley and mint, stir and cook everything for 6 minutes.
4. Add coconut yogurt, salt, pepper and chives, stir, cook for 2 minutes, divide into soup bowls and serve.
5. Enjoy!

Nutrition Value: calories 200, fat 4, fiber 2, carbs 6, protein 10

284. Arugula And Broccoli Soup

Preparation time: 10 minutes
Cooking time: 20 minutes
Servings: 4

Ingredients:

- 1 small yellow onion, chopped
- 1 tablespoon olive oil
- 1 garlic clove, minced
- 1 broccoli head, florets separated
- Salt and black pepper to the taste
- 2 and ½ cups veggie stock
- 1 teaspoon cumin, ground
- Juice from ½ lemon
- 1 cup arugula leaves

Directions:

1. Heat up a pot with the oil over medium high heat, add onions, stir and cook for 4 minutes.
2. Add garlic, stir and cook for 1 minute.
3. Add broccoli, cumin, salt and pepper, stir and cook for 4 minutes.
4. Add stock, stir and cook for 8 minutes.
5. Blend soup using an immersion blender, add half of the arugula and blend again.
6. Ad the rest of the arugula, stir and heat up the soup again.
7. Add lemon juice, stir, ladle into soup bowls and serve.
8. Enjoy!

Nutrition Value: calories 150, fat 3, fiber 1, carbs 3, protein 7

285. Delicious Zucchini Cream

Preparation time: 10 minutes
Cooking time: 25 minutes
Servings: 8

Ingredients:

- 6 zucchinis, cut in halves and then sliced
- Salt and black pepper to the taste
- 1 tablespoon ghee
- 28 ounces veggie stock
- 1 teaspoon oregano, dried
- ½ cup yellow onion, chopped
- 3 garlic cloves, minced
- 2 ounces parmesan, grated
- ¾ cup heavy cream

Directions:

1. Heat up a pot with the ghee over medium high heat, add onion, stir and cook for 4 minutes.
2. Add garlic, stir and cook for 2 minutes more.
3. Add zucchinis, stir and cook for 3 minutes.
4. Add stock, stir, bring to a boil and simmer over medium heat for 15 minutes.
5. Add oregano, salt and pepper, stir, take off heat and blend using an immersion blender.
6. Heat up soup again, add heavy cream, stir and bring to a simmer.
7. Add parmesan, stir, take off heat, ladle into bowls and serve right away.
8. Enjoy!

Nutrition Value: calories 160, fat 4, fiber 2, carbs 4, protein 8

286. Zucchini And Avocado Soup

Preparation time: 10 minutes
Cooking time: 15 minutes
Servings: 4

Ingredients:

- 1 big avocado, pitted, peeled and chopped
- 4 scallions, chopped
- 1 teaspoon ginger, grated
- 2 tablespoons avocado oil

- Salt and black pepper to the taste
- 2 zucchinis, chopped
- 29 ounces veggie stock
- 1 garlic clove, minced
- 1 cup water
- 1 tablespoon lemon juice
- 1 red bell pepper, chopped

Directions:
1. Heat up a pot with the oil over medium heat, add onions, stir and cook for 3 minutes.
2. Add garlic and ginger, stir and cook for 1 minute.
3. Add zucchini, salt, pepper, water and stock, stir, bring to a boil, cover pot and cook for 10 minutes.
4. Take off heat, leave soup aside for a couple of minutes, add avocado, stir, blend everything using an immersion blender and heat up again.
5. Add more salt and pepper, bell pepper and lemon juice, stir, heat up soup again, ladle into soup bowls and serve.
6. Enjoy!

Nutrition Value: calories 154, fat 12, fiber 3, carbs 5, protein 4

287. Swiss Chard Pie
Preparation time: 10 minutes
Cooking time: 45 minutes
Servings: 12

Ingredients:
- 8 cups Swiss chard, chopped
- ½ cup onion, chopped
- 1 tablespoon olive oil
- 1 garlic clove, minced
- Salt and black pepper to the taste
- 3 eggs
- 2 cups ricotta cheese
- 1 cup mozzarella, shredded
- A pinch of nutmeg
- ¼ cup parmesan, grated
- 1 pound sausage, chopped

Directions:
1. Heat up a pan with the oil over medium heat, add onions and garlic, stir and cook for 3 minutes.
2. Add Swiss chard, stir and cook for 5 minutes more.
3. Add salt, pepper and nutmeg, stir, take off heat and leave aside for a few minutes.
4. In a bowl, whisk eggs with mozzarella, parmesan and ricotta and stir well.
5. Add Swiss chard mix and stir well.
6. Spread sausage meat on the bottom of a pie pan and press well.
7. Add Swiss chard and eggs mix, spread well, introduce in the oven at 350 degrees F and bake for 35 minutes.
8. Leave pie aside to cool down, slice and serve it.
9. Enjoy!

Nutrition Value: calories 332, fat 23, fiber 3, carbs 4, protein 23

288. Swiss Chard Salad
Preparation time: 10 minutes
Cooking time: 20 minutes
Servings: 4

Ingredients:
- 1 bunch Swiss chard, cut in strips
- 2 tablespoons avocado oil
- 1 small yellow onion, chopped
- A pinch of red pepper flakes
- ¼ cup pine nuts, toasted
- ¼ cup raisins
- 1 tablespoon balsamic vinegar
- Salt and black pepper to the taste

Directions:
1. Heat up a pan with the oil over medium heat, add chard and onions, stir and cook for 5 minutes.
2. Add salt, pepper and pepper flakes, stir and cook for 3 minutes more.
3. Put raisins in a bowl, add water to cover them, heat them up in your microwave for 1 minute, leave aside for 5 minutes and drain them well.
4. Add raisins and pine nuts to the pan, also add vinegar, stir, cook for 3 minutes more, divide on plates and serve.
5. Enjoy!

Nutrition Value: calories 120, fat 2, fiber 1, carbs 4, protein 8

289. Green Salad
Preparation time: 10 minutes
Cooking time: 0 minutes
Servings: 4

Ingredients:
- 4 handfuls grapes, halved
- 1 bunch Swiss chard, chopped
- 1 avocado, pitted, peeled and cubed
- Salt and black pepper to the taste
- 2 tablespoons avocado oil

- 1 tablespoon mustard
- 7 sage leaves, chopped
- 1 garlic clove, minced

Directions:
1. In a salad bowl, mix Swiss chard with grapes and avocado cubes.
2. In a bowl, mix mustard with oil, sage, garlic, salt and pepper and whisk well.
3. Add this over salad, toss to coat well and serve.
4. Enjoy!

Nutrition Value: calories 120, fat 2, fiber 1, carbs 4, protein 5

290. Catalan Style Greens

Preparation time: 10 minutes
Cooking time: 15 minutes
Servings: 4

Ingredients:
- 1 apple, cored and chopped
- 1 yellow onion, sliced
- 3 tablespoons avocado oil
- ¼ cup raisins
- 6 garlic cloves, chopped
- ¼ cup pine nuts, toasted
- ¼ cup balsamic vinegar
- 5 cups mixed spinach and chard
- Salt and black pepper to the taste
- A pinch of nutmeg

Directions:
1. Heat up a pan with the oil over medium high heat, add onion, stir and cook for 3 minutes.
2. Add apple, stir and cook for 4 minutes more.
3. Add garlic, stir and cook for 1 minute.
4. Add raisins, vinegar and mixed spinach and chard, stir and cook for 5 minutes.
5. Add nutmeg, salt and pepper, stir, cook for a few seconds more, divide on plates and serve.
6. Enjoy!

Nutrition Value: calories 120, fat 1, fiber 2, carbs 3, protein 6

291. Swiss Chard Soup

Preparation time: 10 minutes
Cooking time: 35 minutes
Servings: 12

Ingredients:
- 4 cups Swiss chard, chopped
- 4 cups chicken breast, cooked and shredded
- 2 cups water
- 1 cup mushrooms, sliced
- 1 tablespoon garlic, minced
- 1 tablespoon coconut oil, melted
- ¼ cup onion, chopped
- 8 cups chicken stock
- 2 cups yellow squash, chopped
- 1 cup green beans, cut in medium pieces
- 2 tablespoons vinegar
- ¼ cup basil, chopped
- Salt and black pepper to the taste
- 4 bacon slices, chopped
- ¼ cup sundried tomatoes, chopped

Directions:
1. Heat up a pot with the oil over medium high heat, add bacon, stir and cook for 2 minutes.
2. Add tomatoes, garlic, onions and mushrooms, stir and cook for 5 minutes.
3. Add water, stock and chicken, stir and cook for 15 minutes.
4. Add Swiss chard, green beans, squash, salt and pepper, stir and cook for 10 minutes more.
5. Add vinegar, basil, more salt and pepper if needed, stir, ladle into soup bowls and serve.
6. Enjoy!

Nutrition Value: calories 140, fat 4, fiber 2, carbs 4, protein 18

292. Special Swiss Chard Soup

Preparation time: 10 minutes
Cooking time: 2 hours and 10 minutes
Servings: 4

Ingredients:
- 1 red onion, chopped
- 1 bunch Swiss chard, chopped
- 1 yellow squash, chopped
- 1 zucchini, chopped
- 1 green bell pepper, chopped
- Salt and black pepper to the taste
- 6 carrots, chopped
- 4 cups tomatoes, chopped
- 1 cup cauliflower florets, chopped
- 1 cup green beans, chopped
- 6 cups chicken stock
- 7 ounces canned tomato paste
- 2 cups water
- 1 pound sausage, chopped
- 2 garlic cloves, minced
- 2 teaspoons thyme, chopped
- 1 teaspoon rosemary, dried
- 1 tablespoon fennel, minced
- ½ teaspoon red pepper flakes

- Some grated parmesan for serving

Directions:
1. Heat up a pan over medium high heat, add sausage and garlic, stir and cook until it browns and transfer along with its juices to your slow cooker.
2. Add onion, Swiss chard, squash, bell pepper, zucchini, carrots, tomatoes, cauliflower, green beans, tomato paste, stock, water, thyme, fennel, rosemary, pepper flakes, salt and pepper, stir, cover and cook on High for 2 hours.
3. Uncover pot, stir soup, ladle into bowls, sprinkle parmesan on top and serve.
4. Enjoy!

Nutrition Value: calories 150, fat 8, fiber 2, carbs 4, protein 9

293. Roasted Tomato Cream

Preparation time: 10 minutes
Cooking time: 1 hour
Servings: 8

Ingredients:
- 1 jalapeno pepper, chopped
- 4 garlic cloves, minced
- 2 pounds cherry tomatoes, cut in halves
- 1 yellow onion, cut in wedges
- Salt and black pepper to the taste
- ¼ cup olive oil
- ½ teaspoon oregano, dried
- 4 cups chicken stock
- ¼ cup basil, chopped
- ½ cup parmesan, grated

Directions:
1. Spread tomatoes and onion in a baking dish.
2. Add garlic and chili pepper, season with salt, pepper and oregano and drizzle the oil.
3. Toss to coat and bake in the oven at 425 degrees F for 30 minutes.
4. Take tomatoes mix out of the oven, transfer to a pot, add stock and heat everything up over medium high heat.
5. Bring to a boil, cover pot, reduce heat and simmer for 20 minutes.
6. Blend using an immersion blender, add salt and pepper to the taste and basil, stir and ladle into soup bowls.
7. Sprinkle parmesan on top and serve.
8. Enjoy!

Nutrition Value: calories 140, fat 2, fiber 2, carbs 5, protein 8

294. Eggplant Soup

Preparation time: 10 minutes
Cooking time: 50 minutes
Servings: 4

Ingredients:
- 4 tomatoes
- 1 teaspoon garlic, minced
- ¼ yellow onion, chopped
- Salt and black pepper to the taste
- 2 cups chicken stock
- 1 bay leaf
- ½ cup heavy cream
- 2 tablespoons basil, chopped
- 4 tablespoons parmesan, grated
- 1 tablespoon olive oil
- 1 eggplant, chopped

Directions:
1. Spread eggplant pieces on a baking sheet, mix with oil, onion, garlic, salt and pepper, introduce in the oven at 400 degrees F and bake for 15 minutes.
2. Put water in a pot, bring to a boil over medium heat, add tomatoes, steam them for 1 minutes, peel them and chop.
3. Take eggplant mix out of the oven and transfer to a pot.
4. Add tomatoes, stock, bay leaf, salt and pepper, stir, bring to a boil and simmer fro 30 minutes.
5. Add heavy cream, basil and parmesan, stir, ladle into soup bowls and serve.
6. Enjoy!

Nutrition Value: calories 180, fat 2, fiber 3, carbs 5, protein 10

295. Eggplant Stew

Preparation time: 10 minutes
Cooking time: 30 minutes
Servings: 4

Ingredients:
- 1 red onion, chopped
- 2 garlic cloves, chopped
- 1 bunch parsley, chopped
- Salt and black pepper to the taste
- 1 teaspoon oregano, dried
- 2 eggplants, cut in medium chunks
- 2 tablespoons olive oil
- 2 tablespoons capers, chopped
- 1 handful green olives, pitted and sliced
- 5 tomatoes, chopped

- 3 tablespoons herb vinegar

Directions:
1. Heat up a pot with the oil over medium heat, add eggplant, oregano, salt and pepper, stir and cook for 5 minutes.
2. Add garlic, onion and parsley, stir and cook for 4 minutes.
3. Add capers, olives, vinegar and tomatoes, stir and cook for 15 minutes.
4. Add more salt and pepper if needed, stir, divide into bowls and serve.
5. Enjoy!

Nutrition Value: calories 200, fat 13, fiber 3, carbs 5, protein 7

296. Roasted Bell Peppers Soup

Preparation time: 10 minutes
Cooking time: 15 minutes
Servings: 6

Ingredients:
- 12 ounces roasted bell peppers, chopped
- 2 tablespoons olive oil
- 2 garlic cloves, minced
- 29 ounces canned chicken stock
- Salt and black pepper to the taste
- 7 ounces water
- 2/3 cup heavy cream
- 1 yellow onion, chopped
- ¼ cup parmesan, grated
- 2 celery stalks, chopped

Directions:
1. Heat up a pot with the oil over medium heat, add onion, garlic, celery, some salt and pepper, stir and cook for 8 minutes.
2. Add bell peppers, water and stock, stir, bring to a boil, cover, reduce heat and simmer for 5 minutes.
3. Use an immersion blender to puree the soup, then add more salt, pepper and cream, stir, bring to a boil and take off heat.
4. Ladle into bowls, sprinkle parmesan and serve.
5. Enjoy!

Nutrition Value: calories 176, fat 13, fiber 1, carbs 4, protein 6

297. Delicious Cabbage Soup

Preparation time: 10 minutes
Cooking time: 45 minutes
Servings: 8

Ingredients:
- 1 garlic clove, minced
- 1 cabbage head, chopped
- 2 pounds beef, ground
- 1 yellow onion, chopped
- 1 teaspoon cumin
- 4 bouillon cubes
- Salt and black pepper to the taste
- 10 ounces canned tomatoes and green chilies
- 4 cups water

Directions:
1. Heat up a pan over medium heat, add beef, stir and brown for a few minutes.
2. Add onion, stir, cook for 4 minutes more and transfer to a pot.
3. Heat up, add cabbage, cumin, garlic, bouillon cubes, tomatoes and chilies and water, stir, bring to a boil over high heat, cover, reduce temperature and cook for 40 minutes.
4. Season with salt and pepper, stir, ladle into soup bowls and serve.
5. Enjoy!

Nutrition Value: calories 200, fat 3, fiber 2, carbs 6, protein 8

SOUP RECIPES

298. Creamy Cauliflower Mushroom Soup

Preparation Time: 40 minutes
Servings: 3

Ingredients:

- 1 1/2 cups mushrooms, diced
- 1/2 onion, chopped
- 1/2 tsp olive oil
- 2 cups cauliflower florets
- 1 tsp onion powder
- 1 2/3 cups almond milk, unsweetened
- 1/4 tsp sea salt

Directions:

1. Add cauliflower, pepper, salt, onion powder, and almond milk in a saucepan and stir well.
2. Cover pan with lid and simmer for 8 minutes.
3. Add cauliflower into the blender and blend until smooth
4. Meanwhile, Add onion and mushroom in the pan and cook for 8 minutes.
5. Add cauliflower mixture into the mushroom and bring to boil.
6. Cover pan with lid and simmer for 10 minutes.
7. Serve hot and enjoy.

Nutrition Value:

Calories 348
Fat 32 g
Carbohydrates 13 g
Sugar 7 g
Protein 5 g
Cholesterol 0 mg

299. Avocado Broccoli Soup

Preparation Time: 25 minutes
Servings: 4

Ingredients:

- 1 small avocado, peel and chopped
- 4 cups broccoli florets
- 2 cups vegetable broth
- 1/2 tsp cinnamon

Directions:

1. Add broth in saucepan and heat over medium-high heat.
2. Add broccoli florets in a saucepan and cook for 8 minutes.
3. Reduce heat and add avocado and nutmeg.
4. Continue cook for 4 minutes.
5. Using blender puree the soup until smooth.
6. Serve warm and enjoy.

Nutrition Value:

Calories 153
Fat 10 g
Carbohydrates 11 g
Sugar 2 g
Protein 6 g
Cholesterol 0 mg

300. Healthy Zucchini Soup

Preparation Time: 25 minutes
Servings: 4

Ingredients:

- 2 lbs zucchini, chopped
- 1/4 cup fresh basil leaves
- 3 cups vegetable stock
- 1 tbsp butter
- 3/4 cup onion, chopped
- 2 garlic cloves, minced
- 1 tsp salt

Directions:

1. Melt butter in a saucepan over medium heat.
2. Add garlic and onion to the pan and sauté for 5 minutes.
3. Add zucchini and salt and cook for 5 minutes.
4. Add vegetable stock and simmer for 15 minutes.
5. Add basil leaves and stir well.
6. Using blender puree the soup until smooth and creamy.
7. Serve hot and enjoy.

Nutrition Value:

Calories 80
Fat 4 g
Carbohydrates 11 g
Sugar 6 g
Protein 3 g
Cholesterol 8 mg

301. Coconut Leek Cauliflower Soup

Preparation Time: 1 hour 10 minutes
Servings: 4

Ingredients:

- 1/2 cauliflower, chopped
- 1 large leek, chopped
- 3 cups vegetable broth

- 1/2 cup coconut cream
- Salt

Directions:
1. Add cauliflower, leek, and broth in a saucepan and simmer for 1 hour over medium-low heat.
2. Using blender puree the soup until smooth and creamy.
3. Add coconut cream and salt and stir well.
4. Serve warm and enjoy.

Nutrition Value:
Calories 129
Fat 8 g
Carbohydrates 9 g
Sugar 4 g
Protein 6 g
Cholesterol 0 mg

302. Chilled Mint Avocado Soup

Preparation Time: 10 minutes
Servings: 3

Ingredients:
- 1 medium avocado
- 4 tbsp fresh mint leaves
- 1 tbsp fresh lime juice
- 1 cup coconut milk
- 2 romaine lettuce leaves
- Salt

Directions:
1. Add all ingredients into the blender and blend until smooth.
2. Place soup in refrigerator for 10 minutes.
3. Serve chilled and enjoy.

Nutrition Value:
Calories 325
Fat 32 g
Carbohydrates 11 g
Sugar 3 g
Protein 3 g
Cholesterol 0 mg

303. Pumpkin Tomato Soup

Preparation Time: 25 minutes
Servings: 4

Ingredients:
- 1/2 cup tomato, chopped
- 2 cups pumpkin
- 2 cups vegetable broth, low-sodium
- 1 tsp olive oil
- 1/2 tsp garlic, minced
- 1 1/2 tsp curry powder
- 1/2 tsp paprika
- 1/2 cup onion, chopped

Directions:
1. In a saucepan, add oil, garlic, and onion and sauté for 3 minutes.
2. Add remaining ingredients into the saucepan and bring to boil.
3. Reduce heat and cover saucepan with lid and simmer for 10 minutes.
4. Using blender puree the soup until smooth.
5. Serve hot and enjoy.

Nutrition Value:
Calories 84
Fat 2 g
Carbohydrates 13 g
Sugar 5 g
Protein 4 g
Cholesterol 0 mg

304. Delicious Tomato Herb Soup

Preparation Time: 30 minutes
Servings: 4

Ingredients:
- 3 cups tomatoes, peeled, seeded and chopped
- 1 tbsp basil, chopped
- 1 cup red bell pepper, chopped
- 1 cup onion, chopped
- 2 tbsp tomato paste
- 4 cups vegetable broth, low-sodium
- 1/2 tsp thyme, chopped
- 1 tsp fresh oregano, chopped
- 1 tbsp garlic, minced
- 1 tbsp olive oil
- 1/4 tsp pepper

Directions:
1. Heat oil in large saucepan over medium heat.
2. Add garlic, onion, bell pepper, and tomatoes and sauté for 10 minutes.
3. Add all remaining ingredients and stir well.
4. Increase heat to high and bring to boil.
5. Reduce heat to low and cover and simmer for 10 minutes.
6. Remove from heat and using blender puree the soup until smooth.
7. Serve warm and enjoy.

Nutrition Value:
Calories 125
Fat 5 g

Carbohydrates 13 g
Sugar 8 g
Protein 7 g
Cholesterol 0 mg

305. Healthy Spinach Kale Soup

Preparation Time: 20 minutes
Servings: 8

Ingredients:

- 1/2 lb fresh spinach
- 1/2 lb kale
- 2 avocados
- 1 fresh lime juice
- 3 oz olive oil
- 1 cup water
- 3 1/3 cup coconut milk
- 1/4 tsp pepper
- 1 tsp salt

Directions:

1. Heat olive oil in a pan over medium heat.
2. Add kale and spinach and sauté until spinach wilted.
3. Add water, spices, avocado, and coconut milk. Stir well.
4. Using blender puree the soup until smooth.
5. Add lime juice and stir well.
6. Serve and enjoy.

Nutrition Value:
Calories 438
Fat 43 g
Carbohydrates 13 g
Sugar 3 g
Protein 5 g
Cholesterol 0 mg

306. Simple Celery Soup

Preparation Time: 40 minutes
Servings: 4

Ingredients:

- 6 cups celery, diced
- 1/2 tsp dill
- 2 cups water
- 1 cup coconut milk
- 1 medium onion, diced
- 1/2 tsp sea salt

Directions:

1. Add all ingredients into the saucepan and bring to boil over medium heat.
2. Reduce heat to medium-low and simmer for 30 minutes.
3. Using blender puree the soup until smooth.
4. Stir well and serve.

Nutrition Value:
Calories 174
Fat 14 g
Carbohydrates 10 g
Sugar 5 g
Protein 2 g
Cholesterol 0 mg

307. Broccoli Cheddar Soup

Preparation Time: 25 minutes
Servings: 3

Ingredients:

- 1 cup broccoli, chopped
- 1/2 cup heavy whipping cream
- 1 1/2 cups vegetable broth
- 1/4 cup celery, chopped
- 1/4 cup onion, chopped
- 1/2 tsp xanthan gum
- 2 tbsp butter
- 5 oz cheddar cheese
- Pepper
- Salt

Directions:

1. Melt butter in a saucepan over medium heat.
2. Add celery, onion, pepper and salt in a pan and cook until softened.
3. Add broccoli in pan and cook for 3 minutes.
4. Add heavy whipping cream and vegetable broth and bring to boil.
5. Slowly add cheddar cheese and stir well.
6. Add xanthan gum and stir until thickened.
7. Serve and enjoy.

Nutrition Value:
Calories 362
Fat 31 g
Carbohydrates 4 g
Sugar 1 g
Protein 15 g
Cholesterol 97 mg

398. Onion Mushroom Clear Soup

Preparation Time: 40 minutes
Servings: 4

Ingredients:

- 2 onions, sliced
- 2 carrots peel and sliced
- 2 garlic cloves, minced
- 1/4 cup button mushrooms, sliced

- 6 cups vegetable broth
- 2 celery stalks, chopped
- 1/4 cup scallions, chopped
- Pepper
- Salt

Directions:
1. Heat little oil in a pan over medium heat.
2. Add onion to the pan and sauté until lightly brown.
3. Add garlic, celery, carrot and broth. Bring to boil.
4. Reduce heat to medium-low and simmer for 30 minutes.
5. Season with pepper and salt.
6. Strain all veggies from broth.
7. Add scallions and mushrooms. Stir well.
8. Serve and enjoy.

Nutrition Value:
Calories 99
Fat 2 g
Carbohydrates 10 g
Sugar 5 g
Protein 8 g
Cholesterol 0 mg

309. Lemon Garlic Asparagus Soup

Preparation Time: 35 minutes
Servings: 4

Ingredients:
- 1 lb asparagus, sliced
- 1/4 tsp lemon zest, grated
- 2 cups coconut milk
- 2 cups vegetable broth
- 2 garlic cloves, crushed
- 3/4 tsp fresh thyme, chopped
- 1/2 tbsp fresh lemon juice
- 1 bay leaf
- 1 tsp salt
- Pepper

Directions:
1. In a saucepan add asparagus, garlic, bay leaf, thyme, coconut milk and vegetable broth.
2. Bring to boil over medium-high heat for 10 minutes.
3. Remove bay leaf and using blender puree the soup until smooth.
4. Remove from heat and strain.
5. Add lemon juice, lemon zest, salt and pepper.
6. Serve and enjoy.

Nutrition Value:
Calories 321
Fat 29 g
Carbohydrates 12 g
Sugar 6 g
Protein 7 g
Cholesterol 0 mg

310. Smooth Spinach Cauliflower Soup

Preparation Time: 45 minutes
Servings: 5

Ingredients:
- 5 watercress, chopped
- 8 cups vegetable broth
- 1/2 cup coconut milk
- 1 lb cauliflower, chopped
- 5 oz fresh spinach, chopped
- Salt

Directions:
1. Add broth and cauliflower in a large saucepan and bring to boil.
2. Cover saucepan with lid and simmer for 15 minutes.
3. Add spinach and watercress and cook for another 10 minutes.
4. Remove from heat and using blender puree the soup until smooth.
5. Add coconut milk and stir well.
6. Season with salt and serve.

Nutrition Value:
Calories 153
Fat 8 g
Carbohydrates 8 g
Sugar 4 g
Protein 12 g
Cholesterol 0 mg

311. EZucchini Asparagus Soup

Preparation Time: 40 minutes
Servings: 4

Ingredients:
- 1 lb zucchini, chopped
- 4 cups Vegetable broth
- 1 lb asparagus, trimmed and chopped
- Salt

Directions:
1. Add zucchini, asparagus, and broth in a saucepan and bring to boil.
2. Cover pan and simmer for 20 minutes.
3. Remove soup from heat.

4. Using blender puree the soup until smooth.
5. Season with salt and serve.

Nutrition Value:

Calories 79
Fat 2 g
Carbohydrates 9 g
Sugar 4 g
Protein 8 g

312. Cholesterol 0 mg

Creamy Shallot Onion Soup
Preparation Time: 45 minutes
Servings: 4

Ingredients:

- 1 onion, sliced
- 1 leek, sliced
- 1 garlic clove, chopped
- 1 shallot, sliced
- 1 1/2 tbsp olive oil
- 4 cups vegetable stock
- Salt

Directions:

1. Add vegetable stock and olive oil in a saucepan and bring to boil.
2. Add remaining ingredients and stir well.
3. Cover pan with lid and simmer for 25 minutes.
4. Using blender puree the soup until smooth.
5. Stir well and serve.

Nutrition Value:

Calories 82
Fat 5 g
Carbohydrates 8 g
Sugar 2 g
Protein 1 g
Cholesterol 0 mg

313. Yummy Carrot Tomato Soup

Preparation Time: 1 hour 20 minutes
Servings: 6

Ingredients:

- 1 carrot, peeled and cut into small pieces
- 1 tbsp ginger, grated
- 1 onion, chopped
- 2 tomatoes, chopped
- 4 tbsp olive oil
- 1 cup coriander, chopped
- 2 garlic clove, minced
- 1 tsp pepper
- 1 tsp cumin
- 5 cups vegetable broth, low sodium
- 2 tsp salt

Directions:

1. Heat olive oil in a saucepan over medium heat.
2. Add onion, ginger, garlic and carrots in pan and sauté for 5 minutes over medium heat.
3. Add tomatoes and chopped coriander sauté for further 5 minutes.
4. Add remaining ingredients and bring to boil.
5. Cover pan with lid and simmer over medium-low heat for 60 minutes.
6. Using blender puree the soup until smooth.
7. Serve hot and enjoy.

Nutrition Value:

Calories 138
Fat 10 g
Carbohydrates 6 g
Sugar 3 g
Protein 5 g
Cholesterol 0 mg

314. Garbanzo Bean Tortilla Soup

Ingredients:

- 1 teaspoon extra-virgin olive oil
- 1/2 cup chopped red onions
- 6 cloves garlic, minced
- 1 cup vegetable broth
- 1 cup vegetable stock
- 1 cup salsa
- 1 14-ounce can garbanzo beans
- 5 pcs. black olives
- 5 pcs. capers
- 1 green bell pepper, chopped
- 1/2 teaspoon salt
- 1 avocado, chopped
- 1/2 cup loosely-packed cilantro

Optional:

1. 1/2 cup crumbled corn tortilla chips
2. Add olive oil to a pan and heat it to medium.
3. Add onions and garlic to saucepan and sauté until softened.
4. Add the stock, salsa, bell peppers, capers, olives beans, and salt.
5. Bring to a boil over high heat.
6. Reduce to low and simmer for 5 minutes.
7. Garnish with half of the avocado, cilantro, and tortilla chips.

315. Black Bean and Annatto Seed Tortilla Soup

Ingredients:

- 1 teaspoon extra-virgin olive oil
- 1/2 cup chopped onions
- 4 cloves garlic, minced
- 1 tsp. annatto seeds
- 1 orange, peeled
- 1 cup vegetable broth
- 1 cup vegetable stock
- 1 cup salsa
- 1 14-ounce can black beans
- 1 green bell pepper, chopped
- 1/2 teaspoon salt
- 1 avocado, chopped
- 1/2 cup loosely-packed cilantro

Optional:

1. 1/2 cup crumbled corn tortilla chips
2. Add olive oil to a pan and heat it to medium.
3. Add onions and garlic to saucepan and sauté until softened.
4. Add the stock, salsa, bell peppers, beans, orange, annatto seeds and salt.
5. Bring to a boil over high heat.
6. Reduce to low and simmer for 5 minutes.
7. Garnish with half of the avocado, cilantro, and tortilla chips.
8. Remove the orange

316. Navy Bean Taco Soup

Ingredients:

- 1 teaspoon extra-virgin olive oil
- 1/2 cup chopped red onions
- 8 cloves garlic, minced
- 1 lime, peeled
- 1 cup vegetable broth
- 1 cup vegetable stock
- 1 cup salsa
- 1 14-ounce can navy beans
- 1 green bell pepper, chopped
- 1/2 teaspoon salt
- 1 avocado, chopped
- 1/2 cup loosely-packed cilantro

Optional:

1. 1/2 cup crumbled corn tortilla chips
2. Add olive oil to a pan and heat it to medium.
3. Add red onions and garlic to saucepan and sauté until softened.
4. Add the stock, salsa, bell peppers, beans, lime, and salt.
5. Bring to a boil over high heat.
6. Reduce to low and simmer for 5 minutes.
7. Garnish with half of the avocado, cilantro, and tortilla chips.
8. Remove the lime

317. Habanero Garbanzo Taco Soup

Ingredients:

- 1 teaspoon extra-virgin olive oil
- 1/2 cup chopped onions
- 4 cloves garlic, minced
- 1 cup vegetable broth
- 1 cup vegetable stock
- 1 cup salsa
- 1 14-ounce can garbanzo beans
- 1/4 habanero chili, chopped
- 1/2 teaspoon salt
- 1 tsp. annatto seed powder
- 1 avocado, chopped
- 1/2 cup loosely-packed cilantro

Optional:

1. 1/2 cup crumbled corn tortilla chips
2. Add olive oil to a pan and heat it to medium.
3. Add onions and garlic to saucepan and sauté until softened.
4. Add the stock, salsa, habanero pepper, beans, annatto seed powder and salt.
5. Bring to a boil over high heat.
6. Reduce to low and simmer for 5 minutes.
7. Garnish with half of the avocado, cilantro, and tortilla chips.

318. Jalapeno Taco Soup

Ingredients:

- 1 teaspoon olive oil
- 1/2 cup chopped red onions
- 10 cloves garlic, minced
- 1 cup vegetable broth
- 1 cup vegetable stock
- 1 cup salsa
- 1 14-ounce can white kidney beans
- 1 green bell pepper, chopped
- 1 Anaheim pepper, coarsely chopped
- 2 jalapeno peppers, coarsely chipped
- 1/2 teaspoon salt
- 1 avocado, chopped
- 1/2 cup loosely-packed cilantro

Optional:

1. 1/2 cup crumbled corn tortilla chips
2. Add olive oil to a pan and heat it to medium.

3. Add red onions and garlic to saucepan and sauté until softened.
4. Add the stock, salsa, bell peppers, Anaheim peppers, jalapeno, beans, and salt.
5. Bring to a boil over high heat.
6. Reduce to low and simmer for 5 minutes.
7. Garnish with half of the avocado, cilantro, and tortilla chips.

319. Black Bean Pepper Soup

Ingredients:

- 1 teaspoon extra-virgin olive oil
- 1/2 cup chopped onions
- 4 cloves garlic, minced
- 1 ½ cup vegetable broth
- ½ cup vegetable stock
- 1 cup salsa
- 1 14-ounce can black beans
- 1 red bell pepper, chopped
- 1 green red bell pepper
- ½ tsp. all spice
- ¼ tsp. oregano
- 1/2 teaspoon salt
- 1 avocado, chopped
- 1/2 cup loosely-packed cilantro

Optional:

1. 1/2 cup crumbled corn tortilla chips
2. Add olive oil to a pan and heat it to medium.
3. Add onions and garlic to saucepan and sauté until softened.
4. Add the stock, salsa, red and green bell peppers, beans, all spice, oregano, and salt.
5. Bring to a boil over high heat.
6. Reduce to low and simmer for 5 minutes.
7. Garnish with half of the avocado, cilantro, and tortilla chips.

320. Garbanzo and Jalapeno Pepper Soup

Ingredients:

- 1 teaspoon olive oil
- 1/2 cup chopped red onions
- 4 cloves garlic, minced
- 1 cup vegetable broth
- 1 cup vegetable stock
- 1 cup salsa
- 1 14-ounce can garbanzo beans
- 1 green bell pepper, chopped
- 1 jalapeno pepper, coarsely chopped
- 1/2 teaspoon sea salt
- 1 avocado, chopped
- 1/2 cup loosely-packed cilantro

Optional:

1. 1/2 cup crumbled corn tortilla chips
2. Add olive oil to a pan and heat it to medium.
3. Add red onions and garlic to saucepan and sauté until softened.
4. Add the stock, salsa, bell peppers, jalapeno, beans, and sea salt.
5. Bring to a boil over high heat.
6. Reduce to low and simmer for 5 minutes.
7. Garnish with half of the avocado, cilantro, and tortilla chips.

321. Carrot and Chili Soup

Ingredients

- 1 tablespoon extra virgin olive oil
- 2 teaspoon crushed garlic
- 1 tablespoon chopped fresh cilantro
- 1 teaspoon chili paste
- 1 red onion, chopped
- 3 large carrots, peeled and sliced
- Sea salt to taste
- 1 large potato, peeled and chopped
- 5 cups vegetable broth

Directions

1. Heat oil over medium heat.
2. Cook the garlic, cilantro and chili paste.
3. Stir fry the onion until tender.
4. Add the carrots and potato.
5. Cook for 5 minutes and add the vegetable broth.
6. Simmer until potatoes and carrots are soft.
7. Blend until smooth.

322. Oriental Carrot Soup

Ingredients

- 1 tablespoon sesame seed oil
- 2 teaspoon crushed garlic
- 1 tablespoon chopped fresh cilantro
- 1 teaspoon chili garlic sauce
- 3 red onions, chopped
- 3 large carrots, peeled and sliced
- Sea salt to taste
- 5 cups vegetable broth

Directions

1. Heat oil over medium heat.
2. Cook the garlic, cilantro and chili garlic sauce.
3. Stir fry the onion until tender.
4. Add the carrots and potato.

5. Cook for 5 minutes and add the vegetable broth.
   6. Simmer until potatoes and carrots are soft.
   7. Blend until smooth.

323. Vietnamese Carrot Soup

Ingredients
- 1 tablespoon canola oil
- 2 teaspoon crushed garlic
- 1 tablespoon chopped fresh cilantro
- 1 teaspoon Sriracha sauce
- 1 tbsp. rice wine vinegar
- 1 red onion, chopped
- 3 large carrots, peeled and sliced
- Sea salt to taste
- ½ cup shitake mushrooms, stemmed and coarsely chopped
- 5 cups vegetable broth

Directions
1. Heat oil over medium heat.
2. Cook the garlic, cilantro, rice wine vinegar, mushrooms and Sriracha hot sauce.
3. Stir fry the onion until tender.
4. Add the carrots and potato.
5. Cook for 5 minutes and add the vegetable broth.
6. Simmer until potatoes and carrots are soft.
7. Blend until smooth.

324. Italian Carrot Soup

Ingredients
- 1 tablespoon extra virgin olive oil
- 2 teaspoon crushed garlic
- ½ tsp. dried basil
- 1 teaspoon Italian seasoning
- 1 red onion, chopped
- 3 large carrots, peeled and sliced
- Sea salt to taste
- 1 large potato, peeled and chopped
- 5 cups vegetable broth

Directions
- Heat oil over medium heat.
- Cook the garlic, dried basil and Italian seasoning.
- Stir fry the onion until tender.
- Add the carrots and potato.
- Cook for 5 minutes and add the vegetable broth.
- Simmer until potatoes and carrots are soft.
- Blend until smooth.

325. Potato and Parsnip Soup

Ingredients
- 1 tablespoon non-dairy butter
- 2 teaspoon crushed garlic
- 1 teaspoon dried thyme
- 1 red onion, chopped
- 1 large carrot, peeled and sliced
- 1 large parsnip, peeled and sliced
- Sea salt to taste
- 1 large potato, peeled and chopped
- 5 cups vegetable broth
- Vegan cheese slices, for topping

Directions
1. Heat and melt non-dairy butter over medium heat.
2. Cook the garlic, and thyme.
3. Stir fry the onion until tender.
4. Add the carrot, parsnip and potato.
5. Cook for 5 minutes and add the vegetable broth.
6. Simmer until potatoes and carrots are soft.
7. Blend until smooth.
8. Top with vegan cheese slices

526. Jalapeno Carrot Soup

Ingredients
- 1 tablespoon extra virgin olive oil
- 2 teaspoon crushed garlic
- 1 tablespoon chopped fresh cilantro
- 1 teaspoon chili paste
- 1 teaspoon limejuice
- 1 teaspoon jalapeno, coarsely chopped
- 1 red onion, chopped
- 3 large carrots, peeled and sliced
- *Sea salt to taste*
- 1 large potato, peeled and chopped
- 5 cups vegetable broth

Directions
1. Heat oil over medium heat.
2. Cook the garlic, cilantro, lime, cumin, jalapeno and chili paste.
3. Stir fry the onion until tender.
4. Add the carrots and potato.
5. Cook for 5 minutes and add the vegetable broth.
6. Simmer until potatoes and carrots are soft.
7. Blend until smooth.

327. Mexican Potato and Onion Soup

Ingredients
- 1 tablespoon extra virgin olive oil
- 2 teaspoon crushed garlic

- 1 tablespoon chopped fresh cilantro
- 1 teaspoon ground annatto
- ½ tsp. cumin
- 3 red onions, chopped
- 3 large carrots, peeled and sliced
- Sea salt to taste
- 1 large potato, peeled and chopped
- 5 cups vegetable broth

Directions

1. Heat oil over medium heat.
2. Cook the garlic, annatto, cumin, cilantro and chili paste.
3. Stir fry the onion until tender.
4. Add the carrots and potato.
5. Cook for 5 minutes and add the vegetable broth.
6. Simmer until potatoes and carrots are soft.
7. Blend until smooth.

328. Japanese Sweet Potato Soup

Ingredients

- 1 tablespoon non-dairy butter oil
- 4 teaspoon crushed garlic
- 1 red onion, chopped
- 5 tsp. miso paste
- 3 large carrots, peeled and sliced
- Sea salt to taste
- 1 large sweet potato, peeled and chopped
- 3 cups vegetable broth
- 2 cups almond milk

Directions

1. Heat non-dairy butter over medium heat.
2. Cook the garlic, cilantro and chili paste.
3. Stir fry the onion until tender.
4. Add the carrots and potato.
5. Cook for 5 minutes and add the almond milk, miso paste and vegetable broth.
6. Simmer until potatoes and carrots are soft.
7. Blend until smooth.

329. Creamy Poblano Pepper Soup

Ingredients

- 4 tablespoons non-dairy butter
- 1 small red onion, coarsely chopped
- 1 large leek, white part only, sliced
- 1 green bell pepper, coarsely chopped
- 1 (or two if you like things spicy) small dry-roasted poblano chili, sliced
- 4 cloves garlic, diced
- 1 large red potato, cubed (you can use two if you like your soup thick)
- 4 cups vegetable broth
- 1 cup cashews
- 1-1/4 cup almond milk
- Sea Salt
- Black pepper, to taste

Optional garnish:

1. Sliced jalapeno pepper
2. Soak the cashews in almond milk for half an hour.
3. Melt non-dairy butter in a pan.
4. Cook the onion, leek, chilies, red bell pepper, garlic, and potato over low heat until the onion is translucent.
5. Add the broth into the pan.
6. Simmer until the potatoes are fork tender, about 25 min.
7. Remove from the heat.
8. Pour into a blender and blend until smooth.
9. Clean the blender.
10. Blend cashews with the milk until smooth
11. Stir this into the soup.
12. Heat on medium for a few minutes.
13. Garnish with slices of jalapeno chili.

330. Middle Eastern Inspired Creamy Potato Soup

Ingredients

- 4 tablespoons extra virgin olive oil
- 1 small red onion, coarsely chopped
- 1 large leek, white part only, sliced
- 1 green bell pepper, coarsely chopped
- 1 (or two if you like things spicy) small dry-roasted poblano chili, sliced
- 8 cloves garlic, diced
- ½ tsp. turmeric
- ¾ tsp. cumin
- 1 tbsp. dried parsley
- 1 tbsp lemon juice
- 1 large red potato, cubed (you can use two if you like your soup thick)
- 4 cups vegetable broth
- 1 cup cashews
- 1-1/4 cup almond milk
- Sea Salt
- Black pepper, to taste

Optional garnish:

1. Sliced jalapeno pepper
2. Soak the cashews in almond milk for half an hour.

3. Heat the olive oil in a pan.
4. Cook the onion, leek, chilies, green bell pepper, garlic, and potato over low heat until the onion is translucent.
5. Add the broth, turmeric, cumin, parsley and lemon juice into the pan.
6. Simmer until the potatoes are fork tender, about 25 min.
7. Remove from the heat.
8. Pour into a blender and blend until smooth.
9. Clean the blender.
10. Blend cashews with the milk until smooth
11. Stir this into the soup.
12. Heat on medium for a few minutes.
13. Garnish with slices of jalapeno chili.

331. Lebanese Inspired Potato Soup

Ingredients

- 4 tablespoons non-dairy butter
- 1 small red onion, coarsely chopped
- 1 large leek, white part only, sliced
- 1 green bell pepper, coarsely chopped
- 1 (or two if you like things spicy) small dry-roasted poblano chili, sliced
- 4 cloves garlic, diced
- 1 large red potato, cubed (you can use two if you like your soup thick)
- 4 cups vegetable broth
- 2 tsp. cumin
- 2 tsp. cinnamon
- Juice of 1 lemon
- 1 cup cashews
- 1-1/4 cup almond milk
- Sea Salt
- Black pepper, to taste

Optional garnish:

1. Sliced jalapeno pepper
2. Soak the cashews in almond milk for half an hour.
3. Melt non-dairy butter in a pan.
4. Cook the onion, leek, chilies, red bell pepper, garlic, and potato over low heat until the onion is translucent.
5. Add the broth, cumin, cinnamon and lemon juice into the pan.
6. Simmer until the potatoes are fork tender, about 25 min.
7. Remove from the heat.
8. Pour into a blender and blend until smooth.
9. Clean the blender.
10. Blend cashews with the milk until smooth

11. Stir this into the soup.
12. Heat on medium for a few minutes.
13. Garnish with slices of jalapeno chili.

332. Habanero and Ancho Chili Potato Soup

Ingredients

- 4 tablespoons non-dairy butter
- 1 small yellow onion, coarsely chopped
- 1 large leek, white part only, sliced
- 1 ancho chili, coarsely chopped
- 1 (or two if you like things spicy) small dry-roasted poblano chili, sliced
- 9 cloves garlic, diced
- 1 large red potato, cubed (you can use two if you like your soup thick)
- 4 cups vegetable broth
- 1 cup kidney beans
- 1-1/4 cup almond milk
- ½ tsp. cumin
- 1 habanero pepper, coarsely chopped
- Sea Salt
- Black pepper, to taste

Optional garnish:

1. Sliced jalapeno pepper
2. Soak the cashews in almond milk for half an hour.
3. Melt non-dairy butter in a pan.
4. Cook the onion, leek, chilies, garlic, and potato over low heat until the onion is translucent.
5. Add the broth, cumin and habanero pepper into the pan.
6. Simmer until the potatoes are fork tender, about 25 min.
7. Remove from the heat.
8. Pour into a blender and blend until smooth.
9. Clean the blender.
10. Blend cashews with the milk until smooth
11. Stir this into the soup.
12. Heat on medium for a few minutes.
13. Garnish with slices of jalapeno chili.

333. Thai and Mexican Fusion Potato Soup

Ingredients

- 4 tablespoons non-dairy butter
- 1 small red onion, coarsely chopped
- 1 large leek, white part only, sliced
- 1 green red pepper, coarsely chopped
- 1 (or two if you like things spicy) small dry-

roasted poblano chili, sliced
- 9 cloves garlic, diced
- 1 large red potato, cubed (you can use two if you like your soup thick)
- 4 cups vegetable broth
- 3 pcs. Thai basil, coarsely chopped
- 2 tsp. Sriracha hot sauce
- 5 Thai bird chilies
- 1 tsp. curry powder
- 1 cup almonds
- 1-1/4 cup coconut milk
- Sea Salt
- Black pepper, to taste

Optional garnish:
1. Sliced Thai bird chilies
2. Soak the cashews in almond milk for half an hour.
3. Melt non-dairy butter in a pan.
4. Cook the onion, leek, chilies, red bell pepper, garlic, and potato over low heat until the onion is translucent.
5. Add the broth, basil , Sriracha hot sauce, curry powder & Thai bird chilies into the pan.
6. Simmer until the potatoes are fork tender, about 25 min.
7. Remove from the heat.
8. Pour into a blender and blend until smooth.
9. Clean the blender.
10. Blend cashews with the milk until smooth
11. Stir this into the soup.
12. Heat on medium for a few minutes.
13. Garnish with slices of Thai bird chilies.

334. Spanish Potato and Poblano Pepper Soup

Ingredients:
- 4 tablespoons non-dairy butter
- 1 small red onion, coarsely chopped
- 1 large leek, white part only, sliced
- 1 red bell pepper, coarsely chopped
- 1 (or two if you like things spicy) small dry-roasted poblano chili, sliced
- 4 cloves garlic, diced
- 1 large red potato, cubed (you can use two if you like your soup thick)
- 4 cups vegetable broth
- 2 tsp. cumin
- 1 tsp. oregano
- 1 tsp. Spanish paprika
- 1 dash of cayenne pepper
- 1 cup cashews
- 1-1/4 cup almond milk
- Sea Salt
- Black pepper, to taste

Optional garnish:
1. Sliced jalapeno pepper
2. Soak the cashews in almond milk for half an hour.
3. Melt non-dairy butter in a pan.
4. Cook the onion, leek, chilies, red bell pepper, garlic, and potato over low heat until the onion is translucent.
5. Add the broth , cumin, oregano, paprika and cayenne pepper into the pan.
6. Simmer until the potatoes are fork tender, about 25 min.
7. Remove from the heat.
8. Pour into a blender and blend until smooth.
9. Clean the blender.
10. Blend cashews with the milk until smooth
11. Stir this into the soup.
12. Heat on medium for a few minutes.
13. Garnish with slices of jalapeno chili.

335. Creamy Nutty Potato Soup

Ingredients:
- 4 tablespoons non-dairy butter
- 1 small red onion, coarsely chopped
- 1 large leek, white part only, sliced
- 1 green bell pepper, coarsely chopped
- 1 (or two if you like things spicy) small dry-roasted poblano chili, sliced
- 4 cloves garlic, diced
- 1 large red potato, cubed (you can use two if you like your soup thick)
- 4 cups vegetable broth
- 1 cup cashews
- 1-1/4 cup almond milk
- Sea Salt
- Black pepper, to taste

Optional garnish:
1. Sliced jalapeno pepper
2. Soak the cashews in almond milk for half an hour.
3. Melt non-dairy butter in a pan.
4. Cook the onion, leek, chilies, red bell pepper, garlic, and potato over low heat until the onion is translucent.
5. Add the broth into the pan.
6. Simmer until the potatoes are fork tender, about

25 min.
7. Remove from the heat.
8. Pour into a blender and blend until smooth.
9. Clean the blender.
10. Blend cashews with the milk until smooth
11. Stir this into the soup.
12. Heat on medium for a few minutes.
13. Garnish with slices of jalapeno chili.

336. Squash, Lentil and Fenugreek Soup

Ingredients

- 1 tablespoon extra virgin olive oil
- 1 small red onion, chopped
- 1 tablespoon minced fresh ginger root
- 3 cloves garlic, chopped
- 1 pinch fenugreek seeds
- 1 cup dry red lentils
- 1 cup butternut squash - peeled, seeded, and cubed
- 1/3 cup finely chopped fresh cilantro
- 2 cups water
- 2 tablespoons maple syrup
- 1/8 teaspoon ground cinnamon
- 1 pinch ground nutmeg
- salt and pepper to taste

Directions

1. Heat the pot over medium heat
2. Sauté the onion, ginger, garlic, and fenugreek until onion is tender.
3. Add the lentils, squash, and cilantro into the pot.
4. Add the water, coconut milk, and tomato paste.
5. Add the curry powder, cayenne pepper, nutmeg, salt, and pepper.
6. Boil, reduce the heat to low, and simmer until lentils and squash are tender for 25 min.

337. Sichuan Lentil and Squash Soup

Ingredients

- 1 tablespoon sesame seed oil
- 1 small red onion, chopped
- 1 tablespoon minced fresh ginger root
- 4 cloves garlic, chopped
- 1 pinch Sichuan peppercorns
- 1 cup dry red lentils
- 1 cup butternut squash - peeled, seeded, and cubed
- 1/3 cup finely chopped fresh cilantro
- 2 cups water
- 1/2 (14 ounce) can almond milk
- 1 teaspoon red curry powder
- ¼ tsp. cayenne pepper
- 1 pinch ground nutmeg
- salt and pepper to taste

Directions

1. Heat the pot over medium heat
2. Sauté the onion, ginger, garlic, until onion is tender.
3. Add the lentils, squash, and cilantro into the pot.
4. Add the water, almond milk, and tomato paste.
5. Add the curry powder, cayenne pepper, nutmeg, salt, and pepper.
6. Boil, reduce the heat to low, and simmer until lentils and squash are tender for 25 min.

338. Squash Curry Soup

Ingredients

- 1 tablespoon extra virgin olive oil
- 1 small red onion, chopped
- 1 tablespoon minced fresh ginger root
- 4 cloves garlic, chopped
- 1 cup dry red lentils
- 1 cup butternut squash - peeled, seeded, and cubed
- 1/3 cup finely chopped fresh coriander
- 2 cups water
- 1/2 (14 ounce) can coconut milk
- ½ teaspoon ground cumin
- 1 teaspoon red curry powder
- 1/2 tsp. garam masala
- 1 pinch ground turmeric
- salt and pepper to taste

Directions

1. Heat the pot over medium heat
2. Sauté the onion, ginger, and garlic until onion is tender.
3. Add the lentils, squash, and coriander into the pot.
4. Add the water & coconut milk
5. Add the curry powder, cumin, garam masala, turmeric, salt, and pepper.
6. Boil, reduce the heat to low, and simmer until lentils and squash are tender for 25 min.

339. Squash and Ginger Soup

Ingredients

- 1 tablespoon extra virgin olive oil
- 1 small red onion, chopped

- 1 tablespoon minced fresh ginger root
- 3 cloves garlic, chopped
- 1 pinch fenugreek seeds
- 1 cup dry red lentils
- 1 cup butternut squash - peeled, seeded, and cubed
- 1/3 cup finely chopped fresh cilantro
- 2 cups water
- 1/2 (14 ounce) can coconut milk
- 2 tablespoons tomato paste
- 1 teaspoon red curry powder
- ¼ tsp. cayenne pepper
- 1 pinch ground nutmeg
- salt and pepper to taste

Directions

1. Heat the pot over medium heat
2. Sauté the onion, ginger, garlic, and fenugreek until onion is tender.
3. Add the lentils, squash, and cilantro into the pot.
4. Add the water, coconut milk, and tomato paste.
5. Add the curry powder, cayenne pepper, nutmeg, salt, and pepper.
6. Boil, reduce the heat to low, and simmer until lentils and squash are tender for 25 min.

340. Squash and Kidney Bean Soup

Ingredients

- 3 tablespoons extra virgin olive oil
- 1 small red onion, chopped
- 1 tablespoon minced fresh ginger root
- 4 cloves garlic, chopped
- 1 pinch fenugreek seeds
- 1 cup dry kidney beans
- 1 cup butternut squash - peeled, seeded, and cubed
- 1/3 cup finely chopped fresh cilantro
- 2 ½ cups vegetable broth
- 2 tablespoons tomato paste
- 1 teaspoon Italian seasoning
- ¼ tsp. cayenne pepper
- 1 pinch thyme
- salt and pepper to taste

Directions

1. Heat the pot over medium heat
2. Sauté the red onion, ginger, garlic, and fenugreek until onion is tender.
3. Add the beans, squash, and cilantro into the pot.
4. Add the broth and tomato paste.

5. Add the Italian seasoning, cayenne pepper, thyme, salt, and pepper.
6. Boil, reduce the heat to low, and simmer until lentils and squash are tender for 25 min.

341. Simple Squash and Lentil Soup

Ingredients

- 1 tablespoon vegan margarine
- 1 small red onion, chopped
- 4 cloves garlic, chopped
- 1 cup dry red lentils
- 1 cup butternut squash - peeled, seeded, and cubed
- 2 cups vegetable broth
- 1/2 (14 ounce) can almond milk
- 1 teaspoon thyme
- ¼ tsp. cayenne pepper
- 1 pinch ground nutmeg
- salt and pepper to taste

Directions

1. Heat the pot over medium heat and melt the vegan margarine
2. Sauté the onion, & garlic until onion is tender.
3. Add the lentils & squash into the pot.
4. Add the broth and almond milk.
5. Add the thyme, cayenne pepper, nutmeg, salt, and pepper.
6. Boil, reduce the heat to low, and simmer until lentils and squash are tender for 25 min.

Carrot and Tarragon Soup

Ingredients

- 3 tablespoons extra virgin olive oil
- 1 small red onion, minced
- 1 small carrot, peeled and thinly sliced
- 1 celery rib, thinly sliced
- 1/2 teaspoon dried tarragon
- 2 cups vegetable broth
- 2 tbsp. white wine vinegar

Directions

1. Heat oil over medium-high heat.
2. Sauté onions until tender for about 5 minutes.
3. Add carrots, celery, and tarragon, and cook for another 5 minutes, or until carrots become tender.
4. Add vegetable broth and wine vinegar.
5. Boil and reduce to a simmer, and cook for 15 minutes longer.

343. Creamy Almond Carrot and

Celery Soup

Ingredients

- 3 tablespoons vegan butter/margarine
- 1 small red onion, minced
- 1 small carrot, peeled and thinly sliced
- 1 celery rib, thinly sliced
- 5 cloves garlic, minced
- 1 cup vegetable broth
- 1 cup almond milk
- 2 tbsp. white wine vinegar
- Melt vegan butter over medium-high heat.
- Sauté onions until tender for about 5 minutes.
- Add carrots, celery, and garlic, and cook for another 5 minutes, or until carrots become tender.
- Add vegetable broth, almond milk and wine vinegar.
- Boil and reduce to a simmer, and cook for 15 minutes longer.

344. Thai Carrot and Celery Soup

Ingredients

- 3 tablespoons sesame seed oil
- 1 small red onion, minced
- 1 small carrot, peeled and thinly sliced
- 1 celery rib, thinly sliced
- 1/2 teaspoon Thai bird chilies
- 2 cups vegetable broth
- 2 tbsp. sherry vinegar

Directions

1. Heat sesame oil over medium-high heat.
2. Sauté onions until tender for about 5 minutes.
3. Add carrots, celery, and Thai bird chilies, and cook for another 5 minutes, or until carrots become tender.
4. Add vegetable broth and sherry vinegar.
5. Boil and reduce to a simmer, and cook for 15 minutes longer.

345. Creamy French Carrot Soup

Ingredients

- 3 tablespoons melted vegan butter/margarine
- 1 small yellow onion, minced
- 1 small parsnips, peeled and thinly sliced
- 1 celery rib, thinly sliced
- 1/2 teaspoon herbs de Provence
- 2 cups vegetable broth
- 2 tbsp. white wine vinegar

Directions

1. Heat oil over medium-high heat.
2. Sauté onions until tender for about 5 minutes.
3. Add parsnips, celery, and tarragon, and cook for another 5 minutes, or until carrots become tender.
4. Add vegetable broth and wine vinegar.
5. Boil and reduce to a simmer, and cook for 15 minutes longer.

346. Creamy Lemon Garlic Carrot Soup

Ingredients

- 3 tablespoons melted vegan butter/ margarine
- 1 small red onion, minced
- 1 small carrot, peeled and thinly sliced
- 1 celery rib, thinly sliced
- 8 pcs. kalamata olives
- 2 tsp. lemon juice
- 9 cloves garlic, minced
- 1/2 teaspoon cumin
- 2 cups vegetable broth
- 2 tbsp. white wine vinegar

Directions

1. Heat oil over medium-high heat.
2. Sauté onions and garlic until tender for about 5 minutes.
3. Add carrots, celery, and tarragon, cumin and cook for another 5 minutes, or until carrots become tender.
4. Add vegetable broth, kalamata olives, capers and lemon juice and wine vinegar.
5. Boil and reduce to a simmer, and cook for 15 minutes longer.

347. Italian Carrot Soup

Ingredients

- 3 tablespoons extra virgin olive oil
- 1 small red onion, minced
- 1 small carrot, peeled and thinly sliced
- 1 celery rib, thinly sliced
- 1/2 teaspoon Italian seasoning
- 2 cups vegetable broth
- ¼ cup pesto
- 2 tbsp. white wine vinegar

Directions

1. Heat oil over medium-high heat.
2. Sauté onions until tender for about 5 minutes.
3. Add carrots, celery, and Italian seasoning, and cook for another 5 minutes, or until carrots

become tender.
4. Add vegetable broth and wine vinegar.
5. Boil and reduce to a simmer, add the pesto and cook for 15 minutes longer.

348. Spicy Red Onion Soup

Ingredients

- 3 tablespoons extra virgin olive oil
- 1 large red onion, minced
- 1 small carrot, peeled and thinly sliced
- 1 ancho chili, thinly sliced
- 1/2 teaspoon cumin
- ½ tsp. cayenne pepper
- 1 cup vegetable broth
- 1 cup vegetable stock
- 2 tbsp. white wine vinegar

Directions

1. Heat oil over medium-high heat.
2. Sauté onions until tender for about 5 minutes.
3. Add carrots, ancho chili, cumin and cayenne pepper, and cook for another 5 minutes, or until carrots become tender.
4. Add vegetable broth, vegetable stock and wine vinegar.
5. Boil and reduce to a simmer, and cook for 15 minutes longer.

349. Hungarian Red Onion Soup

Ingredients

- 3 tablespoons vegan butter/margarine
- 1 large red onion, minced
- 1 small carrot, peeled and thinly sliced
- 1 potato, thinly sliced
- 1/2 teaspoon Hungarian paprika
- 1 cup vegetable broth
- 1 cup almond milk
- 2 tbsp. white wine vinegar

Directions

1. Heat melted vegan butter over medium-high heat.
2. Sauté onions until tender for about 5 minutes.
3. Add carrots, potato, and paprika, and cook for another 5 minutes, or until carrots become tender.
4. Add vegetable broth and almond milk.
5. Boil and reduce to a simmer, and cook for 15 minutes longer.

350. Simple French Red Soup

Ingredients

- 3 tablespoons extra virgin olive oil
- 1 small red onion, minced
- 1 small carrot, peeled and thinly sliced
- 1 celery rib, thinly sliced
- 1/2 teaspoon dried tarragon
- 2 cups vegetable broth
- 2 tbsp. white wine vinegar

Directions

1. Heat oil over medium-high heat.
2. Sauté onions until tender for about 5 minutes.
3. Add carrots, celery, and tarragon, and cook for another 5 minutes, or until carrots become tender.
4. Add vegetable broth and wine vinegar.
5. Boil and reduce to a simmer, and cook for 15 minutes longer.

351. Spanish Vegan Chorizo Onion Soup

Ingredients

- 3 tablespoons extra virgin olive oil
- 1 small red onion, minced
- 1 small carrot, peeled and thinly sliced
- 1 vegan chorizo, coarsely chopped (Soyrizo brand)
- 1 tbsp. dried Spanish paprika
- 1 tsp. thyme
- 2 cups vegetable broth
- 2 tbsp. white wine vinegar
- Parsley for garnishing

Directions

1. Heat oil over medium-high heat.
2. Sauté onions until tender for about 5 minutes.
3. Add carrots, vegan chorizo, and tarragon, and cook for another 5 minutes, or until carrots become tender.
4. Add vegetable broth, paprika, thyme and wine vinegar.
5. Boil and reduce to a simmer, and cook for 15 minutes longer.
6. Garnish with parsley

SOUPS

352. Sun-dried Tomato Navy Bean Soup

Ingredients

- 1 pound dry navy beans, sorted and rinsed
- 1 1/2 quarts vegetable stock
- ½ quart water
- 1 medium onion, diced
- 6 cloves of garlic, peeled and smashed
- 2 tsp sea salt
- 1/4 tsp pepper
- 2 medium potatoes, diced
- 1 pound frozen, sliced carrots
- 1 cup chopped sun-dried tomatoes*
- 1-2 tsp dried dill
- 3-4 tbsp fresh, minced parsley

Directions

1. Add the beans, veggie stock and water, onion, garlic, salt and pepper in a pot and cook over low-medium heat.
2. Simmer for 3-4 hours.
3. When the beans become soft, add the potato and simmer until the potatoes become tender.
4. Add the carrots, tomatoes and dill and cook until heated through.
5. Add the parsley.
6. Season with more salt and pepper.

353. Vegan Chorizo and Potato Soup

Ingredients

- 1 pound garbanzo beans, sorted and rinsed
- 1 1/2 quarts vegetable stock
- ½ quart water
- 1 medium onion, diced
- 6 cloves of garlic, peeled and smashed
- 1 vegan chorizo (brand: Soyrizo), coarsely chopped
- 2 tsp sea salt
- 1/4 tsp pepper
- 2 medium potatoes, diced
- 1 pound frozen, sliced carrots
- 1 cup chopped sun-dried tomatoes*
- 1 tsp saffron
- 2 tsp. Spanish Paprika
- 3-4 tbsp fresh, minced parsley

Directions

1. Add the beans, veggie stock and water, onion, garlic, salt and pepper in a pot and cook over low-medium heat.
2. Simmer for 3-4 hours.
3. When the beans become soft, add the potato and simmer until the potatoes become tender.
4. Add the carrots, tomatoes, vegan chorizo, paprika and saffron and cook until heated through.
5. Add the parsley.
6. Season with more salt and pepper.

354. Asian Spinach and Mung Bean Soup

Ingredients

- 3/4 pound mung beans, sorted and rinsed
- 1 1/2 quarts vegetable stock
- ½ quart coconut milk
- ½ quart water
- 1 medium onion, diced
- 6 cloves of garlic, peeled and smashed
- 2 tsp sea salt
- 1/4 tsp pepper
- 1 bunch spinach, diced
- 1 pound frozen, sliced carrots
- 1-2 tsp minced ginger
- 3-4 tbsp fresh, minced parsley

Directions

1. Add the beans, vegetable stock, coconut milk and water, onion, garlic, salt and pepper in a pot and cook over low-medium heat.
2. Simmer for 3-4 hours.
3. When the beans become soft, add the spinach and simmer until the potatoes become tender.
4. Add the carrots, tomatoes and ginger and cook until heated through.
5. Add the parsley.
6. Season with more salt and pepper.

355. Potato and White Bean Soup

Ingredients

- 1 pound dry white dried beans, sorted and rinsed
- 1 1/2 quarts vegetable broth
- ½ quart water
- 1 medium onion, diced

- 6 cloves of garlic, peeled and smashed
- 2 tsp sea salt
- 1/4 tsp pepper
- 2 medium potatoes, diced
- 1 pound frozen, sliced carrots
- 1-2 tsp balsamic vinegar
- 3-4 tbsp fresh, minced parsley

Directions

1. Add the beans, vegetable broth and water,
7.
  onion, garlic, salt and pepper in a pot and cook over low-medium heat.
2. Simmer for 3-4 hours.
3. When the beans become soft, add the potato and simmer until the potatoes become tender.
4. Add the carrots, tomatoes and balsamic vinegar and cook until heated through.
5. Add the parsley.
6. Season with more salt and pepper.

BEAN & GRAIN MAINS

356. Kidney Bean Dinner

Preparation Time: 5-8 min.
Cooking Time: 25 min.
Servings: 4

Ingredients:

- 2 roasted peppers, cut to make strips
- 1 teaspoon ground cumin
- 1/2 teaspoon mustard powder
- 1 pound dried red kidney beans
- 1/2 cup shallots, chopped
- 2 cloves garlic, chopped
- 1 teaspoon celery seeds
- Sea salt and ground black pepper, to taste
- 2 cups roasted vegetable broth

Directions:

1. Take your Instant Pot; open the top lid and plug it on.
2. Add the ingredients; gently stir to combine.
3. Properly close the top lid; make sure that safety valve is properly locked.
4. Press "BEAN/CHILI" cooking function; set timer to 25 minutes. Then, set pressure level to "HIGH".
5. Allow the pressure to build to cook the ingredients.
6. After cooking time is over press "CANCEL" setting. Find and press "NPR" for natural pressure release; it takes around 10 minutes to slowly release pressure.
7. Open the top lid, divide the cooked recipe in serving containers. Serve warm.

Nutritional Values;

Calories: 394
Fat: 4g
Saturated Fat: 0g
Trans Fat: 0g
Carbohydrates: 54g
Fiber: 21g
Sodium: 286mg
Protein: 31g

357. Rice Lentil Meal

Preparation Time: 5-8 min.
Cooking Time: 15 min.
Servings: 5-6

Ingredients:

- 1 cup lentils, soaked overnight
- 1 yellow onion, finely chopped
- 1 celery stalk, finely chopped
- 1 tablespoon extra-virgin olive oil
- 1 cup arborio rice
- Black pepper and salt to the taste
- 1 tablespoon parsley, finely chopped
- 3 ¼ cup veggie stock
- 2 garlic cloves, crushed

Directions:

1. Take your Instant Pot; open the top lid and plug it on.
2. Press "SAUTE" cooking function; add the oil and heat it.
3. In the pot, add the onions; stir-cook using wooden spatula until turns translucent and softened for 3-4 minutes.
4. Add the celery and parsley, stir-cook for 1 minute.
5. Add the garlic, rice, stock, and lentils; stir the mix.
6. Properly close the top lid; make sure that safety valve is properly locked.
7. Press "MANUAL" cooking function; set timer to 10 minutes. Then, set pressure level to "HIGH".
8. Allow the pressure to build to cook the ingredients.
9. After cooking time is over press "CANCEL" setting. Find and press "NPR" for natural pressure release; it takes around 10 minutes to slowly release pressure.
10. Open the top lid, divide the cooked recipe in serving containers. Serve warm.

Nutritional Values;

Calories: 193
Fat: 4g
Saturated Fat: 1g
Trans Fat: 0g
Carbohydrates: 35g
Fiber: 4g
Sodium: 428mg
Protein: 6g

358. Mushroom Quinoa Pilaf

Preparation Time: 5-8 min.
Cooking Time: 5-7 min.
Servings: 4

Ingredients:

- 1 onion, chopped
- 1 bell pepper, chopped
- 2 garlic cloves, chopped
- 2 cups dry quinoa
- 3 cups water
- 2 tablespoons olive oil
- 2 cups Cremini mushrooms, thinly sliced
- 1/3 teaspoon ground black pepper, or more to taste
- 1 teaspoon cayenne pepper
- 1/2 teaspoon sea salt
- 1/2 teaspoon dried dill
- 1/4 teaspoon ground bay leaf

Directions:
1. Take your Instant Pot; open the top lid and plug it on.
2. Add the water and quinoa; gently stir to combine.
3. Properly close the top lid; make sure that safety valve is properly locked.
4. Press "MANUAL" cooking function; set timer to 1 minute. Then, set pressure level to "HIGH".
5. Allow the pressure to build to cook the ingredients.
6. After cooking time is over press "CANCEL" setting. Find and press "NPR" for natural pressure release; it takes around 10 minutes to slowly release pressure.
7. Drain quinoa and set it aside.
8. Press "SAUTE" cooking function; add the oil and heat it.
9. In the pot, add the onions; stir-cook using wooden spatula until turns translucent and softened.
10. Add the bell pepper, garlic, and mushrooms; stir-cook for 1-2 minutes.
11. Add the mix in a bowl; mix in the quinoa and other ingredients. Serve fresh.

Nutritional Values;
Calories: 386
Fat: 12g
Saturated Fat: 2g
Trans Fat: 0g
Carbohydrates: 58g
Fiber: 16g
Sodium: 284mg
Protein: 14g

359. Cabbage Rice Treat

Preparation Time: 5-8 min.
Cooking Time: 10 min.
Servings: 4

Ingredients:
- 1 head purple cabbage, cut to make wedges
- 2 ripe tomatoes, pureed
- 2 tablespoons tomato ketchup
- 2 tablespoons olive oil
- 2 shallots, diced
- 1 garlic clove, minced
- 1 bay leaf
- 1/4 teaspoon marjoram
- 1/2 teaspoon cayenne pepper
- 1 cup basmati rice
- 1 ½ cups water
- Salt and freshly ground black pepper, to taste
- 1/4 cup fresh chives, chopped

Directions:
1. Take your Instant Pot; open the top lid and plug it on.
2. Press "SAUTE" cooking function; add the oil and heat it.
3. In the pot, add the shallots; stir-cook using wooden spatula until turns translucent and softened for 2 minutes.
4. Add the minced garlic and cook until it is lightly browned.
5. Add the cabbage, tomatoes, ketchup, rice, water, bay leaf, marjoram, cayenne pepper, salt, and black pepper; stir the mix.
6. Properly close the top lid; make sure that safety valve is properly locked.
7. Press "MANUAL" cooking function; set timer to 6 minutes. Then, set pressure level to "HIGH".
8. Allow the pressure to build to cook the ingredients.
9. After cooking time is over press "CANCEL" setting. Find and press "NPR" for natural pressure release; it takes around 10 minutes to slowly release pressure.
10. Open the top lid, divide the cooked recipe in serving containers. Top with the chives. Serve warm.

Nutritional Values;
Calories: 257
Fat: 13g
Saturated Fat: 2g
Trans Fat: 0g
Carbohydrates: 34g
Fiber: 11g
Sodium: 354mg
Protein: 9g

360. Almond Quinoa Pilaf

Preparation Time: 5-8 min.
Cooking Time: 8 min.
Servings: 4

Ingredients:

- 1 tablespoon vegan butter or vegetable oil
- 14 ounces canned veggie stock
- 1 celery stalk, finely chopped
- ½ cup yellow onion, finely chopped
- 1 ½ cups quinoa, washed and drained
- Salt to the taste
- ¼ cup water
- 2 tablespoons parsley leaves, chopped
- ½ cup almonds, sliced and toasted

Directions:

1. Take your Instant Pot; open the top lid and plug it on.
2. Press "SAUTE" cooking function; add the oil or butter and heat it.
3. In the pot, add the onions, celery; stir-cook using wooden spatula until turns translucent and softened for 4-5 minutes.
4. Add the stock, water, quinoa, and salt, stir the mix.
5. Properly close the top lid; make sure that safety valve is properly locked.
6. Press "MANUAL" cooking function; set timer to 3 minutes. Then, set pressure level to "HIGH".
7. Allow the pressure to build to cook the ingredients.
8. After cooking time is over press "CANCEL" setting. Find and press "NPR" for natural pressure release; it takes around 10 minutes to slowly release pressure.
9. Open the top lid, divide the cooked recipe in serving containers. Top with the almond and parsley. Serve warm.

Nutritional Values;

Calories: 176
Fat: 6g
Saturated Fat: 0.3g
Trans Fat: 0g
Carbohydrates: 15g
Fiber: 3g
Sodium: 142mg
Protein: 7g

361. Bean Pepper Salad

Preparation Time: 5-8 min.
Cooking Time: 30 min.
Servings: 3-4

Ingredients:

- 1 red bell pepper, seeded and chopped
- 1 green bell pepper, seeded and chopped
- 1 teaspoon ground sumac
- 1 1/2 cup mix of black beans and Northern beans
- 6 cups water
- 1 cucumber, peeled and sliced
- 3 tablespoons extra-virgin olive oil
- 1 tablespoon fresh lime juice
- 1/4 cup fresh parsley leaves, roughly chopped
- 1/4 teaspoon freshly ground black pepper
- 1/2 teaspoon red pepper flakes
- Salt, to taste

Directions:

1. Take your Instant Pot; open the top lid and plug it on.
2. Add the water and beans; gently stir to combine.
3. Properly close the top lid; make sure that safety valve is properly locked.
4. Press "BEAN/CHILI" cooking function; set timer to 30 minutes. Then, set pressure level to "HIGH".
5. Allow the pressure to build to cook the ingredients.
6. After cooking time is over press "CANCEL" setting. Find and press "NPR" for natural pressure release; it takes around 10 minutes to slowly release pressure.
7. Drain the beans and add in a mixing bowl.
8. Mix in the other ingredients and serve fresh or chilled.

Nutritional Values;

Calories: 210
Fat: 5g
Saturated Fat: 1g
Trans Fat: 0g
Carbohydrates: 31g
Fiber: 8g
Sodium: 154mg
Protein: 10g

362. Lentils Tomato Bowl

Preparation Time: 5-8 min.
Cooking Time: 12 min.
Servings: 4

Ingredients:

- 1 teaspoon garlic, minced
- 1 teaspoon turmeric powder
- Sea salt and ground black pepper, to taste

- 1 teaspoon sweet paprika
- 1 tablespoon olive oil
- 2 cups red lentils
- 1/2 cup scallions, finely chopped
- 1 (15-ounce) can tomatoes, crushed
- 1 bay leaf
- 1 handful fresh cilantro leaves, chopped

Directions:
1. Take your Instant Pot; open the top lid and plug it on.
2. Add the olive oil, lentils, scallions, garlic, turmeric, salt, black pepper, paprika, tomatoes, and bay leaf; gently stir to combine.
3. Properly close the top lid; make sure that safety valve is properly locked.
4. Press "MANUAL" cooking function; set timer to 12 minutes. Then, set pressure level to "HIGH".
5. Allow the pressure to build to cook the ingredients.
6. After cooking time is over press "CANCEL" setting. Find and press "NPR" for natural pressure release; it takes around 10 minutes to slowly release pressure.
7. Open the top lid, remove the bay leaf, divide the cooked recipe in serving containers. Top with some cilantro. Serve warm.

Nutritional Values;
Calories: 396
Fat: 5g
Saturated Fat: 1g
Trans Fat: 0g
Carbohydrates: 58g
Fiber: 14g
Sodium: 536mg
Protein: 24g

363. Squash Barley Meal
Preparation Time: 5-8 min.
Cooking Time: 43 min.
Servings: 4

Ingredients:
- 1/2 cup scallions, chopped
- 2 cups butternut squash, peeled and cubed
- 1/2 teaspoon turmeric powder
- 2 tablespoons olive oil divided
- 2 cloves garlic, minced
- 2 cups barley, whole
- 4 ½ cups water
- Sea salt and ground black pepper, to taste

Directions:
1. Take your Instant Pot; open the top lid and plug it on.
2. Press "SAUTE" cooking function; add the oil and heat it.
3. In the pot, add the garlic, scallions; stir-cook using wooden spatula until turns translucent and softened.
4. Add the ingredients; gently stir to combine.
5. Properly close the top lid; make sure that safety valve is properly locked.
6. Press "MANUAL" cooking function; set timer to 40 minutes. Then, set pressure level to "HIGH".
7. Allow the pressure to build to cook the ingredients.
8. After cooking time is over press "CANCEL" setting. Find and press "NPR" for natural pressure release; it takes around 10 minutes to slowly release pressure.
9. Open the top lid, divide the cooked recipe in serving containers. Serve warm.

Nutritional Values;
Calories: 356
Fat: 6g
Saturated Fat: 1g
Trans Fat: 0g
Carbohydrates: 62g
Fiber: 18g
Sodium: 426mg
Protein: 9g

364. Creamed Peas & Rice
Preparation Time: 5-8 min.
Cooking Time: min.
Servings: 3

Ingredients:
- 4 ounces fresh green peas
- 2 fresh green chilies, chopped
- 1 garlic clove, pressed
- 1 cup basmati rice, rinsed
- 1 ¼ cups water
- Kosher salt and white pepper, to taste
- 2 tablespoons fresh coriander
- 1/2 cup small onions, chopped
- 4 whole cloves
- 1/2 cup coconut cream
- 1 tablespoon fresh lime juice

Directions:
1. Take your Instant Pot; open the top lid and plug it on.

2. Add the ingredients except for the lime juice; gently stir to combine.
3. Properly close the top lid; make sure that safety valve is properly locked.
4. Press "MANUAL" cooking function; set timer to 4-6 minutes. Then, set pressure level to "HIGH".
5. Allow the pressure to build to cook the ingredients.
6. After cooking time is over press "CANCEL" setting. Find and press "NPR" for natural pressure release; it takes around 10 minutes to slowly release pressure.
7. Open the top lid, mix in the lime juice, divide the cooked recipe in serving containers. Serve warm.

Nutritional Values;
Calories: 326
Fat: 16g
Saturated Fat: 3g
Trans Fat: 0g
Carbohydrates: 43g
Fiber: 8g
Sodium: 346mg
Protein: 9g

365. Cornmeal Onion Polenta
Preparation Time: 5-8 min.
Cooking Time: 12 min.
Servings: 3

Ingredients:
- 2 cups hot water
- 2 teaspoons garlic, minced
- 1 tablespoon chili powder
- 1 cup cornmeal
- 1 bunch green onion, thinly sliced
- 2 cups veggie stock
- Vegetable oil as required
- ¼ cup cilantro, finely chopped
- Black pepper and salt to the taste
- 1 teaspoon cumin
- 1 teaspoon oregano
- A pinch of cayenne pepper
- ½ teaspoon smoked paprika

Directions:
1. Take your Instant Pot; open the top lid and plug it on.
2. Press "SAUTE" cooking function; add the oil and heat it.
3. In the pot, add the onions, garlic; stir-cook using wooden spatula until turns translucent and softened for 2 minutes.
4. Add the stock, hot water, cornmeal, cilantro, salt, pepper, chili powder, cumin, oregano, paprika and a pinch of cayenne pepper; stir the mix.
5. Properly close the top lid; make sure that safety valve is properly locked.
6. Press "MANUAL" cooking function; set timer to 10 minutes. Then, set pressure level to "HIGH".
7. Allow the pressure to build to cook the ingredients.
8. After cooking time is over press "CANCEL" setting. Find and press "NPR" for natural pressure release; it takes around 10 minutes to slowly release pressure.
9. Open the top lid, divide the cooked recipe in serving containers. Serve warm.

Nutritional Values;
Calories: 285
Fat: 2g
Saturated Fat: 0g
Trans Fat: 0g
Carbohydrates: 42g
Fiber: 4g
Sodium: 364mg
Protein: 9g

GRILLED RECIPES

366. Grilled Zucchinis and Button Mushrooms

Ingredients

- 2 zucchinis, cut into 1/2-inch slices
- 2 red bell peppers, cut into chunks
- 1/2 pound fresh button mushrooms
- 1/2 pound cherry tomatoes1 red onion, cut into 1/2-inch-thick slices
- 1/2 cup olive oil
- sea salt to taste
- freshly ground black pepper to taste
- Preheat your grill for medium-high heat
- Oil the grate.

Directions

1. Mix the zucchinis, green bell peppers, mushrooms, tomatoes, and onion in a bowl.
2. Drizzle some olive oil over vegetables and toss them to coat.
3. Season with sea salt and pepper.
4. Grill the vegetables for 4 minutes per side.

367. Grilled Zucchini and Cremini Mushrooms with Balsamic Glaze

Ingredients

- 3 green bell peppers, seeded and halved
- 3 yellow squash (about 1 pound total), sliced lengthwise into 1/2-inch-thick rectangles
- 3 zucchini (about 12 ounces total), sliced lengthwise into 1/2-inch-thick rectangles
- 3 eggplant (12 ounces total), sliced lengthwise into 1/2-inch-thick rectangles
- 12 cremini mushrooms
- 1 bunch (1-pound) asparagus, trimmed
- 12 green onions, roots cut off
- 6 tablespoons olive oil
- Salt and freshly ground black pepper
- 3 tablespoons balsamic vinegar
- 4 garlic cloves, minced
- 1 teaspoon chopped fresh parsley leaves
- 1 teaspoon chopped fresh basil leaves
- 1/2 teaspoon finely chopped fresh rosemary leaves

Directions

1. Preheat your grill for medium-high heat
2. Lightly brush the vegetables with 1/4 cup of the oil
3. Season the vegetables with salt and pepper.
4. Working in batches, grill them until tender.
5. Combine the 2 tablespoons of oil, balsamic vinegar, garlic, parsley, basil, and rosemary in a bowl.
6. Season with salt and pepper.
7. Drizzle the vinaigrette over the vegetables.

368. Grilled Asparagus Green Pepper and Squash

Marinade Ingredients

- 1/4 cup extra virgin olive oil
- 2 tablespoons honey
- 4 teaspoons balsamic vinegar
- 1 teaspoon dried oregano
- 1 teaspoon garlic powder
- 1/8 teaspoon rainbow peppercorns
- Sea salt

Vegetable Ingredients

- 1 pound fresh asparagus, trimmed
- 3 small carrots, cut in half lengthwise
- 1 large sweet green pepper, cut into 1-inch strips
- 1 medium yellow summer squash, cut into 1/2-inch slices
- 1 medium yellow onion, cut into wedges
- Combine the marinade ingredients.
- Combine the 3 tablespoons marinade and vegetables in a bag.

Directions

1. Marinate 1 1/2 hours at room temperature or overnight in the refrigerator.
2. Grill the vegetables over medium heat for 8-12 minutes or until tender.
3. Sprinkle the remaining marinade.

369. Simple Grilled Zucchini and Red Onions

Ingredients

- 2 large zucchini , cut lengthwise into ½ inch slabs
- 2 large red onions, cut into ½ inch rings but don't separate into individual rings
- 2 tbsp. extra virgin olive oil
- 2 tbsp. ranch dressing mix

Directions

1. Lightly brush each side of the vegetables with olive oil.
2. Season with the ranch dressing mix
3. Grill over 4 minutes over medium heat or until tender.

370. Simple Grilled Corns and Portobello

Ingredients

- 2 large Corn, cut lengthwise
- 5 pcs. Portobello, rinsed and drained
- Marinade Ingredients:
- 6 tbsp. extra virgin olive oil
- Sea salt, to taste
- 3 tbsp. distilled white vinegar
- 1 tsp. Dijon mustard

Directions

1. Marinate the vegetable with the dressing or marinade ingredients for 15 to 30 min.
2. Grill for 4 minutes over medium heat or until the vegetable becomes tender.

371. Grilled Marinated Eggplant and Zucchini

Ingredients

- 2 large Eggplants, cut lengthwise and cut in half
- 2 large Zucchinis, cut lengthwise and cut in half
- Marinade Ingredients:
- 6 tbsp. extra virgin olive oil
- Sea salt, to taste
- 3 tbsp. distilled white vinegar
- 1 tsp. Dijon mustard

Directions

1. Marinate the vegetable with the dressing or marinade ingredients for 15 to 30 min.
2. Grill for 4 minutes over medium heat or until the vegetable becomes tender.

372. Grilled Bell Pepper and Broccolini

Ingredients

- 2 Green Bell Peppers, cut in half
- 10 Broccolini Florets
- Marinade Ingredients:
- 6 tbsp. extra virgin olive oil
- Sea salt, to taste
- 3 tbsp. distilled white vinegar
- 1 tsp. Dijon mustard

Directions

1. Marinate the vegetable with the dressing or marinade ingredients for 15 to 30 min.
2. Grill for 4 minutes over medium heat or until the vegetable becomes tender.

Directions

373. Grilled Cauliflower and Brussel Sprouts

Ingredients

- 10 Cauliflower florets
- 10 pcs. Brussel Sprouts
- Marinade Ingredients:
- 6 tbsp. extra virgin olive oil
- Sea salt, to taste
- 3 tbsp. distilled white vinegar
- 1 tsp. Dijon mustard

Directions

1. Marinate the vegetable with the dressing or marinade ingredients for 15 to 30 min.
2. Grill for 4 minutes over medium heat or until the vegetable becomes tender.

374. Grilled Corn and Crimini Mushrooms

Ingredients

- 2 Corns, cut lengthwise
- 10 Crimini Mushrooms, rinsed and drained
- Marinade Ingredients:
- 6 tbsp. extra virgin olive oil
- Sea salt, to taste
- 3 tbsp. distilled white vinegar
- 1 tsp. Dijon mustard

Directions

1. Marinate the vegetable with the dressing or marinade ingredients for 15 to 30 min.
2. Grill for 4 minutes over medium heat or until the vegetable becomes tender.

Grilled Eggplant, Zucchini and Corn

Ingredients

- 2 large Eggplants, cut lengthwise and cut in half
- 2 large Zucchinis, cut lengthwise and cut in half
- 2 Corns, cut lengthwise
- Marinade Ingredients:
- 6 tbsp. extra virgin olive oil
- Sea salt, to taste
- 3 tbsp. distilled white vinegar
- 1 tsp. Dijon mustard

Grilled Recipes

Directions
1. Marinate the vegetable with the dressing or marinade ingredients for 15 to 30 min.
2. Grill for 4 minutes over medium heat or until the vegetable becomes tender.

376. Grilled Zucchini and Pineapple

Ingredients

- 2 large zucchini, cut lengthwise into ½ inch slabs
- 2 large red onions, cut into ½ inch rings but don't separate into individual rings
- 1 medium Pineapple, cut into 1/2 inch slices
- 10 Green Beans
- Marinade Ingredients:
- 6 tbsp. extra virgin olive oil
- Sea salt, to taste
- 3 tbsp. distilled white vinegar
- 1 tsp. Dijon mustard

Directions
1. Marinate the vegetable with the dressing or marinade ingredients for 15 to 30 min.
2. Grill for 4 minutes over medium heat or until the vegetable becomes tender.

377. Grilled Portobello and Asparagus

Ingredients

- 3 pcs. Portobello, rinsed and drained
- 2 pcs. Eggplant, cut lengthwise and cut in half
- 2 pcs. Zucchini, cut lengthwise and cut in half
- 6 pcs. Asparagus
- Marinade Ingredients:
- 6 tbsp. extra virgin olive oil
- Sea salt, to taste
- 3 tbsp. distilled white vinegar
- 1 tsp. Dijon mustard

Directions
1. Marinate the vegetable with the dressing or marinade ingredients for 15 to 30 min.
2. Grill for 4 minutes over medium heat or until the vegetable becomes tender.

378. Simple Grilled Vegetables Recipe

Ingredients

- 3 pcs. Portobello, rinsed and drained
- 2 pcs. Eggplant, cut lengthwise and cut in half
- 2 pcs. Zucchini, cut lengthwise and cut in half
- 6 pcs. Asparagus
- Dressing Ingredients
- 6 tbsp. extra virgin olive oil
- Sea salt, to taste
- 3 tbsp. apple cider vinegar
- 1 tbsp. honey
- 1 tsp. Egg-free mayonnaise

Directions
1. Marinate the vegetable with the dressing or marinade ingredients for 15 to 30 min.
2. Grill for 4 minutes over medium heat or until the vegetable becomes tender.

379. Grilled Japanese Eggplant and Shitake Mushroom

Ingredients

- Corns, cut lengthwise
- 2 pcs. Japanese Eggplant, cut lengthwise and cut in half
- Shitake Mushroom, rinsed and drained
- Dressing Ingredients
- 6 tbsp. olive oil
- Sea salt, to taste
- 3 tbsp. white wine vinegar
- 1 tsp. Egg-free mayonnaise

Directions
1. Marinate the vegetable with the dressing or marinade ingredients for 15 to 30 min.
2. Grill for 4 minutes over medium heat or until the vegetable becomes tender.

380. Grilled Japanese Eggplant and Broccolini

Ingredients

- 2 Green Bell Peppers, cut in half
- 10 Broccolini Florets
- 2 pcs. Japanese Eggplant, cut lengthwise and cut in half
- Dressing Ingredients
- 6 tbsp. sesame oil
- Sea salt, to taste
- 3 tbsp. distilled white vinegar
- 1 tsp. Egg-free mayonnaise

Directions
1. Marinate the vegetable with the dressing or marinade ingredients for 15 to 30 min.
2. Grill for 4 minutes over medium heat or until the vegetable becomes tender.

381. Grilled Cauliflower and Brussel Sprouts

Ingredients

- 10 Cauliflower florets
- 10 pcs. Brussel Sprouts
- Dressing Ingredients
- 6 tbsp. sesame oil
- Sea salt, to taste
- 3 tbsp. distilled white vinegar
- 1 tsp. Egg-free mayonnaise

Directions

1. Marinate the vegetable with the dressing or marinade ingredients for 15 to 30 min.
2. Grill for 4 minutes over medium heat or until the vegetable becomes tender.

382. Grilled Japanese and Cauliflower Recipe with Balsamic Glaze

Ingredients

- 2 Green Bell Peppers, cut in half lengthwise
- 10 Cauliflower Florets
- 2 pcs. Japanese Eggplant, cut lengthwise and cut in half
- Dressing Ingredients
- 6 tbsp. extra virgin olive oil
- Sea salt, to taste
- 3 tbsp. Balsamic vinegar
- 1 tsp. Dijon mustard

Directions

1. Marinate the vegetable with the dressing or marinade ingredients for 15 to 30 min.
2. Grill for 4 minutes over medium heat or until the vegetable becomes tender.

383. Simple Grilled Vegetables Recipe

Ingredients

- 2 large Eggplants, cut lengthwise and cut in half
- 1 large Zucchini, cut lengthwise and cut in half
- 5 Broccoli Florets
- Marinade Ingredients:
- 6 tbsp. extra virgin olive oil
- Sea salt, to taste
- 3 tbsp. distilled white vinegar
- 1 tsp. Dijon mustard

Directions

1. Marinate the vegetable with the dressing or marinade ingredients for 15 to 30 min.
2. Grill for 4 minutes over medium heat or until the vegetable becomes tender.

384. Grilled Eggplant and Green Bell Peppers

Ingredients

- 2 Green Bell Peppers, cut in half
- 10 Broccolini Florets
- 2 pcs. Eggplant, cut lengthwise and cut in half
- Dressing Ingredients
- 6 tbsp. olive oil
- Sea salt, to taste
- 3 tbsp. white wine vinegar
- 1 tsp. English mustard

Directions

1. Marinate the vegetable with the dressing or marinade ingredients for 15 to 30 min.
2. Grill for 4 minutes over medium heat or until the vegetable becomes tender.

385. Grilled Portobello Asparagus and Green Beans with Apple Cider Vinaigrette

Ingredients

- 3 pcs. Portobello, rinsed and drained
- 2 pcs. Eggplant, cut lengthwise and cut in half
- 2 pcs. Zucchini, cut lengthwise and cut in half
- 6 pcs. Asparagus
- 1 medium Pineapple, cut into 1/2 inch slices
- 10 Green Beans
- Dressing Ingredients
- 6 tbsp. extra virgin olive oil
- Sea salt, to taste
- 3 tbsp. apple cider vinegar
- 1 tbsp. honey
- 1 tsp. Egg-free mayonnaise

Directions

1. Marinate the vegetable with the dressing or marinade ingredients for 15 to 30 min.
2. Grill for 4 minutes over medium heat or until the vegetable becomes tender.

386. Grilled Beans and Portobello Mushrooms

Ingredients

- Corns, cut lengthwise
- 5 pcs. Portobello mushrooms, rinsed and drained
- 10 Green Beans

Grilled Recipes

- Dressing Ingredients
- 6 tbsp. olive oil
- Sea salt, to taste
- 3 tbsp. white wine vinegar
- 1 tsp. Egg-free mayonnaise

Directions
1. Marinate the vegetable with the dressing or marinade ingredients for 15 to 30 min.
2. Grill for 4 minutes over medium heat or until the vegetable becomes tender.

387. Brussel Sprouts and Green Beans

Ingredients
- 10 Cauliflower florets
- 10 pcs. Brussel Sprouts
- 10 Green Beans
- Dressing Ingredients
- 6 tbsp. olive oil
- Sea salt, to taste
- 3 tbsp. white wine vinegar
- 1 tsp. Egg-free mayonnaise

Directions
1. Marinate the vegetable with the dressing or marinade ingredients for 15 to 30 min.
2. Grill for 4 minutes over medium heat or until the vegetable becomes tender.

388. Zucchini and Onion in Ranch Dressing

Ingredients
- 2 large zucchini, cut lengthwise into ½ inch slabs
- 2 large red onions, cut into ½ inch rings but don't separate into individual rings
- 2 tbsp. extra virgin olive oil
- 2 tbsp. ranch dressing mix

Directions
1. Marinate the vegetable with the dressing or marinade ingredients for 15 to 30 min.
2. Grill for 4 minutes over medium heat or until the vegetable becomes tender.

389. Grilled Green Bean and Pineapple in Balsamic Vinaigrette

Ingredients
- 1 medium Pineapple, cut into 1/2 inch slices
- 10 Green Beans
- Dressing Ingredients
- 6 tbsp. extra virgin olive oil
- Sea salt, to taste
- 3 tbsp. Balsamic vinegar
- 1 tsp. Dijon mustard

Directions
1. Marinate the vegetable with the dressing or marinade ingredients for 15 to 30 min.
2. Grill for 4 minutes over medium heat or until the vegetable becomes tender.

390. Grilled Broccolini and Eggplants

Ingredients
- 1 large Eggplants, cut lengthwise and cut in half
- 1 large Zucchinis, cut lengthwise and cut in half
- 10 Green Beans
- 10 Broccolini Florets
- Marinade Ingredients:
- 6 tbsp. extra virgin olive oil
- Sea salt, to taste
- 3 tbsp. distilled white vinegar
- 1 tsp. Dijon mustard

Directions
1. Marinate the vegetable with the dressing or marinade ingredients for 15 to 30 min.
2. Grill for 4 minutes over medium heat or until the vegetable becomes tender.

391. Grilled Broccolini and Green Bell Peppers

Ingredients
- 2 Green Bell Peppers, cut in half
- 8 Broccolini Florets
- Dressing Ingredients
- 6 tbsp. sesame oil
- Sea salt, to taste
- 3 tbsp. distilled white vinegar
- 1 tsp. Egg-free mayonnaise

Directions
1. Marinate the vegetable with the dressing or marinade ingredients for 15 to 30 min.
2. Grill for 4 minutes over medium heat or until the vegetable becomes tender.

392. Grilled Zucchini and Carrots

Ingredients
- 2 large zucchini, cut lengthwise into ½ inch slabs
- 1 large red onion, cut into ½ inch rings but don't separate into individual rings

- 1 large carrot, peeled and cut lengthwise
- Dressing Ingredients
- 6 tbsp. olive oil
- Sea salt, to taste
- 3 tbsp. white wine vinegar
- 1 tsp. English mustard

Directions
1. Marinate the vegetable with the dressing or marinade ingredients for 15 to 30 min.
2. Grill for 4 minutes over medium heat or until the vegetable becomes tender.

393. Grilled Portobello Mushrooms in Apple Cider Vinaigrette

Ingredients
- Corns, cut lengthwise
- 5 pcs. Portobello mushrooms, rinsed and drained
- Dressing Ingredients
- 6 tbsp. extra virgin olive oil
- Sea salt, to taste
- 3 tbsp. apple cider vinegar
- 1 tbsp. honey
- 1 tsp. Egg-free mayonnaise

Directions
1. Marinate the vegetable with the dressing or marinade ingredients for 15 to 30 min.
2. Grill for 4 minutes over medium heat or until the vegetable becomes tender.

394. Grilled Carrots with Brussel Sprouts

Ingredients
- 10 Cauliflower florets
- 10 pcs. Brussel Sprouts
- 1 large carrot, peeled and cut lengthwise
- Dressing Ingredients
- 6 tbsp. olive oil
- Sea salt, to taste
- 3 tbsp. white wine vinegar
- 1 tsp. Egg-free mayonnaise

Directions
1. Marinate the vegetable with the dressing or marinade ingredients for 15 to 30 min.
2. Grill for 4 minutes over medium heat or until the vegetable becomes tender.

395. Grilled Parsnip and Zucchini Recipe

Ingredients
- 1 large parsnip, peeled and cut lengthwise
- 1 large zucchini, cut lengthwise into ½ inch slabs
- 2 large red onions, cut into ½ inch rings but don't separate into individual rings
- Marinade Ingredients:
- 6 tbsp. extra virgin olive oil
- Sea salt, to taste
- 3 tbsp. distilled white vinegar
- 1 tsp. Dijon mustard

Directions
1. Marinate the vegetable with the dressing or marinade ingredients for 15 to 30 min.
2. Grill for 4 minutes over medium heat or until the vegetable becomes tender.

396. Grilled Turnip in Oriental Vinaigrette

Ingredients
- 1 large turnip, peeled and cut lengthwise
- 2 Green Bell Peppers, cut in half
- 10 Broccolini Florets
- Dressing Ingredients
- 6 tbsp. sesame oil
- Sea salt, to taste
- 3 tbsp. distilled white vinegar
- 1 tsp. Egg-free mayonnaise

Directions
1. Marinate the vegetable with the dressing or marinade ingredients for 15 to 30 min.
2. Grill for 4 minutes over medium heat or until the vegetable becomes tender.

397. Grilled Carrot, Turnip and Portobello with Balsamic Glaze

Ingredients
- 1 large carrots, peeled and cut lengthwise
- 1 large turnip, peeled and cut lengthwise
- 1 Corn, cut lengthwise
- 2 pcs. Portobello mushrooms, rinsed and drained
- Dressing Ingredients
- 6 tbsp. extra virgin olive oil
- Sea salt, to taste
- 3 tbsp. Balsamic vinegar
- 1 tsp. Dijon mustard

Directions

Grilled Recipes

1. Marinate the vegetable with the dressing or marinade ingredients for 15 to 30 min.
2. Grill for 4 minutes over medium heat or until the vegetable becomes tender.

398. Grilled Zucchinis and Mangoes

Ingredients

- 2 large Zucchinis, cut lengthwise and cut in half
- 2 large mangoes, cut lengthwise and pitted
- Dressing Ingredients
- 6 tbsp. sesame oil
- Sea salt, to taste
- 3 tbsp. distilled white vinegar
- 1 tsp. Egg-free mayonnaise

Directions

1. Marinate the vegetable with the dressing or marinade ingredients for 15 to 30 min.
2. Grill for 4 minutes over medium heat or until the vegetable becomes tender.
3. For the mango, grill only until you start seeing brown grill marks.

399. Grilled Baby Corn and Green Beans

Ingredients

- ½ cup baby corn
- 1 medium Pineapple, cut into 1/2 inch slices
- 10 Green Beans
- 2 large red onions, cut into ½ inch rings but don't separate into individual rings
- Dressing Ingredients
- 6 tbsp. olive oil
- Sea salt, to taste
- 3 tbsp. white wine vinegar
- 1 tsp. English mustard

Directions

1. Marinate the vegetable with the dressing or marinade ingredients for 15 to 30 min.
2. Grill for 4 minutes over medium heat or until the vegetable becomes tender.

400. Grilled Artichoke Hearts and Brussel Sprouts

Ingredients

- ½ cup canned artichoke hearts
- 5 Broccoli Florets
- 10 pcs. Brussel Sprouts
- Dressing Ingredients
- 6 tbsp. olive oil
- Sea salt, to taste
- 3 tbsp. white wine vinegar
- 1 tsp. Egg-free mayonnaise

Directions

1. Marinate the vegetable with the dressing or marinade ingredients for 15 to 30 min.
2. Grill for 4 minutes over medium heat or until the vegetable becomes tender.

401. Grilles Bell Peppers Broccolini and Brussel Sprouts with Honey Apple Cider Glaze

Ingredients

- 10 Broccolini Florets
- ½ cup canned artichoke hearts
- 10 Brussel Sprouts
- Dressing Ingredients
- 6 tbsp. extra virgin olive oil
- Sea salt, to taste
- 3 tbsp. apple cider vinegar
- 1 tbsp. honey
- 1 tsp. Egg-free mayonnaise

Directions

1. Marinate the vegetable with the dressing or marinade ingredients for 15 to 30 min.
2. Grill for 4 minutes over medium heat or until the vegetable becomes tender.

402. Grilled Assorted Bell Peppers with Broccolini Florets Recipe

Ingredients

- 1 Green Bell Pepper, cut in half
- 1 Yellow Bell Pepper, cut in half
- 1 Red Bell Pepper, cut in half
- 10 Broccolini Florets
- Marinade Ingredients:
- mustard 6 tbsp. extra virgin olive oil
- Sea salt, to taste
- 3 tbsp. distilled white vinegar
- 1 tsp. Dijon

Directions

1. Marinate the vegetable with the dressing or marinade ingredients for 15 to 30 min.
2. Grill for 4 minutes over medium heat or until the vegetable becomes tender.

403. Grilled Eggplant, Zucchini with Assorted Bell Peppers

Ingredients

- 1 small Eggplant, cut lengthwise and cut in half
- 1 small Zucchini, cut lengthwise and cut in half
- 1 Green Bell Pepper, cut in half
- 1 Yellow Bell Pepper, cut in half
- 1 Red Bell Pepper, cut in half
- Dressing Ingredients
- 6 tbsp. sesame oil
- Sea salt, to taste
- 3 tbsp. distilled white vinegar
- 1 tsp. Egg-free mayonnaise

Directions

1. Marinate the vegetable with the dressing or marinade ingredients for 15 to 30 min.
2. Grill for 4 minutes over medium heat or until the vegetable becomes tender.

404. Grilled Portobello and Red Onion

Ingredients

- 1 Corn, cut lengthwise
- 5 pcs. Portobello mushrooms, rinsed and drained
- 1 medium red onion, cut into ½ inch rings but don't separate into individual rings
- Dressing Ingredients
- 6 tbsp. extra virgin olive oil
- Sea salt, to taste
- 3 tbsp. Balsamic vinegar
- 1 tsp. Dijon mustard

Directions

1. Marinate the vegetable with the dressing or marinade ingredients for 15 to 30 min.
2. Grill for 4 minutes over medium heat or until the vegetable becomes tender.

405. Grilled Corn and Red Onions

Ingredients

- 2 large zucchini, cut lengthwise into ½ inch slabs
- 2 large red onions, cut into ½ inch rings but don't separate into individual rings
- 1 Corn, cut Lengthwise
- Dressing Ingredients
- 6 tbsp. sesame oil
- Sea salt, to taste
- 3 tbsp. distilled white vinegar
- 1 tsp. Egg-free mayonnaise

Directions

1. Marinate the vegetable with the dressing or marinade ingredients for 15 to 30 min.
2. Grill for 4 minutes over medium heat or until the vegetable becomes tender.

ROASTED RECIPES

406. Roasted Napa Cabbage Baby Carrots and Spinach

Extra Ingredients

- cooking spray
- 1 tablespoon extra virgin olive oil
- 1/2 teaspoon sea salt
- 1/4 teaspoon ground black pepper
- Main Ingredients
- 1/2 medium Napa cabbage, sliced thinly
- 5 baby carrots
- 1 bunch of spinach, rinsed and drained

Directions

1. Preheat your oven to 450 degrees F.
2. Line a baking sheet with foil and grease with olive oil.
3. Mix the extra ingredients thoroughly.
4. Add in the main ingredients
5. Combine until well coated.
6. Spread them out in a single layer on the baking sheet.
7. Roast in the oven until vegetables become caramelized, for about 25 minutes.

407. Roasted Spinach Watercress and Carrots

Extra Ingredients

- cooking spray
- 1 tablespoon extra virgin olive oil
- 1/2 teaspoon sea salt
- 1/4 teaspoon ground black pepper
- Main Ingredients
- 5 baby carrots
- 1 bunch of spinach, rinsed and drained
- 1 bunch of watercress, rinsed and drained

Directions

1. Preheat your oven to 450 degrees F.
2. Line a baking sheet with foil and grease with olive oil.
3. Mix the extra ingredients thoroughly.
4. Add in the main ingredients
5. Combine until well coated.
6. Spread them out in a single layer on the baking sheet.
7. Roast in the oven until vegetables become caramelized, for about 25 minutes.

408. Roasted Artichoke Hearts and Red Cabbage

Extra Ingredients

- cooking spray
- 1 tablespoon extra virgin olive oil
- 1/2 teaspoon sea salt
- 1/4 teaspoon ground black pepper

Main Ingredients

- 1/2 medium red cabbage, sliced thinly
- 1 cup canned artichoke hearts

Directions

1. Preheat your oven to 450 degrees F.
2. Line a baking sheet with foil and grease with olive oil.
3. Mix the extra ingredients thoroughly.
4. Add in the main ingredients
5. Combine until well coated.
6. Spread them out in a single layer on the baking sheet.
7. Roast in the oven until vegetables become caramelized, for about 25 minutes.

409. Roasted kale and Red Cabbage

Extra Ingredients

- cooking spray
- 1 tablespoon extra virgin olive oil
- 1/2 teaspoon sea salt
- 1/4 teaspoon ground black pepper

Main Ingredients

- 1 bunch of kale, rinsed and drained
- 1/2 medium red cabbage, sliced thinly

Directions

1. Preheat your oven to 450 degrees F.
2. Line a baking sheet with foil and grease with olive oil.
3. Mix the extra ingredients thoroughly.
4. Add in the main ingredients
5. Combine until well coated.
6. Spread them out in a single layer on the baking sheet.
7. Roast in the oven until vegetables become caramelized, for about 25 minutes.

410. Roasted Napa Cabbage and Kale

Extra Ingredients

- cooking spray
- 1 tablespoon extra virgin olive oil
- 1/2 teaspoon sea salt
- 1/4 teaspoon ground black pepper

Main Ingredients

- 1/2 medium Napa cabbage, sliced thinly
- 1 bunch of kale, rinsed and drained

Directions

1. Preheat your oven to 450 degrees F.
2. Line a baking sheet with foil and grease with olive oil.
3. Mix the extra ingredients thoroughly.
4. Add in the main ingredients
5. Combine until well coated.
6. Spread them out in a single layer on the baking sheet.
7. Roast in the oven until vegetables become caramelized, for about 25 minutes.

411. Roasted Butterbeans and Butternut Squash

Ingredients

- 2 (15 ounce) cans butterbeans, rinsed and drained
- 1/2 butternut squash - peeled, seeded, and cut into 1-inch pieces
- 1 red onion, diced
- 1 sweet potato, peeled and cut into 1-inch cubes
- 2 large carrots, cut into 1 inch pieces
- 3 medium potatoes, cut into 1-inch pieces
- 3 tablespoons sesame oil

Seasoning ingredients

- 1 teaspoon salt
- 1/2 teaspoon ground black pepper
- 1 teaspoon onion powder
- 2 teaspoon garlic powder
- 1 teaspoon ground fennel seeds
- 1 teaspoon dried rubbed sage
- Garnishing Ingredients
- 2 green onions, chopped (optional)

Directions

1. Preheat your oven to 350 degrees F.
2. Grease your baking pan.
3. Combine the chickpeas, butternut squash, onion, sweet potato, carrots, and russet potatoes on the prepared sheet pan.
4. Drizzle with the oil and toss to coat.
5. Combine the seasoning ingredients in a bowl
6. Sprinkle them over the vegetables on the pan and toss to coat with seasonings.
7. Bake in the oven for 25 minutes.
8. Stir frequently until vegetables are soft and lightly browned and chickpeas are crisp, for about 20 to 25 minutes more.
9. Season with more salt and black pepper to taste, top with the green onion before serving.

412. Roasted Black Bean and Squash

Ingredients

- 2 (15 ounce) cans black beans, rinsed and drained
- 1/2 butternut squash - peeled, seeded, and cut into 1-inch pieces
- 1 red onion, diced
- 1 sweet potato, peeled and cut into 1-inch cubes
- 2 large carrots, cut into 1 inch pieces
- 3 medium potatoes, cut into 1-inch pieces
- 3 tablespoons extra virgin oil
- Seasoning ingredients
- 1 teaspoon salt
- 1/2 teaspoon ground black pepper
- 1 teaspoon onion powder
- 2 teaspoon garlic powder
- 1 teaspoon cumin
- 1 teaspoon chili powder
- Garnishing Ingredients
- 2 green onions, chopped (optional)

Directions

1. Preheat your oven to 350 degrees F.
2. Grease your baking pan.
3. Combine the black beans, butternut squash, onion, sweet potato, carrots, and russet potatoes on the prepared sheet pan.
4. Drizzle with the oil and toss to coat.
5. Combine the seasoning ingredients in a bowl
6. Sprinkle them over the vegetables on the pan and toss to coat with seasonings.
7. Bake in the oven for 25 minutes.
8. Stir frequently until vegetables are soft and lightly browned and chickpeas are crisp, for about 20 to 25 minutes more.
9. Season with more salt and black pepper to taste, top with the green onion before serving.

413. Roasted Kidney Beans and Potato

Ingredients

- 2 (15 ounce) cans kidney beans, rinsed and drained

- 1/2 butternut squash - peeled, seeded, and cut into 1-inch pieces
- 1 red onion, diced
- 1 sweet potato, peeled and cut into 1-inch cubes
- 2 large carrots, cut into 1 inch pieces
- 3 medium potatoes, cut into 1-inch pieces
- 4 tablespoons extra virgin oil
- Seasoning ingredients
- 1 teaspoon salt
- 1/2 teaspoon ground black pepper
- 1 teaspoon onion powder
- 1 teaspoon dried basil
- 1 teaspoon Italian seasoning
- Garnishing Ingredients
- 2 green onions, chopped (optional)

Directions

1. Preheat your oven to 350 degrees F.
2. Grease your baking pan.
3. Combine the kidney beans, butternut squash, onion, sweet potato, carrots, and russet potatoes on the prepared sheet pan.
4. Drizzle with the oil and toss to coat.
5. Combine the seasoning ingredients in a bowl
6. Sprinkle them over the vegetables on the pan and toss to coat with seasonings.
7. Bake in the oven for 25 minutes.
8. Stir frequently until vegetables are soft and lightly browned and chickpeas are crisp, for about 20 to 25 minutes more.
9. Season with more salt and black pepper to taste, top with the green onion before serving.

414. Roasted Potato and Parsnips

Main Ingredients

- 2 (15 ounce) cans great northern beans, rinsed and drained
- 1/2 butternut squash - peeled, seeded, and cut into 1-inch pieces
- 1 yellow onion, diced
- 1 potato, peeled and cut into 1-inch cubes
- 2 large parsnips, cut into 1 inch pieces
- 3 medium potatoes, cut into 1-inch pieces
- 3 tablespoons extra virgin olive oil
- Seasoning ingredients
- 1 teaspoon sea salt
- 1/2 teaspoon ground rainbow peppercorns
- 1 teaspoon onion powder
- 2 teaspoon garlic powder
- 1 teaspoon ground fennel seeds
- 1 teaspoon dried rubbed sage
- Garnishing Ingredients
- 2 green onions, chopped (optional)

Directions

1. Preheat your oven to 350 degrees F.
2. Grease your baking pan.
3. Combine the main ingredients on the prepared sheet pan.
4. Drizzle with the oil and toss to coat.
5. Combine the seasoning ingredients in a bowl
6. Sprinkle them over the vegetables on the pan and toss to coat with seasonings.
7. Bake in the oven for 25 minutes.
8. Stir frequently until vegetables are soft and lightly browned and chickpeas are crisp, for about 20 to 25 minutes more.
9. Season with more salt and black pepper to taste, top with the green onion before serving.

415. Oriental Roasted Butterbeans and Butternut Squash

Ingredients

- 2 (15 ounce) cans mushrooms, sliced and drained
- 1/2 butternut squash - peeled, seeded, and cut into 1-inch pieces
- 1 red onion, diced
- 1 potato, peeled and cut into 1-inch cubes
- 2 large carrots, cut into 1 inch pieces
- 3 medium potatoes, cut into 1-inch pieces
- 3 tablespoons sesame oil
- Seasoning ingredients
- 1 teaspoon salt
- 1/2 teaspoon ground black pepper
- 1 teaspoon onion powder
- 2 teaspoon garlic powder
- 1 teaspoon Sichuan peppercorns
- 1 teaspoon Chinese five-spice powder
- Garnishing Ingredients
- 2 green onions, chopped (optional)

Directions

1. Preheat your oven to 350 degrees F.
2. Grease your baking pan.
3. Combine the main ingredients on the prepared sheet pan.
4. Drizzle with the oil and toss to coat.
5. Combine the seasoning ingredients in a bowl
6. Sprinkle them over the vegetables on the pan and toss to coat with seasonings.
7. Bake in the oven for 25 minutes.
8. Stir frequently until vegetables are soft and

lightly browned and chickpeas are crisp, for about 20 to 25 minutes more.
9. Season with more salt and black pepper to taste, top with the green onion before serving.

416. Smoky Roasted Kidney Beans and Potatoes

Ingredients

- 2 (15 ounce) cans kidney beans, rinsed and drained
- 1/2 butternut squash - peeled, seeded, and cut into 1-inch pieces
- 1 red onion, diced
- 1 sweet potato, peeled and cut into 1-inch cubes
- 2 large carrots, cut into 1 inch pieces
- 3 medium potatoes, cut into 1-inch pieces
- 3 tablespoons sesame oil
- Seasoning ingredients
- 1 teaspoon salt
- 1/2 teaspoon ground black pepper
- 1 teaspoon onion powder
- 2 teaspoon garlic powder
- 1 teaspoon ground annatto seeds
- 1 teaspoon cumin
- ½ teaspoon cayenne pepper
- Garnishing Ingredients
- 2 cilantro, chopped (optional)

Directions

1. Preheat your oven to 350 degrees F.
2. Grease your baking pan.
3. Combine the main ingredients on the prepared sheet pan.
4. Drizzle with the oil and toss to coat.
5. Combine the seasoning ingredients in a bowl
6. Sprinkle them over the vegetables on the pan and toss to coat with seasonings.
7. Bake in the oven for 25 minutes.
8. Stir frequently until vegetables are soft and lightly browned and chickpeas are crisp, for about 20 to 25 minutes more.
9. Season with more salt and black pepper to taste, top with the cilantro before serving.

417. Roasted Mushrooms and Potatoes

Ingredients

- 2 (15 ounce) cans mushrooms, rinsed and drained
- 1/2 butternut squash - peeled, seeded, and cut into 1-inch pieces
- 1 red onion, diced
- 1 sweet potato, peeled and cut into 1-inch cubes
- 2 large carrots, cut into 1 inch pieces
- 3 medium potatoes, cut into 1-inch pieces
- 3 tablespoons vegan butter/margarine oil
- Seasoning ingredients
- 1 teaspoon salt
- 1/2 teaspoon ground black pepper
- 1 teaspoon onion powder
- 2 teaspoon garlic powder
- 1 teaspoon Herbs de Provence
- Garnishing Ingredients
- 2 sprigs of thyme, chopped (optional)

Directions

1. Preheat your oven to 350 degrees F.
2. Grease your baking pan.
3. Combine the main ingredients on the prepared sheet pan.
4. Drizzle with the melted vegan butter or margarine and toss to coat.
5. Combine the seasoning ingredients in a bowl
6. Sprinkle them over the vegetables on the pan and toss to coat with seasonings.
7. Bake in the oven for 25 minutes.
8. Stir frequently until vegetables are soft and lightly browned and chickpeas are crisp, for about 20 to 25 minutes more.
9. Season with more salt and black pepper to taste, top with thyme before serving.

418. Roasted Potatoes and Sweet Potato

Ingredients

- ¼ cups capers
- ½ cup olives
- 1/2 butternut squash - peeled, seeded, and cut into 1-inch pieces
- 1 red onion, diced
- 1 sweet potato, peeled and cut into 1-inch cubes
- 2 large carrots, cut into 1 inch pieces
- 3 medium potatoes, cut into 1-inch pieces
- 3 tablespoons sesame oil
- Seasoning ingredients
- 1/2 teaspoon sea salt
- 1/2 teaspoon ground black pepper
- 1 teaspoon onion powder
- 2 teaspoon garlic powder
- 1 teaspoon ground fennel seeds
- 1 teaspoon dried rubbed sage

- Garnishing Ingredients
- 2 green onions, chopped (optional)

Directions
1. Preheat your oven to 350 degrees F.
2. Grease your baking pan.
3. Combine the main ingredients on the prepared sheet pan.
4. Drizzle with the oil and toss to coat.
5. Combine the seasoning ingredients in a bowl
6. Sprinkle them over the vegetables on the pan and toss to coat with seasonings.
7. Bake in the oven for 25 minutes.
8. Stir frequently until vegetables are soft and lightly browned and chickpeas are crisp, for about 20 to 25 minutes more.
9. Season with more salt and black pepper to taste, top with the green onion before serving.

419. Roasted Butterbeans and Butternut Squash

Ingredients

- 3 medium tomatoes, cut into 1-inch pieces
- 1/2 butternut squash - peeled, seeded, and cut into 1-inch pieces
- 1 red onion, diced
- 1 turnip, peeled and cut into 1-inch cubes
- 2 large carrots, cut into 1 inch pieces
- 3 medium potatoes, cut into 1-inch pieces
- 3 tablespoons extra virgin olive oil
- Seasoning ingredients
- 1 teaspoon salt
- 1/2 teaspoon ground black pepper
- 1 teaspoon onion powder
- 2 teaspoon garlic powder
- 1 teaspoon dried thyme
- Garnishing Ingredients
- 2 sprigs fresh thyme, chopped (optional)

Directions
1. Preheat your oven to 350 degrees F.
2. Grease your baking pan.
3. Combine the main ingredients on the prepared sheet pan.
4. Drizzle with the oil and toss to coat.
5. Combine the seasoning ingredients in a bowl
6. Sprinkle them over the vegetables on the pan and toss to coat with seasonings.
7. Bake in the oven for 25 minutes.
8. Stir frequently until vegetables are soft and lightly browned and chickpeas are crisp, for about 20 to 25 minutes more.
9. Season with more salt and black pepper to taste, top with the thyme before serving.

420. Roasted Tomatoes and Bean Sprouts

Ingredients

- 3 large tomatoes, cut into 1-inch pieces
- 1/2 butternut squash - peeled, seeded, and cut into 1-inch pieces
- 1 red onion, diced
- 1 cup bean sprouts
- 3 large carrots, cut into 1 inch pieces
- 3 tablespoons sesame oil
- Seasoning ingredients
- 1 teaspoon salt
- 1/2 teaspoon ground black pepper
- 1 teaspoon onion powder
- 2 teaspoon garlic powder
- 1 teaspoon Thai chili paste
- 1 teaspoon Fresh Thai Basil, chopped
- Garnishing Ingredients
- 2 green onions, chopped (optional)

Directions
1. Preheat your oven to 350 degrees F.
2. Grease your baking pan.
3. Combine the main ingredients on the prepared sheet pan.
4. Drizzle with the oil and toss to coat.
5. Combine the seasoning ingredients in a bowl
6. Sprinkle them over the vegetables on the pan and toss to coat with seasonings.
7. Bake in the oven for 25 minutes.
8. Stir frequently until vegetables are soft and lightly browned and chickpeas are crisp, for about 20 to 25 minutes more.
9. Season with more salt and black pepper to taste, top with the green onion before serving.

421. Roasted Carrot Turnip and Parsnips

Main Ingredients

- 3 large tomatoes, cut into 1-inch pieces
- 3 red onion, diced
- 1 sweet turnips, peeled and cut into 1-inch cubes
- 2 large carrots, cut into 1 inch pieces
- 3 medium parsnips, cut into 1-inch pieces
- 3 tablespoons extra virgin olive oil
- Seasoning ingredients
- 1 teaspoon salt

- 1/2 teaspoon ground black pepper
- 1 teaspoon onion powder
- 2 teaspoon garlic powder
- 1 teaspoon Spanish paprika
- 1 teaspoon cumin
- Garnishing Ingredients
- 2 sprigs parsley, chopped (optional)

Directions

1. Preheat your oven to 350 degrees F.
2. Grease your baking pan.
3. Combine the main ingredients on the prepared sheet pan.
4. Drizzle with the oil and toss to coat.
5. Combine the seasoning ingredients in a bowl
6. Sprinkle them over the vegetables on the pan and toss to coat with seasonings.
7. Bake in the oven for 25 minutes.
8. Stir frequently until vegetables are soft, for about 20 to 25 minutes more.
9. Season with more salt and black pepper to taste, top with the parsley before serving.

422. Roasted Aromatic Tomatoes

Ingredients

- 3 large tomatoes, cut into 1-inch pieces
- 1/2 butternut squash - peeled, seeded, and cut into 1-inch pieces
- 2 red onion, diced
- 1 sweet potato, peeled and cut into 1-inch cubes
- 12 cherry tomatoes, sliced in half
- 3 medium potatoes, cut into 1-inch pieces
- 3 tablespoons extra virgin olive oil
- Seasoning ingredients
- 1 teaspoon salt
- 1/2 teaspoon ground black pepper
- 1 teaspoon onion powder
- 2 teaspoon garlic powder
- 2 tablespoons lemon grass, finely chopped
- Garnishing Ingredients
- 2 sprigs parsley, chopped (optional)

Directions

1. Preheat your oven to 350 degrees F.
2. Grease your baking pan.
3. Combine the main ingredients on the prepared sheet pan.
4. Drizzle with the oil and toss to coat.
5. Combine the seasoning ingredients in a bowl
6. Sprinkle them over the vegetables on the pan and toss to coat with seasonings.
7. Bake in the oven for 25 minutes.
8. Stir frequently until vegetables are soft and lightly browned and chickpeas are crisp, for about 20 to 25 minutes more.
9. Season with more salt and black pepper to taste, top with the parsley before serving.

423. Oriental Roasted Bean Sprouts and Broccoli

Ingredients

- 1 large broccoli, sliced
- 1 cup bean sprouts
- 1/2 butternut squash - peeled, seeded, and cut into 1-inch pieces
- 2 red onions, diced
- 2 large carrots, cut into 1 inch pieces
- 4 medium potatoes, cut into 1-inch pieces
- 3 tablespoons sesame oil
- Seasoning ingredients
- 1 teaspoon sea salt
- 1/2 teaspoon ground black pepper
- 1 teaspoon onion powder
- 2 teaspoon garlic powder
- 1 teaspoon Sichuan peppercorns
- Garnishing Ingredients
- 2 green onions, chopped (optional)

Directions

1. Preheat your oven to 350 degrees F.
2. Grease your baking pan.
3. Combine the main ingredients on the prepared sheet pan.
4. Drizzle with the oil and toss to coat.
5. Combine the seasoning ingredients in a bowl
6. Sprinkle them over the vegetables on the pan and toss to coat with seasonings.
7. Bake in the oven for 25 minutes.
8. Stir frequently until vegetables are soft and lightly browned and chickpeas are crisp, for about 20 to 25 minutes more.
9. Season with more salt and black pepper to taste, top with the green onion before serving.

424. Roasted Broccoli and Onion

Ingredients

- 1 large broccoli, sliced
- 1 cup bean sprouts
- 1 large red onion, diced
- 1 sweet potato, peeled and cut into 1-inch cubes
- 2 large carrots, cut into 1 inch pieces
- 3 medium potatoes, cut into 1-inch pieces

- 3 tablespoons canola oil
- Seasoning ingredients
- 1 teaspoon salt
- 1/2 teaspoon ground black pepper
- 1 teaspoon cayenne pepper
- 2 teaspoon garlic powder
- Garnishing Ingredients
- 2 green onions, chopped (optional)

Directions

1. Preheat your oven to 350 degrees F.
2. Grease your baking pan.
3. Combine the main ingredients on the prepared sheet pan.
4. Drizzle with the oil and toss to coat.
5. Combine the seasoning ingredients in a bowl
6. Sprinkle them over the vegetables on the pan and toss to coat with seasonings.
7. Bake in the oven for 25 minutes.
8. Stir frequently until vegetables are soft and lightly browned and chickpeas are crisp, for about 20 to 25 minutes more.
9. Season with more salt and black pepper to taste, top with the green onion before serving.

425. Roasted Brussel Sprouts and Bean Sprouts

Ingredients

- 1 large broccoli, sliced
- 1 cup bean sprouts
- 1 red onion, diced
- 8 pcs. brussel sprouts
- 2 large carrots, cut into 1 inch pieces
- 3 medium potatoes, cut into 1-inch pieces
- 3 tablespoons extra virgin olive oil
- Seasoning ingredients
- 1 teaspoon salt
- 1/2 teaspoon ground black pepper
- 1 teaspoon onion powder
- 2 teaspoon garlic powder
- 1 teaspoon ground fennel seeds
- 1 teaspoon dried rubbed sage
- Garnishing Ingredients
- 2 green onions, chopped (optional)

Directions

1. Preheat your oven to 350 degrees F.
2. Grease your baking pan.
3. Combine the main ingredients on the prepared sheet pan.
4. Drizzle with the oil and toss to coat.
5. Combine the seasoning ingredients in a bowl
6. Sprinkle them over the vegetables on the pan and toss to coat with seasonings.
7. Bake in the oven for 25 minutes.
8. Stir frequently until vegetables are soft and lightly browned and chickpeas are crisp, for about 20 to 25 minutes more.
9. Season with more salt and black pepper to taste, top with the green onion before serving.

426. Roasted Butterbeans and Broccoli

Ingredients

- 2 (15 ounce) cans butterbeans, rinsed and drained
- 1/2 butternut squash - peeled, seeded, and cut into 1-inch pieces
- 1 red onion, diced
- 1 large broccoli, sliced
- 2 large carrots, cut into 1 inch pieces
- 3 medium potatoes, cut into 1-inch pieces
- 3 tablespoons canola oil
- Seasoning ingredients
- 1 teaspoon salt
- 1/2 teaspoon ground black pepper
- 1 teaspoon onion powder
- 2 teaspoon garlic powder
- 1 teaspoon herbs de Provence
- Garnishing Ingredients
- 2 green onions, chopped (optional)

Directions

1. Preheat your oven to 350 degrees F.
2. Grease your baking pan.
3. Combine the main ingredients on the prepared sheet pan.
4. Drizzle with the oil and toss to coat.
5. Combine the seasoning ingredients in a bowl
6. Sprinkle them over the vegetables on the pan and toss to coat with seasonings.
7. Bake in the oven for 25 minutes.
8. Stir frequently until vegetables are soft and lightly browned and chickpeas are crisp, for about 20 to 25 minutes more.
9. Season with more salt and black pepper to taste, top with the green onion before serving.

427. Lemon Garlic Roasted Potatoes

Ingredients

- 1 large broccoli, sliced
- 1 cup bean sprouts
- 1 red onion, diced

- 1 sweet potato, peeled and cut into 1-inch cubes
- 2 large carrots, cut into 1 inch pieces
- 3 medium potatoes, cut into 1-inch pieces
- 3 tablespoons melted vegan butter/ margarine
- Seasoning ingredients
- 1 teaspoon lemon salt
- 1/2 teaspoon ground black pepper
- 1 teaspoon onion powder
- 2 teaspoon garlic powder
- Garnishing Ingredients
- 2 green onions, chopped (optional)

Directions

1. Preheat your oven to 350 degrees F.
2. Grease your baking pan.
3. Combine the main ingredients on the prepared sheet pan.
4. Drizzle with the oil and toss to coat.
5. Combine the seasoning ingredients in a bowl
6. Sprinkle them over the vegetables on the pan and toss to coat with seasonings.
7. Bake in the oven for 25 minutes.
8. Stir frequently until vegetables are soft and lightly browned and chickpeas are crisp, for about 20 to 25 minutes more.
9. Season with more salt and black pepper to taste, top with the green onion before serving.

428. Buttery Roasted Broccoli

Ingredients

- 1 large broccoli, sliced
- 1 cup bean sprouts
- 1 red onion, diced
- 1 sweet potato, peeled and cut into 1-inch cubes
- 2 large parsnips, cut into 1 inch pieces
- 3 medium potatoes, cut into 1-inch pieces
- 3 tablespoons melted vegan butter/ margarine
- Seasoning ingredients
- 1 teaspoon salt
- 1/2 teaspoon rainbow peppercorns
- 1 teaspoon onion powder
- 2 teaspoon garlic powder
- 1 teaspoon annatto seeds
- 1 teaspoon cumin
- Garnishing Ingredients
- 2 green onions, chopped (optional)

Directions

1. Preheat your oven to 350 degrees F.
2. Grease your baking pan.
3. Combine the main ingredients on the prepared sheet pan.
4. Drizzle with the oil and toss to coat.
5. Combine the seasoning ingredients in a bowl
6. Sprinkle them over the vegetables on the pan and toss to coat with seasonings.
7. Bake in the oven for 25 minutes.
8. Stir frequently until vegetables are soft and lightly browned and chickpeas are crisp, for about 20 to 25 minutes more.
9. Season with more salt and black pepper to taste, top with the green onion before serving.

429. Roasted Broccoli and Bean Sprouts

Ingredients

- 1 large broccoli, sliced
- 1 cup bean sprouts
- 1 yellow onion, diced
- 1 sweet potato, peeled and cut into 1-inch cubes
- 2 large carrots, cut into 1 inch pieces
- 3 medium potatoes, cut into 1-inch pieces
- 3 tablespoons canola oil
- Seasoning ingredients
- 1 teaspoon salt
- 1/2 teaspoon ground black pepper
- 1 teaspoon onion powder
- 2 teaspoon garlic powder
- Garnishing Ingredients
- 2 green onions, chopped (optional)

Directions

1. Preheat your oven to 350 degrees F.
2. Grease your baking pan.
3. Combine the main ingredients on the prepared sheet pan.
4. Drizzle with the oil and toss to coat.
5. Combine the seasoning ingredients in a bowl
6. Sprinkle them over the vegetables on the pan and toss to coat with seasonings.
7. Bake in the oven for 25 minutes.
8. Stir frequently until vegetables are soft and lightly browned and chickpeas are crisp, for about 20 to 25 minutes more.
9. Season with more salt and black pepper to taste, top with the green onion before serving.

430. Simple and Easy Roasted Parsnips and Potato

Ingredients

- 1 large broccoli, sliced
- 1 cup bean sprouts
- 1 red onion, diced

- 1 sweet potato, peeled and cut into 1-inch cubes
- 2 large parsnips, cut into 1 inch pieces
- 3 medium potatoes, cut into 1-inch pieces
- 3 tablespoons macadamia nut oil
- Seasoning ingredients
- 1 teaspoon salt
- 1/2 teaspoon ground black pepper
- 1 teaspoon onion powder
- 2 teaspoon garlic powder
- Garnishing Ingredients
- 2 green onions, chopped (optional)

Directions
1. Preheat your oven to 350 degrees F.
2. Grease your baking pan.
3. Combine the main ingredients on the prepared sheet pan.
4. Drizzle with the oil and toss to coat.
5. Combine the seasoning ingredients in a bowl
6. Sprinkle them over the vegetables on the pan and toss to coat with seasonings.
7. Bake in the oven for 25 minutes.
8. Stir frequently until vegetables are soft and lightly browned and chickpeas are crisp, for about 20 to 25 minutes more.
9. Season with more salt and black pepper to taste, top with the green onion before serving.

431. Baked Beets and Potato

Ingredients
- 1 ½ cups Brussels sprouts, trimmed
- 1 cup large potato chunks
- 1 cup large rainbow carrot chunks
- 1 ½ cup cauliflower florets
- 1 cup cubed red beets
- 1/2 cup red onion chunks
- 2 tablespoons extra-virgin olive oil
- salt and ground black pepper to taste

Directions
1. Preheat your oven to 425 degrees F (220 degrees C).
2. Set the rack to the second-lowest level in the oven.
3. Pour some lightly salted water in a bowl.
4. Submerge the Brussels sprouts in salted water for 15 minutes and drain.
5. Place the rest of the ingredients together in a bowl.
6. Spread the vegetables in a single layer onto a baking pan.
7. Roast in the oven until the vegetables start to brown and cook through, for about 45 minutes.

432. Roasted Carrots and Sweet Potato

Ingredients
- 3/4 cup Brussels sprouts, trimmed
- cup large sweet potato chunks
- cup large rainbow carrot chunks
- 1 ½ cup broccoli florets
- 1 cup cubed red beets
- 1/2 cup red onion chunks
- 2 tablespoons extra-virgin olive oil
- Sea salt
- ground black pepper to taste

Directions
2. Preheat your oven to 425 degrees F (220 degrees C).
3. Set the rack to the second-lowest level in the oven.
4. Pour some lightly salted water in a bowl.
5. Submerge the Brussels sprouts in salted water for 15 minutes and drain.
6. Place the rest of the ingredients together in a bowl.
7. Spread the vegetables in a single layer onto a baking pan.
8. Roast in the oven until the vegetables start to brown and cook through, for about 45 minutes.

433. Roasted Broccoli and Red Beets

Ingredients
- 1 ½ cups Brussels sprouts, trimmed
- 1 cup large potato chunks
- 1 cup large carrot chunks
- 1 ½ cup broccoli florets
- 1 cup cubed red beets
- 1/2 cup yellow onion chunks
- 2 tablespoons sesame seed oil
- salt and ground black pepper to taste

Directions
1. Preheat your oven to 425 degrees F (220 degrees C).
2. Set the rack to the second-lowest level in the oven.
3. Pour some lightly salted water in a bowl.
4. Submerge the Brussels sprouts in salted water for 15 minutes and drain.
5. Place the rest of the ingredients together in a bowl.
6. Spread the vegetables in a single layer onto a

434. Roasted Cauliflower and Parsnip

Ingredients

- 1 ½ cups mini cabbage, trimmed
- 1 cup large potato chunks
- 1 cup large parsnip, chunks
- 1 ½ cup cauliflower florets
- 1 cup cubed red beets
- 1/2 cup red onion chunks
- 2 tablespoons extra-virgin olive oil
- salt and ground black pepper to taste

Directions

1. Preheat your oven to 425 degrees F (220 degrees C).
2. Set the rack to the second-lowest level in the oven.
3. Pour some lightly salted water in a bowl.
4. Submerge the mini cabbage in salted water for 15 minutes and drain.
5. Place the rest of the ingredients together in a bowl.
6. Spread the vegetables in a single layer onto a baking pan.
7. Roast in the oven until the vegetables start to brown and cook through, for about 45 minutes.

435. Roasted Carrot and Beets

Ingredients

- 1 ½ cups purple cabbage, trimmed
- 1 cup large sweet potato chunks
- 1 cup large carrot chunks
- 1 ½ cup cauliflower florets
- 1 cup cubed red beets
- 1/2 cup red onion chunks
- 2 tablespoons extra-virgin olive oil
- salt and ground black pepper to taste

Directions

1. Preheat your oven to 425 degrees F (220 degrees C).
2. Set the rack to the second-lowest level in the oven.
3. Pour some lightly salted water in a bowl.
4. Submerge the purple cabbage in salted water for 15 minutes and drain.
5. Place the rest of the ingredients together in a bowl.
6. Spread the vegetables in a single layer onto a baking pan.
7. Roast in the oven until the vegetables start to brown and cook through, for about 45 minutes.

436. Roasted Cabbage and Beets

Ingredients

- ½ cup Brussels sprouts, trimmed
- ½ cup cabbage, trimmed
- ½ cup purple cabbage
- 1 cup large potato chunks
- 1 cup large rainbow carrot chunks
- 1 ½ cup cauliflower florets
- 1 cup cubed red beets
- 1/2 cup red onion chunks
- 2 tablespoons extra-virgin olive oil
- salt and ground black pepper to taste

Directions

1. Preheat your oven to 425 degrees F (220 degrees C).
2. Set the rack to the second-lowest level in the oven.
3. Pour some lightly salted water in a bowl.
4. Submerge the Brussels sprouts and cabbages in salted water for 15 minutes and drain.
5. Place the rest of the ingredients together in a bowl.
6. Spread the vegetables in a single layer onto a baking pan.
7. Roast in the oven until the vegetables start to brown and cook through, for about 45 minutes.

VEGAN

437. Vegan Tzatziki Tofu

Servings: 4
Preparation and Cooking: 40 minutes

Ingredients

- 12 ounces 1/4-inch thick sliced and pressed tofu.
- 1 cup chopped scallions.
- 1 minced garlic clove.
- 2tbs. Champagne Vinegar.
- 2tbs. Sesame oil.
- 1tbs. Sriracha sauce.
- For Vegan Tzatziki:
- 2 cloves pressed garlic.
- 2tbs. fresh lemon juice.
- 1 shredded cucumber.
- 1tbs. fresh or dried dill weed.
- 1cup non-dairy yogurt.
- Sea salt and ground black pepper to taste.

Directions

1. In a bowl, Combine the tofu slices, scallions, garlic, vinegar, and Sriracha sauce and let it rise for 30 minutes.
2. In a nonstick skillet, heat the oil over medium-high heat, and then cook tofu until it is golden brown on each side for about 5 minutes.
3. To make vegan tzatziki, mix garlic, lemon juice, salt, black pepper, dill and yogurt in a mixing bowl.
4. Pour in shredded cucumber and stir thoroughly until everything is well incorporated.
5. Place the tzatziki in the refrigerator until ready to serve.
6. Divide tofu among serving plates and serve with a dollop of tzatziki. Enjoy!

Nutrition Value: 162 Calories; 10.9g Fat; 5.8g Carbs; 9.5g Protein; 3.3g Sugars

438. Avocado with Low-carb Mushrooms

Servings: 8
Preparation and Cooking: 10 minutes

Ingredients

- 4 pitted and halved avocados.
- 2 cups chopped button mushrooms.
- 1 chopped onion.
- 1 chopped tomato.
- 1 tbs. deli mustard.
- 1 tbs. crushed garlic.
- 2tbs. olive oil.
- Salt and black pepper to taste.

Directions

1. Scoop about 2tbs. of avocado flesh from each half and then reserve scooped avocado flash until ready for use.
2. Preheat a sauté pan over a moderately high flame, then heat up the oil in the preheated pan.
3. Cook the mushrooms, onion, and garlic until the mushrooms are tender and the onion is translucent.
4. Incorporate the reserved avocado flash to the mushroom mixture and combine. Put the salt, black pepper, mustard, and tomato.
5. Divide the mushroom mixture among avocado halves and serve immediately. Enjoy!

Nutrition Value: 245 Calories; 23.2g Fat; 6.2g Carbs; 2.4g Protein; 1.5g Sugars

439. Stir-Fried Tofu and Peppers

Servings: 2
Preparation and Cooking: 40 minutes

Ingredients

- 12 ounces pressed and cubed extra firm tofu.
- 1 deveined and sliced red bell pepper.
- 1 deveined and sliced green bell pepper.
- 1 deveined and sliced serrano pepper.
- 1/2 teaspoon paprika.
- 1/2 teaspoon ground bay leaf.
- 1 teaspoon garlic paste.
- 1 teaspoon shallot powder.
- 1 ½tbs. flaxseed meal.
- 1tbs. olive oil.
- Salt and ground black pepper to taste.

Directions

1. Carefully combine the tofu, flaxseed meal, salt, black pepper, garlic paste, paprika, shallot powder, and ground bay leaf in a container.
2. Cover the container firmly, then toss to coat. Let it marinate at least 30 minutes.
3. Pour olive oil in a saucepan and heat over a moderate flame.
4. Cook your tofu along with peppers for between 5 and 7 minutes; gently stirring.
5. Serve immediately and enjoy!

Nutrition Value: 223 Calories; 15.9g Fat; 5.1g Carbs; 15.6g Protein; 2g Sugars

440. Pecans-Spiced Cubed Tofu

Servings: 4
Preparation and Cooking: 13 minutes

Ingredients

- 1cup pressed and cubed extra firm tofu.
- 1/4 cup coarsely chopped pecans.
- 2 teaspoons sunflower seeds.
- 1 teaspoon cayenne pepper.
- 3tbs. vegetable broth.
- 1 ½tbs. soy sauce.
- 1/2tbs. granulated garlic.
- 1/2tbs. turmeric powder.
- 3tbs. olive oil
- Sea salt and ground black pepper to taste.

Directions

1. In a frying pan that is preheated over a moderate heat, pour the oil and let it heat up.
2. Put the tofu cubes in the heated oil and fry them until both sides are golden brown while carefully stirring periodically.
3. Carefully stir in the pecans and then increase the temperature. Cook on high for 2 minutes or more until fragrant.
4. Combine the remaining ingredients, and then cook on medium-low heat for an additional 5 minutes.
5. Serve drizzled with hot sauce and enjoy!

Nutrition Value: 232 Calories; 21.6g Fat; 5.3g Carbs; 8.3g Protein; 1.4g Sugars

441. Kale Dip with Crudités Platter

Servings: 6
Preparation and Cooking: 25minutes

Ingredients

- 2cups kale.
- 2 minced garlic cloves.
- 2tbs. nutritional yeast.
- 1cup pressed, drained and crumbled tofu.
- 1/2cup soy milk.
- 1/2tbs. paprika.
- 1/2tbs. dried dill weed.
- 2 tbs. olive oil.
- 1tbs. sea salt.
- 1tbs. dried basil.
- 1/4tbs. ground black pepper or more to taste.

Directions

1. Preheat your oven to 400 degree F. and then lightly apply oil to a casserole dish with a nonstick cooking spray.
2. Parboil the kale leaves until it is just wilted. Puree the remaining ingredients in your food processor or blender.
3. Put the kale and then stir until the mixture is homogeneous. Firmly lock your oven then bake for approximately 13 minutes.
4. Serve with a crudités platter. Serve!!

442. Stuffed Mushrooms topped with Vegan Parmesan

Servings: 4
Preparation and Cooking: 35 minutes

Ingredients

- 1 pound cleaned medium-sized brown cremini mushrooms.
- 1 finely chopped onion.
- 1 chopped bell pepper.
- 1 cup vegan parmesan
- 1/2 head cauliflower.
- 1 teaspoon Italian seasoning mix
- 1tbs. minced garlic.
- 2tbs. vegetable oil.
- Salt and black pepper to taste.

Directions

1. Cook the cauliflower in a large pot of salted water until tender for about 6 minutes and then cut into florets.
2. Pulse cauliflower florets in your food processor until they resemble small rice-like granules.
3. Preheat an oven to 360 degrees F. Bake mushroom caps for 8 to 12 minutes or more until they are just tender.
4. Heat the oil in a heavy-bottomed skillet. Sauté the onion, garlic and bell pepper until they are softened.
5. Carefully combine the Italian seasoning mix along with salt and pepper. Taste to adjust seasonings, and then fold in cauliflower rice.
6. Divide the filling mixture among mushroom caps. Top with vegan parmesan and bake 17 minutes longer.
7. Serve warm. Ready to eat.

Nutrition Value: 206 Calories; 13.4g Fat; 5.6g Carbs; 12.7g Protein; 3.6g Sugars

443. Healthy Zucchini Avocado Soup

Servings: 4
Preparation and Cooking: 45 minutes

Ingredients

- 3cups peeled and chopped zucchini.
- 4cups water.
- 1 chopped yellow onion.

- 1 sliced carrot.
- 1 sliced parsnip.
- 1 pureed tomato.
- 1 peeled and diced avocado pitted.
- 1tbs. vegetable bouillon powder.
- 3tbs. vegetable oil.
- 1/4tbs. ground black pepper.

Directions
1. Preheated a heavy-bottomed pot over a moderate heat. Pour the oil and heat it up. Sweat the onions until they are softened.
2. Carefully combine the carrot, parsnip, and zucchini in the pot and cook for 7 more minutes. Season with black pepper.
3. Pour the water, vegetable bouillon powder, and pureed tomato, and then boil quickly. Turn the heat to medium-low and let it simmer for 18 minutes.
4. Incorporate the reserved vegetables and simmer for a further 18 minutes. Remove from heat and stir in the avocado. Blend the soup in batches until smooth and creamy.
5. Serve hot!

Nutrition Value: 165 Calories; 13.4g Fat; 6.7g Carbs; 2.2g Protein; 3.3g Sugars

444. Sautéed Stuffed Mushrooms
Servings: 4
Preparation and Cooking: 30 minutes

Ingredients
- 1 minced garlic clove.
- 1pound clean white mushrooms.
- 1cup chopped onions.
- 1/4cup crushed raw walnuts.
- 2tbs. chopped cilantro.
- 2tbs. sesame oil.
- Salt and black pepper to taste.

Directions
1. Preheat an oven to 360 degrees F. Lightly grease a large baking sheet with a nonstick cooking spray.
2. Heat sesame oil in a frying pan that is preheated over medium-high heat. Sauté the onions and garlic until aromatic.
3. Carefully chop the mushroom stems and cook until they are tender. Season with salt and pepper, and then stir in walnuts.
4. Stuff the mushroom caps with walnut/mushroom mixture and arrange them on the prepared baking sheet. Bake for 25 minutes and transfer to a wire rack to cool

slightly.
5. Garnish with fresh cilantro and serve. Serve!!

Nutrition Value: 139 Calories; 11.2g Fat; 5.4g Carbs; 4.8g Protein; 2.6g Sugars

445. Dark Chocolate Almond Butter Smoothie
Servings: 2
Preparation and Cooking: 10 minutes

Ingredients
- 8 walnuts.
- 4 pitted fresh dates.
- 1/4 cup water.
- 1 ½ cups lettuce.
- 3/4cup almond milk.
- 2tbs. zero carb vegan protein powder.
- 1tbs chia seeds.
- 1tbs. Unsweetened cocoa powder.

Directions
1. Carefully combine all ingredients and process all in your blender until everything is uniform and creamy.
2. Divide between two glasses and serve well-chilled.

Nutrition Value: 335 Calories; 31.7g Fat; 5.7g Carbs; 7g Protein; 3.9g Sugars

446. Chanterelle Leek Stew
Servings: 4
Preparation and Cooking: 25 minutes

Ingredients
- 2 chopped rosemary sprigs.
- 2 pressed garlic cloves.
- 2 chopped carrots.
- 2 pureed ripe tomatoes.
- 1 chopped thyme sprig.
- 3 ½cups roasted vegetable stock.
- 1cup chopped leeks.
- 1cup sliced fresh Chanterelle.
- 1/2cup chopped celery with leaves.
- 1tbs. Hungarian paprika.
- 1tbs. flaxseed meal.
- 2tbs. dry red wine.
- 2tbs. olive oil.
- 1/2tbs. cayenne pepper.

Directions
1. In a stockpot, heat the oil over a moderate flame and cook the leeks on low until they are tender.
2. Put the garlic, celery, and carrots and cook for a

further 4 minutes or more until they are softened.
3. Put the Chanterelle mushrooms, then cook until they are dry. Reserve the vegetables until ready for use.
4. Pour the wine to deglaze the bottom of the stockpot.
5. Combine the rosemary, thyme, roasted vegetable stock, cayenne pepper, Hungarian paprika, and tomatoes. Stir in the reserved vegetables and then boil on medium heat.
6. Reduce heat to a simmer. With the stockpot firmly sealed, let it simmer for an additional 15 minutes. Put the flaxseed meal to thicken the soup.
7. Serve in individual soup bowls with a few sprinkles of Hungarian paprika.

Nutrition Value: 114 Calories; 7.3g Fat; 5.2g Carbs; 2.1g Protein; 2.3g Sugars

447. Parmesan Tomato Chips Bakes

Servings 6
Preparation and Cooking: 5 hours

Ingredients

- 1 ½pounds sliced tomatoes.
- 1/4cup extra-virgin olive oil.
- 1tbs. Italian seasoning mix.
- For Vegan Parmesan:
- 1/2cup pumpkin seeds.
- 1 tablespoon nutritional yeast.
- 1tbs. garlic powder.
- Salt and black pepper to taste.

Directions

1. Drizzle sliced tomatoes with olive oil.
2. Preheat your oven to 200 degrees F. Coat a baking pan with Silpat mat.
3. Pulse all the parmesan ingredients in your food processor until you reach a Parmesan cheese consistency.
4. Combine parmesan with Italian seasoning mix. Then, toss seasoned tomato slices with parmesan mixture until they are well coated.
5. Arrange tomato slices on the baking pan and bake for 5 hours.
6. Store in an airtight container until it is ready to be served.

Nutrition Value: 161 Calories; 14g Fat; 6.2g Carbs; 4.6g Protein; 3g Sugars

448. Roasted Asparagus topped Baba Ghanoush

Servings: 6
Preparation and Cooking: 45 minutes

Ingredients

- 1 ½pounds asparagus spears.
- 1/2tbs. paprika.
- 1/4cup olive oil.
- 1tbs. sea salt.
- 1/2tbs. ground black pepper to taste.
- For Baba Ghanoush:
- 2 minced cloves garlic.
- 3/4 pound eggplant.
- 2tbs. olive oil.
- 2tbs. fresh lemon juice.
- 1/2cup chopped scallions.
- 1tbs. tahini.
- 1/2tbs cayenne pepper.
- 1/4cup chopped fresh parsley leaves.
- Salt and ground black pepper to taste.

Directions

1. Preheat your oven to 390 degrees F. Line a baking sheet with parchment paper, and then place the asparagus spears on the baking sheet.
2. Carefully toss asparagus spears with the oil, salt, pepper, and paprika. Bake for about 9 minutes or more until thoroughly cooked.
3. To make Baba Ghanoush, Preheat your oven to 425 degrees F.
4. Place the eggplants on a lined cookie sheet. Set under the broiler approximately 30 minutes. Allow eggplants to cool, then peel the eggplants and remove the stems.
5. Heat 2tbs. of olive oil in a frying pan over a moderately high flame. Sauté the scallions and garlic until tender and aromatic.
6. Combine the roasted eggplant, scallion mixture, tahini, lemon juice, cayenne pepper, salt and black pepper and pour in your food processor.
7. Pulse until ingredients are evenly mixed and garnish with parsley.
8. Serve with roasted asparagus spears. Serve!!

Nutrition Value: 149 Calories; 12.1g Fat; 6.3g Carbs; 3.6g Protein; 3.3g Sugars

449. Homemade Creamy Broccoli Soup

Servings: 4
Preparation and Cooking:15 minutes

Ingredients

- 1pound broccoli cut into small florets.
- 8ounces kale leaves torn into small pieces.
- 2 finely chopped shallots.

- 4cups vegetable broth
- 1/2cup almond milk
- 1tbs. minced garlic.
- 1/2tbs. crushed red pepper flakes
- 1/2tbs. kosher salt
- 2tbs. coarsely chopped chives.
- 2tbs.cool coconut oil.

Directions

1. Preheat your pot over a moderate flame. Pour the coconut oil in the pot and let it heat up. Sauté the shallots and garlic until they're fragrant and slightly browned.
2. Combine the broccoli, kale and vegetable broth and then boil for 5 minutes.
3. Carefully pour in the almond milk, salt and pepper. With the pot firmly sealed, let your soup simmer over a moderate flame.
4. Blend the soup with an immersion blender.
5. Serve right away garnished with fresh chopped chives.

Nutrition Value: 252 Calories; 20.3g Fat; 5.8g Carbs; 8.1g Protein; 2.4g Sugars

450. Orange Pecans Stuffed Avocado

Servings: 4
Preparation: 10 minutes

Ingredients

- 2 peeled and pitted avocados.
- 2 chopped carrots.
- 5ounces ground pecans.
- 1 garlic clove
- 1tbs. lemon juice.
- 1tbs. soy sauce.
- Salt and freshly ground black pepper to taste

Directions

1. In a mixing bowl, thoroughly combine avocado pulp with pecans, carrots, garlic, lemon juice, and soy sauce.
2. Season with salt and black pepper to taste.
3. Divide the mixture among avocado halves.
4. You can add some extra pecans for garnish. Serve!!

Nutrition Value: 263 Calories; 24.8g Fat; 6.5g Carbs; 3.5g Protein; 2.5g Sugars

451. Pepper-Spiced Roasted Curried Cauliflower

Servings: 4
Preparation and Cooking: 35 minutes

Ingredients

- 1 pound cauliflower broken into florets
- 2 halved bell peppers.
- 2 halved pasilla peppers.
- 1tbs. curry powder.
- 1/2tbs. cayenne pepper.
- 1/2tbs. nigella seeds.
- 1/2tbs. sea salt.
- 1/4cup extra-virgin olive oil.
- 1/4tbs. freshly ground black pepper or more to taste.

Directions

1. Preheat your oven to 425 degrees F. Line a large baking sheet with a piece of parchment paper.
2. Drizzle cauliflower and peppers with extra-virgin olive oil. Sprinkle with salt, black pepper, cayenne pepper, curry powder and nigella seeds.
3. Arrange the vegetables on the prepared baking sheet.
4. Roast the vegetables while tossing periodically until they are slightly browned for about 30 minutes.
5. Serve with a homemade tomato dip or mushroom pate. Serve!!

Nutrition Value: 166 Calories; 13.9g Fat; 5.4g Carbs; 3g Protein; 2.4g Sugars

452. Cashew Nuts Baked Tofu Stuffed Zucchini

Servings: 4
Preparation and Cooking: 50 minutes

Ingredients

- 2 12-ounce packages drained and crumbled firm tofu.
- 2ounces lightly salted and chopped cashew nuts.
- 4 scooped halved zucchinis.
- 1/2cup chopped scallions.
- 2 pressed garlic cloves.
- 2cups tomato puree.
- 1tbs nutritional yeast.
- 1/4tbs chili powder.
- 1/4tbs. turmeric.
- 1tbs. olive oil.
- Sea salt and cayenne pepper to taste.

Directions

1. In a pan that is preheated over a moderate heat, pour the oil and let it heat up and then cook the tofu, garlic, and scallions on low for 4 to 6 minutes.
2. Put 1 cup of tomato puree and scooped zucchini flesh. Carefully combine all seasonings

and cook an additional 6 minutes until tofu is slightly browned.
3. Preheat your oven to 360 degrees F.
4. Divide the tofu mixture among zucchini shells. Place stuffed zucchini shells in a baking dish that is previously greased with a cooking spray.
5. Pour in the remaining 1 cup of tomato puree. Bake approximately 30 minutes. Sprinkle with nutritional yeast and cashew nuts, and then bake for an additional 5 to 6 minutes.
6. Serve and Enjoy!

Nutrition Value: 148 Calories; 10g Fat; 4.8g Carbs; 7.5g Protein; 2.5g Sugars

453. Garlic-Avocado Spinach Chips

Servings: 6
Preparation and Cooking: 20 minutes

Ingredients

- 3 pitted ripe avocados.
- 2tbs. lime juice.
- Salt and black pepper to taste
- 2 finely minced garlic cloves
- 2tbs extra-virgin olive oil
- 1/2tbs red pepper flakes.
- For Spinach Chips:
- 2cups washed and dried baby spinach, washed and dried
- 1tbs. olive oil
- Sea salt and garlic powder to taste

Directions

1. Mash avocado pulp with a fork. Pour the fresh lime juice, salt, pepper, garlic, and 2tbs. of olive oil.
2. Thoroughly mix until everything is well incorporated. Transfer to a serving bowl and sprinkle with red pepper flakes.
3. Preheat your oven to 300 degrees F. Line a baking sheet with a Silpat mat.
4. Arrange spinach leaves on the baking sheet, then toss with 1 tablespoon of olive oil, salt, and garlic powder.
5. Bake for 8 to 12 minutes so the leaves have dried up.
6. Serve with well-chilled avocado dip. Serve!!

Nutrition Value: 269 Calories; 26.7g Fat; 3.4g Carbs; 2.3g Protein; 0.6g Sugars

454. Brussels Sprouts and Tempeh Hash with Soy Dressing

Servings: 4
Preparation and Cooking: 20 minutes

Ingredients

- 2 minced garlic cloves.
- 10ounces crumbled tempeh.
- 1/2pound quartered Brussels sprouts.
- 1/2cup chopped leeks.
- 1tbs. tomato puree
- 2tbs. water.
- 2tbs. soy sauce.
- 2tbs olive oil.
- Sea salt and ground black pepper to taste

Directions

1. Heat the oil in a saucepan that is preheated over a moderate heat. Cook the garlic and leeks until tender and aromatic.
2. Pour the water, tempeh, and soy sauce. Cook until the tempeh just beginning to brown, about 5 minutes.
3. Stir in shredded cabbage and season with salt and pepper. Turn the heat to low and cook, stirring often for about 13 minutes.
4. Serve warm.

Nutrition Value: 179 Calories; 11.7g Fat; 2.1g Carbs; 10.5g Protein; 0.7g Sugars

455. Spicy Garam Masala Broccoli

Servings: 4
Preparation and Cooking: 15 minutes

Ingredients

- 3/4pound broccoli broken into florets
- 1 smashed garlic clove.
- 1tbs sesame paste.
- 1/2 teaspoon Garam Masala.
- 1tbs. fresh lime juice.
- 1/4cup extra-virgin olive oil
- Seasoned salt and ground black pepper to taste.

Directions

1. Steam broccoli for 7 minutes until it is crisp-tender but still vibrant green. Pulse in your blender or a food processor until rice-like consistency is achieved.
2. Pour the oil and then combine with salt, black paper, garlic, sesame paste, fresh lime juice and Garam Masala.
3. Blend until everything is well incorporated. Drizzle with some extra olive oil.
4. You may serve immediately. Otherwise, keep in your refrigerator until ready to serve.

Nutrition Value: 100 Calories; 8.2g Fat; 4.7g Carbs; 3.7g Protein; 0.9g Sugars

456. Cashew Parmesan Zoodles

Servings: 4

Preparation and Cooking: 15 minutes

Ingredients

For Zoodles:
- 4 peeled zucchinis.
- 1/2 cup water.
- 2tbs. olive oil.
- Salt and cayenne pepper to taste

For Cashew Parmesan:
- 1/2 cup raw cashews.
- 2tbs. nutritional yeast.
- 1/2tbs. garlic powder.
- 1/4tbs. shallot powder.
- Sea salt and black pepper to taste.

Directions

1. Slice the zucchinis into long strips i.e. noodle-shape strands.
2. Heat the oil in a pan over medium heat, and then cook zucchini for about 1 minute; stirring continuously.
3. Pour in water and cook 6 more minutes. Season with salt and cayenne pepper to taste.
4. Pulse all parmesan ingredients in your food processor until you reach a Parmesan cheese consistency.
5. Top cooked zoodles with cashew parmesan and enjoy!

Nutrition Value: 145 Calories; 10.6g Fat; 5.9g Carbs; 5.5g Protein; 3.3g Sugars

457. Summer Salad dressed with Sunflower Seed.

Servings: 4
Preparation and Cooking: 3 hours 15 minutes

Ingredients

For Sunflower Seed Dressing:
- 1cup raw and hulled sunflower seeds.
- 1 chopped garlic clove.
- 2cups water.
- 1 freshly squeezed lime.
- 2tbs. chopped scallions.
- 2tbs. coconut milk.
- 1/2tbs. crushed red pepper flakes.
- 1/4tbs. minced rosemary.
- Salt and black pepper to taste.

For the salad:
- 1head fresh lettuce separated into leaves
- 3 diced tomatoes.
- 3 sliced cucumbers.
- 2tbs. pitted Kalamata olives.

Directions

1. In a bowl filled with water, soak the sunflower seeds at least 3 hours, then drain the sunflower seeds.
2. Transfer them to your blender and put the remaining ingredients for the dressing.
3. Puree until creamy, smooth and uniform. Put all the salad ingredients into four serving bowls.
4. Toss with dressing and serve immediately. Serve!!

Nutrition Value: 208 Calories; 15.6g Fat; 6.2g Carbs; 7.6g Protein; 3.2g Sugars

458. Cozy Rainbow Vegan Soup

Servings: 6
Preparation and Cooking: 25 minutes

Ingredients

- 2 minced cloves garlic.
- 2 chopped thyme sprigs.
- 2 chopped ripe tomatoes.
- 2 bay leaves
- 1 chopped shallot.
- 1 chopped celery stalk.
- 1 chopped zucchini.
- 1 chopped rosemary sprig.
- 1 sliced carrot.
- 6cups vegetable stock.
- 1cup kale torn into pieces.
- 1cup mustard greens torn into pieces.
- 1cup unflavored almond milk.
- 1/2cup watercress.
- 2tbs. olive oil.
- 1tbs. white miso paste.
- Sea salt and ground black pepper to taste.

Directions

1. In a large pot that is preheated over a moderately high heat, heat the olive oil. Sauté the shallots, garlic, celery, zucchini, and carrots until they're softened.
2. Carefully combine the kale, mustard greens, salt, ground black pepper, thyme, rosemary, bay leaves, vegetable stock and tomatoes.
3. Reduce the heat to simmer and with the lid slightly ajar, let it simmer another 15 minutes.
4. Pour the almond milk, white miso paste, and watercress. Cook an additional 5 minutes, stirring periodically.
5. Prepare in Servings. Ready to eat.

Nutrition Value: 142 Calories; 11.4g Fat; 5.6g Carbs; 2.9g Protein; 3.3g Sugars

459. Protein Quickie Smoothie

Servings: 4
Preparation: 5 minutes

Ingredients

- 1 peeled and sliced banana.
- 1 ½ cups almond milk.
- 1/2cup water.
- 1/3cup frozen cherries.
- 1/3cup fresh blueberries.
- 1/4tbs. vanilla extract.
- 1tbs. zero carb vegan protein powder.

Directions

1. Combine all ingredients in your blender or a smoothie maker until creamy and uniform.
2. Serve in individual glasses and enjoy!

Nutrition Value: 247 Calories; 21.7g Fat; 4.9g Carbs; 2.6g Protein; 3g Sugars

460. Africana Carrot Salad

Servings: 4
Preparation: 10 minutes

Ingredients

- 1pound coarsely shredded carrot.
- 1/4cup chopped fresh cilantro.
- For the Vinaigrette:
- 3 smashed garlic cloves.
- 1 freshly squeezed lime.
- 2tbs. balsamic vinegar.
- 1/2tbs. ground cumin
- 1/2tbs. harissa.
- 1/3 cup extra-virgin olive oil.
- Sea salt and ground black pepper to taste.

Directions

1. Place shredded carrots and freshly chopped cilantro in a salad bowl.
2. Combine all ingredients for the vinaigrette, and then mix until everything is well incorporated.
3. Add the vinaigrette to the carrot salad and toss to coat well. Serve!!

Nutrition Value: 196 Calories; 17.2g Fat; 6g Carbs; 1.2g Protein; 2.3g Sugars

461. Sesame-Spiced Roasted Cabbage

Servings: 6
Preparation and Cooking: 45 minutes

Ingredients

- Nonstick cooking spray.
- 2 pounds green cabbage cut into wedges.
- 2tbs. chopped fresh chives.
- 1tbs. sesame seeds.
- 1/4cup olive oil.
- Coarsely salt and freshly ground black pepper to taste.

Directions

1. Preheat your oven to 390 degrees F. Brush a rimmed baking sheet with a nonstick cooking spray.
2. Carefully put the cabbage wedges to the baking sheet. Toss with olive oil, salt, black pepper and sesame seeds.
3. Roast for 40 to 45 minutes until cabbage is softened.
4. Serve garnished with fresh chopped chives. Serve!!

Nutrition Value: 186 Calories; 17g Fat; 5.3g Carbs; 2.1g Protein; 2.9g Sugars

462. Low-Carb Winter Mushroom Stew

Servings: 4
Preparation and Cooking: 50 minutes

Ingredients

- 2 chopped ripe tomatoes.
- 2 chopped thyme sprigs.
- 1 chopped yellow onion.
- 1 chopped rosemary sprig.
- 1 chopped green bell pepper.
- 1 chopped jalapeno pepper.
- 1 finely minced garlic clove.
- 2 bay leaves.
- 2 ½cups thinly sliced Chanterelle mushrooms.
- 1 ½cups vegetable stock.
- 1/2cup chopped celery.
- 1/2cup chopped carrot.
- 1/4tbs. grated nutmeg.
- 2tbs. apple cider vinegar.
- 1/2tbs. salt.
- 2tbs. olive oil.
- 1/4tbs. ground black pepper or more to taste.

Directions

1. In a pot that is preheated over a moderately high heat, heat the oil. Sauté the onions and garlic until tender and fragrant.
2. Stir in the celery, carrots, pepper, and mushrooms. Cook for 12 minutes more; stirring periodically.

3. Put a splash of vegetable stock to prevent sticking. Pour the remaining ingredients except for apple cider vinegar.
4. Turn the heat to medium-low. Put the lid firmly, and then let it simmer for 25 to 35 minutes or more until everything is thoroughly cooked.
5. Ladle into individual bowls, drizzle each serving with apple cider vinegar and eat warm.

Nutrition Value: 65 Calories; 2.7g Fat; 6g Carbs; 2.7g Protein; 3.9g Sugars

463. Garlic-Spiced Sautéed Savoy Cabbage

Servings: 4
Preparation and Cooking: 25 minutes

Ingredients

- 2 pounds Savoy cabbage, torn into pieces
- 1tbs. minced garlic.
- 1/2tbs. dried basil.
- 1/2tbs. crushed red pepper flakes.
- 2tbs. almond oil
- Salt and ground black pepper to the taste.

Directions

1. In a pot of a lightly salted water, cook the Savoy cabbage for approximately 20 minutes over a moderate heat. Drain and reserve until ready for use.
2. Get your sauté pan and heat the oil over a medium-high heat and then cook the garlic until just aromatic.
3. Combine the reserved Savoy cabbage, basil, red pepper, salt and black pepper, then stir thoroughly until everything is heated through.
4. Taste to adjust the seasonings and serve warm over a cauliflower rice.

Nutrition Value: 118 Calories; 7g Fat; 3.4g Carbs; 2.9g Protein; 1.3g Sugars

464. Tasty Noodles with Avocado Sauce

Servings: 4
Preparation and Cooking: 15 minutes

Ingredients

- 1/2pound carrots.
- 1/2pound bell peppers.
- 1 chopped shallot.
- 1 deveined and minced jalapeno pepper.
- 1 peeled and pitted avocado.
- 1 juiced and zested lemon.
- 2tbs. sesame oil.
- 2tbs. chopped cilantro.
- 1tbs. olive oil.
- Salt and black pepper to taste.

Directions

1. Spiralize carrots and bell peppers by using a spiralizer or a julienne peeler.
2. Heat olive oil in a wok or a large nonstick skillet. Sauté carrots and peppers in hot olive oil for about 8 minutes.
3. Carefully combine all remaining ingredients until creamy. Pour avocado sauce over noodles and serve immediately.

Nutrition Value: 233 Calories; 20.2g Fat; 6g Carbs; 1.9g Protein; 1g Sugars

465. Creamy Sautéed Cauliflower Soup

Servings: 4
Preparation and Cooking: 20 minutes

Ingredients

- 2 heads of cauliflower broken into florets.
- 4cups water
- 1 ½tbs. vegetable bouillon granules.
- 1/2tbs. red pepper flakes.
- 1/4tbs. ground bay leaves.
- 1/4tbs. ground cloves.
- 2tbs. extra-virgin olive oil.

Directions

1. In a heavy-bottomed pot, bring the water to a boil over a moderately high heat.
2. Stir in the cauliflower florets; cook for 10 minutes.
3. Pour the bouillon granules, ground bay leaves, and ground cloves. Reduce the heat to medium-low, then continue to cook for 5 minutes longer.
4. Puree this mixture by using a food processor or an immersion blender. Divide among four soup bowl.
5. Drizzle each serving with olive oil and sprinkle with red pepper. Eat warm.

Nutrition Value: 94 Calories; 7.2g Fat; 7g Carbs; 2.7g Protein; 3.2g Sugars

466. Ethiopian Stewed Cauliflower Rice

Servings: 4
Preparation and Cooking: 40 minutes

Ingredients

- 1 small head cauliflower
- 4 bell peppers
- 1 chopped onion.

- 1 minced garlic cloves.
- 2 pureed ripe tomatoes.
- 1tbs. chipotle powder.
- 1tbs. Berbera.
- 1 ½tbs. oil
- Sea salt and pepper to taste.

Directions

1. To make cauliflower rice, grate the cauliflower into the size of rice. Place on a kitchen towel to soak up any excess moisture.
2. Preheat your oven to 360 degrees F. Lightly grease a casserole dish.
3. Cut off the top of the bell peppers. Discard the seeds and core.
4. Roast the peppers in a parchment lined baking pan for 18 minutes until the skin is slightly browned.
5. In the meantime, heat the oil over medium-high heat. Sauté the onion and garlic until tender and fragrant.
6. Put the cauliflower rice, chipotle powder, and Berbera spice. Cook until the cauliflower rice is tender, about 6 minutes.
7. Divide the cauliflower mixture among bell peppers. Place in the casserole dish.
8. Mix the tomatoes, salt, and pepper. Pour the tomato mixture over the peppers.
9. Bake about 10 minutes, depending on desired tenderness. Serve immediately.

Nutrition Value: 77 Calories; 4.8g Fat; 5.4g Carbs; 1.6g Protein; 2.2g Sugars

467. Cauliflower and Almond Soup

Servings: 4
Preparation and Cooking: 25 minutes

Ingredients

- 1 head cauliflower broken into florets.
- 2 minced cloves garlic.
- 1 chopped celery with leaves.
- 1cup chopped shallots.
- 1/4 cup ground almonds.
- 1tbs. chopped fresh parsley.
- 4cups water.
- 1tbs. almond oil.
- Salt and white pepper to taste.

Directions

1. Heat the oil in a stockpot that is preheated over a moderate heat. Sauté the shallots, celery and garlic until tender for about 6 minutes.
2. Pour the cauliflower, water, salt, and white pepper, and then put the ground almonds.
3. Bring to a boil. Reduce the heat to low, and then continue to simmer for about 17 minutes.
4. Next, puree the soup with an immersion blender.
5. Serve garnished with fresh parsley. Serve!!

Nutrition Value: 114 Calories; 6.5g Fat; 6.4g Carbs; 3.8g Protein; 2g Sugars

468. Crisp Vegan Tofu

Servings: 4
Preparation and Cooking: 25 minutes

Ingredients

- 1 14-ounce pressed and cubed block tofu.
- 1 chopped celery stalk.
- 1 bunch chopped scallions.
- 1 pound trimmed and quartered Brussels sprouts.
- 1 teaspoon cayenne pepper.
- 1 teaspoon garlic powder.
- 1/2 teaspoon turmeric powder.
- 1/2 teaspoon dried sill weed.
- 1/4 teaspoon dried basil.
- 2tbs. olive oil.
- 2tbs. Worcestershire sauce.
- Salt and black pepper to taste.

Directions

1. Heat 1 tablespoon of olive oil in a large-sized skillet over a moderately high flame. Put tofu cubes and cook; stirring gently, for 8 minutes.
2. Pour the celery and scallions, and then cook until they are softened for about 5 minutes
3. Combine the cayenne pepper, garlic powder, Worcestershire sauce, salt, and pepper. Cook for 3 more minutes, then reserve.
4. Heat the remaining 1tbs. of oil in the same pan. Cook Brussels sprouts along with the remaining seasonings for 4 minutes.
5. Put tofu mixture to Brussels sprouts and serve warm. Enjoy!

Nutrition Value: 128 Calories; 8.3g Fat; 6.5g Carbs; 5.1g Protein; 3g Sugars

469. Low fat Chocolate berry Smoothie

Servings: 2
Preparation: 5 minutes

Ingredients

- 1cup blackberries.
- 1cup water.
- 1tbs. chia seeds

- 1tbs. cocoa.
- 1tbs. peanut butter.
- 1/4teaspoon ground nutmeg.
- Liquid Stevia to taste

Directions
1. Combine all ingredients in your blender or a food processor.
2. Mix until creamy and uniform.
3. Pour into two tall glasses and serve immediately. Enjoy!

Nutrition Value: 103 Calories; 5.9g Fat; 6.1g Carbs; 4.1g Protein; 3.4g Sugars

470. Healthy Granola
Servings: 8
Preparation and Cooking: 1 hour

Ingredients
- 1 ½cups coconut milk.
- 1/3cup coconut flakes.
- 1/2teaspoon ground cinnamon.
- 1/8teaspoon Himalayan salt.
- 1teaspoon orange zest.
- 1/8teaspoon freshly grated nutmeg.
- 1/2 cup chopped walnuts.
- 1/2cup slivered almonds.
- 1/4cup flax seed.
- 2tbs. sugar.
- 2tbs. coconut oil.
- 2tbs. pepitas
- 2tbs. sunflower seeds.

Directions
1. In a deep pan that is preheated over a moderately high flame, warm coconut oil. Toast coconut flakes for 1 to 2 minutes.
2. Put the remaining ingredients and stir to combine.
3. Preheat your oven to 300 degrees F. Spread mixture out in an even layer onto a parchment lined baking sheet.
4. Bake for 1 hour as you gently toss every 15 minutes.
5. Serve with some extra coconut milk. Serve!!

Nutrition Value: 262 Calories; 24.3g Fat; 5.2g Carbs; 5.1g Protein; 3.1g Sugars

471. Cauliflower Salad Delight
Servings: 4
Preparation and Chilling: 15 minutes

Ingredients

- 1 head fresh cauliflower cut into florets.
- 4 ounces chopped bottled roasted peppers.
- 1cup chopped spring onions.
- 1/2cup pitted and chopped green olives.
- 1/2cup coarsely pecans.
- 1teaspoon yellow mustard
- 1 tbs. wine vinegar
- 1/4cup extra-virgin olive oil
- Coarse salt and black pepper to your liking

Directions
1. Steam the cauliflower florets for 4 to 6 minutes, then set aside to cool.
2. In a salad bowl, place spring onions and roasted peppers.
3. In a mixing dish, whisk olive oil, vinegar, mustard, salt and pepper. Drizzle over the veggies in the salad bowl.
4. Pour the reserved cauliflower and toss to combine well. Scatter green olives and pecans over the top and serve.

Nutrition Value: 281 Calories; 26.8g Fat; 5.6g Carbs; 4.2g Protein; 2.3g Sugars

472. Strawberry Overnight Oats
Servings: 4
Preparation: 5 minutes

Ingredients
- 1/2cup water.
- 16 drops of liquid stevia.
- 1/2cup unsweetened almond milk.
- 3/4cup hemp hearts.
- 1/4 teaspoon ground cloves.
- 1/4 teaspoon ground cinnamon.
- 1cup halved strawberries.

Directions
1. Combine all ingredients except for strawberries in an airtight container.
2. Cover tightly and place in your refrigerator overnight.
3. In the morning, top with fresh strawberries and serve immediately.

Nutrition Value: 176 Calories; 12.7g Fat; 6g Carbs; 9.7g Protein; 1.8g Sugars

473. 10 minutes Nuts "Cereals"
Servings: 4
Preparation and Cooking: 10 minutes

Ingredients
- 16 roughly chopped hazelnuts.
- 2 ½ cups full-fat coconut milk.

- 1/3 cup coconut shreds.
- 1/2 cup flax seed.
- 1/2 cup water.
- 2 tbs. confectioners' erythritol
- 1/2 teaspoon vanilla paste.
- 2 tbs. coconut oil.
- 1/8 teaspoon salt.

Directions

1. Melt coconut oil in a pan over a moderate heat. Carefully combine the coconut shreds, coconut milk, water, confectioners' erythritol, salt, vanilla paste, and flax seed.
2. Simmer for 5 minutes; stirring periodically, then allow it to cool down slightly.
3. Ladle into four individual bowls. Serve topped with chopped hazelnuts. Serve!!

Nutrition Value: 279 Calories; 23.6g Fat; 5.9g Carbs; 7.2g Protein; 3g Sugars

474. Fresh and Authentic Guacamole

Servings: 8
Preparation and Chilling time: 10 minutes

Ingredients

- 2 peeled, pitted, and mashed Haas avocados.
- 1 chopped yellow onion.
- 2 minced garlic cloves.
- 1 cup chopped fresh tomatoes.
- 1/2 teaspoon ground cumin.
- 2 tbs. fresh lime juice.
- 2 tbs. chopped coriander leaves.
- 1 deseeded and finely chopped red chili.
- Sea salt and ground black pepper to taste.

Directions

1. In a bowl, thoroughly combine the avocados, lime juice, salt and black pepper.
2. Stir in the onion, cilantro, tomatoes, and garlic; sprinkle with paprika.
3. Keep in your refrigerator until ready to serve. Serve!!

Nutrition Value: 112 Calories; 9.9g Fat; 6.5g Carbs; 1.3g Protein; 1.4g Sugars

475. Healthy homemade Granola

Servings: 6
Preparation and Cooking: 1 hour

Ingredients

- 8 drops stevia
- 1 cup chopped walnuts.
- 1/2 cup chopped pecans.
- 1/3 cup flax meal.
- 1/3 cup coconut milk.
- 1/3 cup sesame seeds.
- 1/3 cup pumpkin seeds.
- 1 ½ teaspoons vanilla paste.
- 1 teaspoon orange zest.
- 1 teaspoon ground cloves.
- 1 teaspoon freshly grated nutmeg.
- 1/3 cup melted coconut oil.
- 1/3 cup water.

Directions

1. Preheat your oven to 300 degrees F. Line a baking sheet with parchment paper.
2. Mix all ingredients until well combined. Spread this mixture out in an even layer onto the prepared baking sheet.
3. Bake about 55 minutes; stirring every 15 minutes. Allow it to cool down at room temperature.
4. Transfer to an airtight container or serve immediately. Serve!!

Nutrition Value: 449 Calories; 44.9g Fat; 6.9g Carbs; 9.3g Protein; 1.4g Sugars

476. Baked Tofu with Asian Tomato Sauce

Servings: 4
Preparation and Cooking: 20 minutes

Ingredients

- 10 ounces pressed and drained smoked tofu.
- 2 tbs. olive oil.
- 1 cup chopped leeks.
- 1 teaspoon minced garlic.
- 1/2 cup vegetable broth.
- 1/2 teaspoon turmeric powder.
- Sea salt and ground black pepper to taste.
- For the Sauce:
- 1 cup tomato sauce.
- 2 tbs. red wine
- 1 teaspoon chopped fresh rosemary.
- 1 teaspoon Asian chili garlic sauce.
- 1/2 tbs. olive oil.

Directions

1. Pat dry the tofu and cut it into 1-inch cubes. Heat 2 tbs. of olive oil in a frying pan over a medium heat.
2. Fry the tofu cubes until they are slightly browned on all sides. Carefully combine the leeks, garlic, broth, turmeric powder, salt and

pepper. Cook until almost all liquid has evaporated.
3. Meanwhile, make the sauce. Heat 1/2 tablespoon of olive oil in a pan over a medium heat. Add the tomato sauce and cook until heated through.
4. Add the remaining ingredients and simmer over a medium-low heat approximately 10 minutes.
5. Serve with prepared tofu cubes. Enjoy!

Nutrition Value: 336 Calories; 22.2g Fat; 5.8g Carbs; 27.6g Protein; 2.5g Sugars

477. Plums and Chia Pudding

Servings: 3
Preparation: 5 minutes

Ingredients

- 2cups unsweetened almond milk.
- 8 pitted and halved plums.
- 2teaspoons powdered Swerve.
- 1/2cup chia seeds.
- 1/2teaspoon vanilla extract.
- 1/4teaspoon cardamom.
- 1/4teaspoon ground cinnamon.
- A pinch of salt.

Directions

1. Place all of the above ingredients, except for Swerve and plums, in an airtight container.
2. Allow it to stand, covered, in your refrigerator overnight.
3. Sweeten with powdered Swerve and serve well-chilled with fresh plums. Enjoy!

Nutrition Value: 153 Calories; 8g Fat; 6.7g Carbs; 6.7g Protein; 4g Sugars

478. Sautéed Fennel with Tomato Basil Sauce

Servings: 4
Preparation and Cooking: 20 minutes

Ingredients

- 1 crushed garlic clove.
- 1 thinly sliced fennel.
- 1/4cup vegetable stock.
- 2tbs. olive oil.
- Sea salt and ground black pepper to taste.
- For the Sauce:
- 2 halved tomatoes.
- 1 bunch fresh basil.
- 1/2cup chopped scallions.
- 1 minced cloves garlic.
- 1 minced ancho chili.
- 1tbs. roughly chopped fresh cilantro.
- 2tbs. extra-virgin olive oil.
- Salt and pepper to taste.

Directions

1. Heat olive oil in a pan over a moderately high heat. Sauté the garlic for 1 to 2 minutes or until aromatic.
2. Throw the slices of fennel into the pan; Put vegetable stock and continue to cook until the fennel is softened.
3. Season with salt and black pepper to taste, and then Heat off.
4. Brush the tomato halves with extra-virgin olive oil. Microwave for 15 minutes on HIGH. Be sure to pour off any excess liquid.
5. Transfer cooked tomatoes to a food processor; Combine the remaining ingredients for the sauce. Puree until your desired consistency is reached.
6. Serve with sautéed fennel. Serve!!

Nutrition Value: 135 Calories; 13.6g Fat; 3g Carbs; 0.9g Protein; 1.1g Sugars

479. Oven-Roasted Autumn Vegetables

Servings: 4
Preparation and Cooking: 45 minutes

Ingredients

- 1 deveined and sliced red bell pepper.
- 1 deveined and sliced green bell pepper.
- 1 deveined and sliced orange bell pepper.
- 2 zucchinis cut into thick slices.
- 1/2 head of cauliflower broken into large florets.
- 2 quartered medium-sized leeks.
- 4 halved garlic cloves.
- 2 chopped thyme sprigs.
- 1teaspoon mixed whole peppercorns.
- 1teaspoon crushed dried sage.
- 4tbs. tomato puree.
- 4tbs. olive oil.
- Sea salt and cayenne pepper to taste.

Directions

1. Preheat your oven to 425 degrees F. Sprits a rimmed baking sheet with a nonstick cooking spray.
2. Toss all of the above vegetables with seasonings, oil and apple cider vinegar.
3. Roast about 40 minutes. Flip vegetables halfway through cook time. Serve!!

Nutrition Value: 165 Calories; 14.3g Fat; 5.6g Carbs; 2.1g Protein; 2.7g Sugars

480. Creamy Eggplant Cashew Soup

Servings: 4

Preparation and Cooking: 1 hour 20 minutes

Ingredients

- 1 pound eggplant cut it in half.
- 2 chopped ripe tomatoes.
- 2 chopped shallots.
- 2 peeled garlic cloves.
- 3 vegan bouillon cubes.
- 1/2teaspoon dried oregano.
- 1/2teaspoon dried basil.
- 1/2teaspoon dried marjoram.
- 3cups water.
- 1/3 cup soaked raw cashews.
- 1tbs. olive oil.
- Salt and pepper to taste.

Directions

1. Preheat your oven to 390 degrees F. Arrange the eggplant on a parchment lined baking sheet. Drizzle olive oil over eggplant.
2. Roast about 35 to 40 minutes or until tender. Scoop eggplant from the skin and transfer to a pot.
3. Combine the remaining ingredient except for cashews. Let it simmer, covered, for 40 minutes. Puree the soup with a hand blender.
4. Drain your cashews and blend them with 1 cup water in a blender until smooth.
5. Slowly pour the cashew cream in the soup, stir well and serve immediately.

Nutrition Value: 159 Calories; 9.4g Fat; 7.1g Carbs; 4.2g Protein; 3.6g Sugars

481. Chocolate Butternut Squash Smoothie

Servings: 2

Preparation: 5 minutes

Ingredients

- 2 ½cups almond milk
- 1/2cup baby spinach.
- 1/2cup roasted butternut squash.
- 1/2teaspoon ground cinnamon.
- 2tbs. cocoa powder.
- A pinch of grated nutmeg.
- A pinch of salt.

Directions

1. In a blender or a food processor, combine all ingredients.
2. Serve well-chilled in tall glasses. Enjoy!

Nutrition Value: 71 Calories; 2.3g Fat; 4.1g Carbs; 4.3g Protein; 2g Sugars

482. Peanut Butter Raspberry Smoothie

Servings: 1

Preparation: 5 minutes

Ingredients

- 1/2cup baby spinach leave.
- 1/3cup raspberries.
- 3/4cup unsweetened almond milk.
- 1tbs. peanut butter.
- 1teaspoon Swerve.

Directions

1. Place all ingredients in your blender and puree until creamy, uniform and smooth.
2. Pour into a tall glass. Serve well-chilled.

Nutrition Value: 114 Calories; 8.2g Fat; 5.9g Carbs; 4.2g Protein; 3.1g Sugars

483. Roasted Cremini Mushroom and Broccoli

Servings: 4

Preparation and Cooking: 30 minutes

Ingredients

- Nonstick cooking spray
- 1 head broccoli cut into florets
- 8ounces halved cremini mushrooms.
- 2 smashed garlic cloves.
- 2 ripe pureed tomatoes.
- 1teaspoon hot paprika paste
- 1/2teaspoon curry powder.
- 1/4teaspoon marjoram
- 1/4cup melted vegan butter.
- Coarse salt and black pepper to taste

Directions

1. Preheat your oven to 390 degrees F. Brush a baking dish with a nonstick cooking oil.
2. Arrange broccoli and mushrooms in the baking dish. Scatter smashed garlic around the vegetables. Put the pureed tomatoes.
3. Drizzle with melted butter and add hot paprika paste, marjoram, curry, salt, and black pepper.
4. Roast for 25 minutes; turning your baking dish once.
5. Serve with a fresh salad of choice. Serve!!

Nutrition Value: 113 Calories; 6.7g Fat; 6.6g Carbs;

5g Protein; 3.2g Sugars

484. Crisp Topped Vegetable Bake

Servings: 4
Preparation and Cooking: 40 minutes

Ingredients

- 1/2 pound quartered Brussels sprout.
- 1cup chopped shallots.
- 1 chopped celery.
- 2 grated carrots.
- 1 cup vegan parmesan.
- 1 cup roasted vegetable broth.
- 2tbs. roughly chopped fresh chives.
- 1teaspoon turmeric.
- 1teaspoon paprika powder.
- 1/2 teaspoon liquid smoke.
- 2tbs. olive oil.
- Sea salt and ground black pepper to taste.

Directions

1. Start by preheating your oven to 360 degrees F. Brush a baking dish with olive oil.
2. In a heavy-bottomed skillet, heat olive oil over a moderately high heat. Sweat the shallots until they are softened.
3. Combine the celery, carrots and Brussels sprouts. Cook an additional 4 minutes or more until just tender. Transfer the vegetable mixture to the baking dish.
4. Mix roasted vegetable broth with turmeric, salt, black pepper, paprika, and liquid smoke. Pour this mixture over the vegetables.
5. Top with vegan parmesan cheese and bake approximately 30 minutes. Serve garnished with fresh chives.

Nutrition Value: 242 Calories; 16.3g Fat; 6.7g Carbs; 16.3g Protein; 2.3g Sugars

485. Stir Fry Artichoke Tofu

Servings: 4
Preparation and Cooking: 30 minutes

Ingredients

- 1 pound whole baby artichokes cut off stems and tough outer leaves.
- 2 pressed and cubed blocks tofu.
- 2 minced garlic cloves.
- 1 chopped bell pepper.
- 1/4cup vegetable broth.
- 1teaspoon Cajun spice mix.
- 1teaspoon deli mustard.
- 2tbs. olive oil.
- Salt and pepper to your liking.

Directions

1. In a large saucepan of lightly salted water, cook artichokes for 15 minutes or until they're tender, and then drain.
2. Heat olive oil in a wok that is preheated over medium-high heat. Put tofu cubes and cook about 6 minutes, gently stirring.
3. Put garlic and cook until aromatic or 30 seconds or so.
4. Combine the remaining ingredients, including reserved artichokes, and then continuc to cook 4 more minutes or until heated through.
5. Serve warm on individual plates. Serve!!

Nutrition Value: 138 Calories; 8.9g Fat; 6.8g Carbs; 6.4g Protein; 2.6g Sugars

SMOOTHIES & JUICE

486. Almonds & Blueberries Smoothie

Servings: 2
Preparation: 5 minutes

Ingredients

- 1/4 cup ground almonds, unsalted
- 1 cup fresh blueberries
- Fresh juice of the 1 lemon
- 1 cup fresh Kale leaves
- 1/2 cup coconut water
- 1 cup water
- 2 Tbsp plain yogurt (optional)

Directions:

1. Dump all ingredients with your high-speed blender, and blend until your smoothie is smooth.
2. Pour a combination in the chilled glass.
3. Serve and enjoy!

Nutrition Value:

Calories: 110 Carbohydrates: 8g Proteins: 2g Fat: 7g Fiber: 2g

487. Almonds and Zucchini Smoothie

Servings: 2
Preparation: 5 minutes

Ingredients

- 1 cup zucchini, cooked and mashed - unsalted
- 1 1/2 cups almond milk
- 1 Tbsp almond butter (plain, unsalted)
- 1 tsp pure almond extract
- 2 Tbsp ground almonds or Macadamia almonds
- 1/2 cup water
- 1 cup Ice cubes crushed (optional, for serving)

Directions:

1. Dump all ingredients from your list above within your fast-speed blender; blend for 45 - 60 seconds or to taste.
2. Serve with crushed ice.

Nutrition Value:

Calories: 322 Carbohydrates: 6g Proteins: 6g Fat: 30g Fiber: 3.5g

488. bAvocado with Walnut Butter Smoothie

Servings: 2
Preparation: 5 minutes

Ingredients

- 1 avocado (fresh diced)
- 1 cup baby spinach
- 1 cup coconut milk (canned)
- 1 Tbsp walnut butter, unsalted
- 2 Tbsp natural sweetener including Stevia, Erythritol, Truvia...etc.

Directions:

1. Place all ingredients into blender or perhaps a blender; blend until smooth or to taste.
2. Add more or less walnut butter.
3. Drink and get!

Nutrition Value:

Calories: 364 Carbohydrates: 7g Proteins: 8g Fat: 35g Fiber: 5.5g

489. Baby Spinach and Dill Smoothie

Servings: 2
Preparation: 5 minutes

Ingredients

- 1 cup of fresh baby spinach leaves
- 2 Tbsp of fresh dill, chopped
- 1 1/2 cup of water
- 1/2 avocado, chopped into cubes
- 1 Tbsp chia seeds (optional)
- 2 Tbsp of natural sweetener Stevia or Erythritol (optional)

Directions:

1. Place all ingredients into fast-speed blender. Beat until smooth and all sorts of ingredients united well.
2. Serve and enjoy!

Nutrition Value:

Calories: 136 Carbohydrates: 8g Proteins: 7g Fat: 10g Fiber: 9g

490. Blueberries and Coconut Smoothie

Servings: 5
Preparation: 5 minutes

Ingredients

- 1 cup of frozen blueberries, unsweetened
- 1 cup Stevia or Erythritol sweetener
- 2 cups coconut milk (canned)

- 1 cup of fresh spinach leaves
- 2 Tbsp shredded coconut (unsweetened)
- 3/4 cup water

Directions:
1. Place all ingredients from the list in food-processor or in your strong blender.
2. Blend for 45 - one minute as well as to taste.
3. Ready for drink! Serve!

Nutrition Value:
Calories: 190 Carbohydrates: 8g Proteins: 3g Fat: 18g Fiber: 2g

491. Chocolate Lettuce Salad Smoothie

Servings: 2
Preparation: 15 minutes

Ingredients

- 2 servings of fresh lettuce salad
- 1 stalk of celery
- 1 cup almond milk unsweetened
- 1/2 tsp of powered cocoa, unsweetened
- 2 Tbsp chocolate bars chips
- 1/2 tsp cinnamon powder
- 1 tsp pure chocolate extract
- 1 cup of water

Directions:
1. Rinse and thoroughly clean lettuce salad from any dirt.
2. Place lettuce salad leaves in a very blender along effortlessly remaining ingredients from your list above.
3. Blend for 45 - one minute or until done.
4. Serve, drink and revel in!

Nutrition Value:
Calories: 73 Carbohydrates: 5g Proteins: 2g Fat: 6g Fiber: 2g

492. Collard Greens, Peppermint and Cucumber Smoothie

Servings: 2
Preparation: quarter-hour

Ingredients

- 1 cup Collard greens
- A few fresh peppermint leaves
- 1 big cucumber
- 1 lime, freshly juiced
- 1/2 cups avocado sliced
- 1 1/2 cup water
- 1 cup crushed ice
- 1/4 cup of natural sweetener Erythritol or Stevia (optional)

Directions:
1. Rinse and clean your Collard greens from any dirt.
2. Place all ingredients inside a blender or blender,
3. Blend until all ingredients within your smoothie is combined well.
4. Pour inside a glass and drink. Enjoy!

Nutrition Value:
Calories: 123 Carbohydrates: 8g Proteins: 4g Fat: 11g Fiber: 6g

493. Creamy Dandelion Greens and Celery Smoothie

Servings: 2
Preparation: 10 mins

Ingredients

- 1 handful of raw dandelion greens
- 2 celery sticks
- 2 Tbsp chia seeds
- 1 small part of ginger, minced
- 1/2 cup almond milk
- 1/2 cup of water
- 1/2 cup plain yogurt

Directions:
1. Rinse and clean dandelion leaves from any dirt; add in the high-speed blender.
2. Clean the ginger; keep only inner part, and cut in small slices; add in a very blender.
3. Add all remaining ingredients and blend until smooth.
4. Serve and enjoy!

Nutrition Value:
Calories: 58 Carbohydrates: 5g Proteins: 3g Fat: 6g Fiber: 3g

494. Dark Turnip Greens Smoothie

Servings: 2
Preparation: ten mins

Ingredients

- 1 cup of raw turnip greens
- 1 1/2 cup of almond milk
- 1 Tbsp of almond butter
- 1/2 cup of water
- 1/2 tsp of hot chocolate mix, unsweetened
- 1 Tbsp of chocolate bars chips
- 1/4 tsp of cinnamon
- A pinch of salt

- 1/2 cup of crushed ice

Directions:
1. Rinse and clean turnip greens from any dirt.
2. Place the turnip greens within your blender along wonderful other ingredients.
3. Blend it for 45 - 60 seconds or until done; smooth and creamy.
4. Serve with or without crushed ice.

Nutrition Value:
Calories: 131 Carbohydrates: 6g Proteins: 4g Fat: 10g Fiber: 2.5g

495. Ever Butter Pecan and Coconut Smoothie
Servings: 2
Preparation: 5 minutes

Ingredients
- 1 cup coconut milk canned
- 1 scoop Butter Pecan powdered creamer
- 2 cups fresh spinach leaves, chopped
- 1/2 banana frozen or fresh
- 2 Tbsp stevia granulated sweetener to taste
- 1/2 cup water
- 1 cup ice cubes crushed

Directions:
1. Place ingredients in the list above within your high-speed blender.
2. Blend for 35 - 50 seconds or until all ingredients combined well.
3. Add less or more crushed ice.
4. Drink and get!

Nutrition Value:
Calories: 268 Carbohydrates: 7g Proteins: 6g Fat: 26g Fiber: 1.5g

496. Fresh Cucumber, Kale and Raspberry Smoothie
Servings: 3
Preparation: 10 mins

Ingredients
- 1 1/2 servings of cucumber peeled
- 1/2 cup raw kale leaves
- 1 1/2 cups fresh raspberries
- 1 cup of almond milk
- 1 cup of water
- Ice cubes crushed (optional)
- 2 Tbsp natural sweetener (Stevia, Erythritol...etc.)

Directions:
1. Place all ingredients through the list in a food processor or high-speed blender; blend for 35 - 40 seconds.
2. Serve into chilled glasses.
3. Add more natural sweeter if you like. Enjoy!

Nutrition Value:
Calories: 70 Carbohydrates: 8g Proteins: 3g Fat: 6g Fiber: 5g

497. Fresh Lettuce and Cucumber-Lemon Smoothie
Servings: 2
Preparation: 10 minutes

Ingredients
- 2 cups fresh lettuce leaves, chopped
- 1 cup of cucumber
- 1 lemon, cleaned and sliced
- 1/2 avocado
- 2 Tbsp chia seeds
- 1 1/2 cup water or coconut water
- 1/4 cup stevia granulate sweetener (as well as to taste)

Directions:
1. Add all ingredients through the list above inside high-speed blender; blend until completely smooth.
2. Pour your smoothie into chilled glasses and luxuriate in!

Nutrition Value:
Calories: 51 Carbohydrates: 4g Proteins: 2g Fat: 4g Fiber: 3.5g

498. Green Coconut Smoothie
Servings: 2
Preparation: ten minutes

Ingredients
- 1 1/4 cup coconut milk (canned)
- 2 Tbsp chia seeds
- 1 cup of fresh kale leaves
- 1 cup of spinach leaves
- 1 scoop vanilla protein powder
- 1 cup ice cubes
- Granulated stevia sweetener (to taste; optional)
- 1/2 cup water

Directions:
1. Rinse and clean kale and the spinach leaves from any dirt.
2. Add all ingredients in your blender.
3. Blend and soon you obtain a nice smoothie.

4. Serve into chilled glass.

Nutrition Value:
Calories: 179 Carbohydrates: 5g Proteins: 4g Fat: 18g Fiber: 2.5g

Instant Coffee Smoothie
Servings: 2
Preparation: twenty minutes

Ingredients
- 2 glasses of instant coffee
- 1 cup almond milk (or coconut milk)
- 1/4 cup heavy cream
- 2 Tbsp hot chocolate mix (unsweetened)
- 1 or 2 Handful of fresh spinach leaves
- 10 drops liquid stevia

Directions:
1. Make a coffee; put aside.
2. Place all remaining ingredients within your fast-speed blender; blend for 45 - 60 seconds or until done.
3. Pour your instant coffee in the blender and then blend for further 30 - 45 seconds.
4. Serve immediately.

Nutrition Value:
Calories: 142 Carbohydrates: 6g Proteins: 5g Fat: 14g Fiber: 3g

500. Keto Blood Sugar Adjuster Smoothie
Servings: 2
Preparation: ten mins

Ingredients
- 2 servings of green cabbage
- 1/2 avocado
- 1 Tbsp Apple cider vinegar
- Juice a single lemon
- 1 cup of water
- 1 cup of crushed ice cubes for serving

Directions:
1. Place all ingredients within your high-speed blender or inside a blender and blend until smooth and soft.
2. Serve in chilled glasses with crushed ice.
3. Enjoy!

Nutrition Value:
Calories: 74 Carbohydrates: 7g Proteins: 2g Fat: 6g Fiber: 4g

501. Lime Spinach Smoothie
Servings: 2
Preparation: 5 minutes

Ingredients
- 1 cup water
- 1 lime juice (2 limes)
- 1 green apple cut into chunks, core discarded
- 2 cups fresh spinach, roughly chopped
- 1/2 cup fresh chopped fresh mint
- 1/2 avocado
- Ice crushed
- 1/4 tsp ground cinnamon
- 1 Tbsp natural sweetener of one's choice (optional)

Directions:
1. Place all ingredients inside your high-speed blender.
2. Blend for 45 - 60 seconds or until your smoothie is smooth and creamy.
3. Serve in the chilled glass.
4. Adjust sweetener to taste.

Nutrition Value:
Calories: 112 Carbohydrates: 8g Proteins: 4g Fat: 10g Fiber: 5.5g

502. Protein Coconut Smoothie
Servings: 2
Preparation: quarter-hour

Ingredients
- 1 1/2 cup of coconut milk canned
- 1 cup of fresh spinach finely chopped
- 1 scoop vanilla protein powder
- 2 Tbsp chia seeds
- 1 cup of ice cubes crushed
- 2 to 3 Tbsp Stevia granulated natural sweetener (optional)

Directions:
1. Rinse and clean your spinach leaves from any dirt.
2. Place all ingredients from the list above in the blender.
3. Blend until you have a smoothie like consistently.
4. Serve into chilled glass and yes it is willing to drink.

Nutrition Value:
Calories: 377 Carbohydrates: 7g Proteins: 10g Fat: 38g Fiber: 2g

503. Strong Spinach and Hemp Smoothie

Servings: 3
Preparation: ten minutes

Ingredients

- 1 cup almond milk
- 1 small ripe banana
- 2 Tbsp hemp seeds
- 2 handful fresh spinach leaves
- 1 tsp pure vanilla flavoring
- 1 cup of water
- 2 Tbsp of natural sweetener such Stevia, Truvia...etc.

Directions:

1. First, rinse and clean your spinach leaves from any dirt.
2. Place the spinach in the blender or mixer in addition to remaining ingredients.
3. Blend for 45 - a minute or until done.
4. Add approximately sweetener.
5. Serve.

Nutrition Value:

Calories: 75 Carbohydrates: 7g Proteins: 4g Fat: 6g Fiber: 3g

304. Total Almond Smoothie

Servings: 2
Preparation: quarter-hour

Ingredients

- 1 1/2 servings of almond milk
- 2 Tbsp of almond butter
- 2 Tbsp ground almonds
- 1 cup of fresh kale leaves (or to taste)
- 1/2 tsp of powered cocoa
- 1 Tbsp chia seeds
- 1/2 cup of water

Directions:

1. Rinse and carefully clean kale leaves from any dirt.
2. Add almond milk, almond butter and ground almonds with your blender; blend for 45 - 60 seconds.
3. Add kale leaves, hot chocolate mix and chia seeds; blend for more 45 seconds.
4. If your smoothie is to thick, pour more almond milk or water.
5. Serve.

Nutrition Value:

Calories: 228 Carbohydrates: 7g Proteins: 8g Fat: 11g Fiber: 6g

505. Ultimate Green Mix Smoothie

Servings: 2
Preparation: 15 minutes

Ingredients

- Handful of spinach leaves
- Handful of collards greens
- Handful of lettuce, cos or romain
- 1 1/2 cup of almond milk
- 1/2 cup of water
- 1/4 cup of stevia granulated sweetener
- 1 tsp pure vanilla extract
- 1 cup crushed ice cubes (optional)

Directions:

1. Rinse and carefully clean your greens from any dirt.
2. Place all ingredients from your list above with your blender or mixer.
3. Blend until done or 45 - a few seconds.
4. Serve with or without crushed ice.

Nutrition Value:

Calories: 73 Carbohydrates: 4g Proteins: 5g Fat: 7g Fiber: 1g

SNACKS

506. Chipotle Tacos
Preparation time: 10 minutes
Cooking time: 4 hours
Servings: 4

Ingredients:
- 30 ounces canned pinto beans, drained
- ¾ cup chili sauce
- 3 ounces chipotle pepper in adobo sauce, chopped
- 1 cup corn
- 6 ounces tomato paste
- 1 tablespoon cocoa powder
- ½ teaspoon cinnamon, ground
- 1 teaspoon cumin, ground
- 8 vegan taco shells
- Chopped avocado, for serving

Directions:
1. Put the beans in your slow cooker.
2. Add chili sauce, chipotle pepper, corn, tomato paste, cocoa powder, cinnamon and cumin.
3. Stir, cover and cook on Low for 4 hours. Divide beans and chopped avocado into taco shells and serve them.
4. Enjoy!

Nutrition Value: calories 342, fat 3, fiber 6, carbs 12, protein 10

507. Tasty Spinach Dip
Preparation time: 10 minutes
Cooking time: 4 hours
Servings: 12

Ingredients:
- 8 ounces baby spinach
- 1 small yellow onion, chopped
- 8 ounces vegan cashew mozzarella, shredded
- 8 ounces tofu, cubed
- 1 cup vegan cashew parmesan cheese, grated
- 1 tablespoon garlic, minced
- A pinch of cayenne pepper
- A pinch of sea salt
- Black pepper to the taste

Directions:
1. Put spinach in your slow cooker.
2. Add onion, cashew mozzarella, tofu, cashew parmesan, salt, pepper, cayenne and garlic.
3. Stir, cover and cook on Low for 2 hours.
4. Stir your dip well, cover and cook on Low for 2 more hours.
5. Divide your spinach dip into bowls and serve.
6. Enjoy!

Nutrition Value: calories 200, fat 3, fiber 4, carbs 6, protein 8

508. Candied Almonds
Preparation time: 10 minutes
Cooking time: 4 hours
Servings: 10

Ingredients:
- 3 tablespoons cinnamon powder
- 3 cups palm sugar
- 4 and ½ cups almonds, raw
- ¼ cup water
- 2 teaspoons vanilla extract

Directions:
1. In a bowl, mix water with vanilla extract and whisk.
2. In another bowl, mix cinnamon with sugar and stir.
3. Dip almonds in water, then add them to the bowl with the cinnamon sugar.
4. Toss to coat really well, add almonds to your slow cooker, cover and cook on Low for 4 hours, stirring often.
5. Divide into bowls and serve as a snack.
6. Enjoy!

Nutrition Value: calories 150, fat 3, fiber 4, carbs 6, protein 8

509. Eggplant Tapenade
Preparation time: 10 minutes
Cooking time: 7 hours
Servings: 6

Ingredients:
- 1 and ½ cups tomatoes, chopped
- 3 cups eggplant, chopped
- 2 teaspoons capers
- 4 garlic cloves, minced
- 1 tablespoon basil, chopped
- 2 teaspoons balsamic vinegar
- A pinch of sea salt
- Black pepper to the taste
- 6 ounces green olives, pitted and sliced

Directions:
1. Put tomatoes and eggplant pieces in your slow cooker.
2. Add garlic, capers, basil and olives, stir, cover and cook on Low for 7 hours.
3. Add salt, pepper, vinegar, stir gently, divide into small bowls and serve as an appetizer.
4. Enjoy!

Nutrition Value: calories 140, fat 3, fiber 5, carbs 7, protein 5

510. Almond and Beans Fondue

Preparation time: 10 minutes
Cooking time: 8 hours
Servings: 4

Ingredients:
- ½ cup almonds
- 1 and ¼ cups water
- 1 teaspoon nutritional yeast flakes
- ¼ cup great northern beans
- A pinch of sea salt
- Black pepper to the taste
- Baby carrots, steamed for serving
- Tofu cubes for serving

Directions:
1. Put the water in your slow cooker.
2. Add almonds and beans, stir, cover and cook on Low for 8 hours.
3. Transfer these to your blender, add yeast flakes, a pinch of salt and black pepper and pulse really well.
4. Transfer to bowls and serve with baby carrots and tofu cubes on the side.
5. Enjoy!

Nutrition Value: calories 200, fat 4, fiber 4, carbs 8, protein 10

511. Beans in Rich Tomato Sauce

Preparation time: 10 minutes
Cooking time: 8 hours and 10 minutes
Servings: 6

Ingredients:
- 1 pound lima beans, soaked for 6 hours and drained
- 2 celery ribs, chopped
- 2 tablespoons olive oil
- 2 onions, chopped
- 2 carrots, chopped
- 4 tablespoons tomato paste
- 3 garlic cloves, minced
- A pinch of sea salt
- Black pepper to the taste
- 7 cups water
- 1 bay leaf
- 1 teaspoon oregano, dried
- ½ teaspoon thyme, dried
- A pinch of red pepper, crushed
- ¼ cup parsley, chopped
- 1 cup cashew cheese, shredded

Directions:
1. Heat up a pan with the oil over medium high heat, add onions, stir and cook for 4 minutes.
2. Add garlic, celery, carrots, salt and pepper, stir, cook for 4-5 minutes more and transfer to your slow cooker.
3. Add beans, tomato paste, water, bay leaf, oregano, thyme and red pepper, stir, cover and cook on Low for 8 hours.
4. Add parsley, stir, divide into bowls and serve cold with cashew cheese on top.
5. Enjoy!

Nutrition Value: calories 160, fat 3, fiber 7, carbs 9, protein 12

512. Tasty Onion Dip

Preparation time: 10 minutes
Cooking time: 8 hours
Servings: 6

Ingredients:
- 3 cups yellow onions, chopped
- A pinch of sea salt
- 2 tablespoons olive oil
- 1 tablespoon coconut butter
- 1 cup coconut milk
- ½ cup avocado mayonnaise
- A pinch of cayenne pepper

Directions:
1. Put the onions in your slow cooker.
2. Add a pinch of salt, oil and coconut butter, stir well, cover and cook on High for 8 hours.
3. Drain excess liquid, transfer onion to a bowl, add coconut milk, avocado mayo and cayenne, stir really well and serve with potato chips on the side.
4. Enjoy!

Nutrition Value: calories 200, fat 4, fiber 4, carbs 9, protein 7

513. Special Beans Dip

Preparation time: 10 minutes

Cooking time: 2 hours
Servings: 20

Ingredients:

- 16 ounces canned beans, drained
- 1 cup mild hot sauce
- 2 cups cashew cheese, shredded
- ¾ cup coconut milk
- ¼ teaspoon cumin, ground
- 1 tablespoon chili powder
- 3 ounces tofu, cubed

Directions:

1. Put beans in your slow cooker.
2. Add hot sauce, cashew cheese, coconut milk, cumin, tofu and chili powder.
3. Stir, cover and cook for 2 hours.
4. Stir halfway.
5. Transfer to bowls and serve with corn chips on the side.
6. Enjoy!

Nutrition Value: calories 230, fat 4, fiber 6, carbs 8, protein 10

514. Sweet and Spicy Nuts

Preparation time: 10 minutes
Cooking time: 2 hours
Servings: 20

Ingredients:

- 1 cup almonds, toasted
- 1 cup cashews
- 1 cup pecans, halved and toasted
- 1 cup hazelnuts, toasted and peeled
- ½ cup palm sugar
- 1 teaspoon ginger, grated
- 1/3 cup coconut butter, melted
- ½ teaspoon cinnamon powder
- ¼ teaspoon cloves, ground
- A pinch of salt
- A pinch of cayenne pepper

Directions:

1. Put almonds, pecans, cashews and hazelnuts in your slow cooker.
2. Add palm sugar, coconut butter, ginger, salt, cayenne, cloves and cinnamon.
3. Stir well, cover and cook on Low for 2 hours.
4. Divide into bowls and serve as a snack.
5. Enjoy!

Nutrition Value: calories 110, fat 3, fiber 2, carbs 5, protein 5

515. Delicious Corn Dip

Preparation time: 10 minutes
Cooking time: 2 hours and 15 minutes
Servings: 8

Ingredients:

- 2 jalapenos, chopped
- 45 ounces canned corn kernels, drained
- ½ cup coconut milk
- 1 and ¼ cups cashew cheese, shredded
- A pinch of sea salt
- Black pepper to the taste
- 2 tablespoons chives, chopped

8 ounces tofu, cubed

Directions:

1. In your slow cooker, mix coconut milk with cashew cheese, corn, jalapenos, tofu, salt and pepper, stir, cover and cook on Low for 2 hours.
2. Stir your corn dip really well, cover slow cooker again and cook on High for 15 minutes.
3. Divide into bowls, sprinkle chives on top and serve as a vegan snack!
4. Enjoy!

Nutrition Value: calories 150, fat 3, fiber 2, carbs 8, protein 10

516. Butternut Squash Spread

Preparation time: 10 minutes
Cooking time: 6 hours
Servings: 4

Ingredients:

- ½ cup butternut squash, peeled and cubed
- ½ cup canned white beans, drained
- 1 tablespoon water
- 2 tablespoons coconut milk
- A pinch of rosemary, dried
- A pinch of sage, dried
- A pinch of salt and black pepper

Directions:

1. In your slow cooker, mix beans with squash, water, coconut milk, sage, rosemary, salt and pepper, toss, cover and cook on Low for 6 hours.
2. Blend using an immersion blender, divide into bowls and serve cold as a party spread.
3. Enjoy!

Nutrition Value: calories 182, fat 5, fiber 7, carbs 12, protein 5

517. Cashew And White Bean Spread

Preparation time: 10 minutes
Cooking time: 7 hours
Servings: 4

Ingredients:

- ½ cup white beans, dried
- 2 tablespoons cashews, soaked for 12 hours and blended
- 1 teaspoon apple cider vinegar
- 1 cup veggie stock
- 1 tablespoon water

Directions:

1. In your slow cooker, mix beans with cashews and stock, stir, cover and cook on Low for 6 hours.
2. Drain, transfer to your food processor, add vinegar and water, pulse well, divide into bowls and serve as a spread.
3. Enjoy!

Nutrition Value: calories 221, fat 6, fiber 5, carbs 19, protein 3

518. Artichoke Spread

Preparation time: 10 minutes
Cooking time: 20 minutes
Servings: 8

Ingredients:

- 28 ounces canned artichokes, drained and chopped
- 10 ounces spinach
- 8 ounces coconut cream
- 1 yellow onion, chopped
- 2 garlic cloves, minced
- ¾ cup coconut milk
- ½ cup tofu, pressed and crumbled
- 1/3 cup vegan avocado mayonnaise
- 1 tablespoon red vinegar
- A pinch of salt and black pepper

Directions:

1. In a pan that fits your air fryer, mix artichokes with spinach, coconut cream, onion, garlic, coconut milk, tofu, avocado mayo, vinegar, salt and pepper, stir well, introduce in the fryer and cook at 365 degrees F for 20 minutes.
2. Divide into bowls and serve as an appetizer.
3. Enjoy!

Nutrition Value: calories 215, fat 4, fiber 4, carbs 19, protein 13

519. Olives and Eggplant Dip

Preparation time: 10 minutes
Cooking time: 10 minutes
Servings: 6

Ingredients:

- 2 pounds eggplant, sliced
- Salt and black pepper to the taste
- 1 tablespoon olive oil
- 4 garlic cloves, chopped
- ½ cup water
- Juice of 1 lemon
- ¼ cup black olives, pitted
- 1 tablespoon sesame paste
- 4 thyme springs, chopped

Directions:

1. In a pan that fits your air fryer, combine oil with eggplants, salt, pepper, garlic, water, lemon juice, olives and thyme, stir, introduce in your fryer and cook at 370 degrees F for 10 minutes.
2. Blend your dip with an immersion blender, add sesame paste, blend again, divide into bowls and serve.
3. Enjoy!

Nutrition Value: calories 205, fat 11, fiber 4, carbs 14, protein 2

520. Veggie Cakes

Preparation time: 10 minutes
Cooking time: 20 minutes
Servings: 8

Ingredients:

- 2 teaspoons ginger, grated
- 1 cup yellow onion, chopped
- 1 cup mushrooms, minced
- 1 cup canned red lentils, drained
- ¼ cup veggie stock
- 1 sweet potato, chopped
- ¼ cup parsley, chopped
- ¼ cup hemp seeds
- 1 tablespoon curry powder
- ¼ cup cilantro, chopped
- A drizzle of olive oil
- 1 cup quick oats
- 2 tablespoons rice flour

Directions:

1. Heat up a pan with the oil over medium-high heat, add ginger, onion and mushrooms, stir and cook for 2-3 minutes.
2. Add lentils, potato and stock, stir, cook for 5-6 minutes, take off heat, cool the whole mixture

and mash it with a fork.
3. Add parsley, cilantro, hemp, oats, curry powder and rice flour, stir well and shape medium cakes out of this mix.
4. Place veggie cakes in your air fryer's basket and cook at 375 degrees F for 10 minutes, flipping them halfway.
5. Serve them as an appetizer.
6. Enjoy!

Nutrition Value: calories 212, fat 4, fiber 3, carbs 8, protein 10

521. Tomatoes Salsa
Preparation time: 10 minutes
Cooking time: 7 minutes
Servings: 6

Ingredients:
- 1 and ½ cups tomatoes, chopped
- 3 cups cucumber, chopped
- 1 teaspoons capers
- 1 garlic clove, minced
- 2 teaspoons lemon juice
- 1 tablespoon parsley, chopped
- 1 tablespoon basil, chopped
- Salt and black pepper to the taste

Directions:
1. In a pan that fits your air fryer, combine tomatoes with capers, garlic, lemon juice, parsley, salt and pepper, toss, introduce in the fryer, cook at 320 degrees F for 7 minutes, transfer to a bowl and cool the mixture down.
2. Add cucumbers and basil, toss, divide into small appetizer bowls and serve cold.
3. Enjoy!

Nutrition Value: calories 161, fat 3, fiber 1, carbs 8, protein 12

522. Chard Party Spread
Preparation time: 10 minutes
Cooking time: 7 minutes
Servings: 4

Ingredients:
- 2 garlic cloves, minced
- 2 cup chard leaves
- ½ cup veggie stock
- ¼ cup sesame paste
- Salt and black pepper to the taste
- A drizzle of olive oil
- Juice of 1 lemon

Directions:
1. In a pan that fits your air fryer, mix stock with chard, salt and pepper, stir, introduce in the fryer and cook at 320 degrees F for 7 minutes.
2. Drain chard, transfer to your food processor, add garlic, sesame paste, lemon juice, olive oil and parsley, pulse well and divide into bowls and serve.
3. Enjoy!

Nutrition Value: calories 202, fat 4, fiber 3, carbs 7, protein 8

523. Tomato and Bell Pepper Dip
Preparation time: 10 minutes
Cooking time: 10 minutes
Servings: 4

Ingredients:
- 1 tablespoon olive oil
- 1 cup yellow onion, chopped
- 2 garlic cloves, minced
- 2 cups sweet bell pepper, chopped
- ¼ cup sun-dried tomatoes, minced
- 2 tablespoons tomato paste
- ¼ cup veggie stock
- Salt and black pepper to the taste

Directions:
1. In a pan that fits your air fryer, combine oil with onion, garlic, bell pepper, tomatoes, tomato paste, stock, salt and pepper, toss, introduce in the fryer and cook at 365 degrees F for 10 minutes.
2. Stir, divide into bowls and serve.
3. Enjoy!

Nutrition Value: calories 173, fat 4, fiber 3, carbs 7, protein 8

524., Apple Dip
Preparation time: 10 minutes
Cooking time: 15 minutes
Servings: 4

Ingredients:
- 8 apples, cored and chopped
- 1 teaspoon cinnamon oil
- ¼ cup water
- 1 teaspoon cinnamon powder

Directions:
1. Put apples in a pan that fits your air fryer, add water and cinnamon powder, stir, introduce in the fryer and cook at 365 degrees F for 15 minutes.
2. Add oil, toss, blend using an immersion blender, divide into bowls and serve as a snack.

3. Enjoy!

Nutrition Value: calories 121, fat 3, fiber 3, carbs 8, protein 1

525. Orange and Cranberry Spread

Preparation time: 10 minutes
Cooking time: 15 minutes
Servings: 4

Ingredients:
- 2 and ½ teaspoons orange zest, grated
- 12 ounces cranberries
- ¼ cup orange juice
- 2 tablespoons maple syrup
- 1 cup stevia

Directions:
1. In a pan that fits your air fryer, combine orange juice with maple syrup, orange zest, cranberries and stevia, toss, introduce in your air fryer and cook at 365 degrees F for 15 minutes.
2. Stir your spread again, divide it into bowls and serve cold.
3. Enjoy!

Nutrition Value: calories 152, fat 1, fiber 4, carbs 7, protein 2

526. Mexican Chili Dip

Preparation time: 10 minutes
Cooking time: 12 minutes
Servings: 8

Ingredients:
- 5 ancho chilies, dried, seedless and chopped
- 2 garlic cloves, crushed
- Salt and black pepper to the taste
- ½ cups water
- 1 and ½ teaspoons stevia
- ½ teaspoon oregano, dried
- ½ teaspoon cumin, ground
- 2 tablespoons apple cider vinegar

Directions:
1. In a pan that fits your air fryer pot mix water with chilies, garlic, salt, pepper, stevia, cumin and oregano, stir, introduce in your air fryer and cook at 365 degrees F for 12 minutes.
2. Transfer this mix to your blender, add vinegar, pulse well, divide into bowls and serve cold.
3. Enjoy!

Nutrition Value: calories 162, fat 2, fiber 6, carbs 8, protein 2

527. Hot Tomato and Plums Dip

Preparation time: 10 minutes
Cooking time: 15 minutes
Servings: 8

Ingredients:
- 1 tablespoon sesame oil
- ½ cup tomato puree
- 1 yellow onion, chopped
- ½ cup water
- 4 tablespoons white wine vinegar
- 4 tablespoons stevia
- ½ teaspoon garlic powder
- 1 teaspoon liquid smoke
- 1 teaspoon Tabasco sauce
- 1/8 teaspoon cumin powder
- 5 ounces plums, dried and seedless

Directions:
1. In a pan that fits your air fryer, combine oil with onion, tomato puree, stevia, water, vinegar, garlic, Tabasco sauce, liquid smoke, cumin and plums, stir, introduce in the fryer and cook at 365 degrees F for 15 minutes.
2. Blend everything with an immersion blender, transfer dip to a bowl and serve.
3. Enjoy!

Nutrition Value: calories 100, fat 2, fiber 4, carbs 5, protein 2

528. Carrots and Beets Dip

Preparation time: 10 minutes
Cooking time: 20 minutes
Servings: 8

Ingredients:
- 1 yellow onion, chopped
- 1 tablespoon olive oil
- 5 celery ribs
- 8 carrots, chopped
- 4 beets, chopped
- 1 butternut squash, chopped
- 8 garlic cloves, minced
- ¼ cup veggie stock
- ¼ cup lemon juice
- 1 bunch basil, chopped
- Salt and black pepper to the taste

Directions:
- In a pan that fits your air fryer, combine oil with onion, celery, beets, carrots, squash, garlic, stock, lemon juice, salt and pepper, toss, introduce in the fryer and cook at 367 degrees F for 20 minutes.

- Blend using an immersion blender, add basil, blend again, divide into bowls and serve as a dip.
- Enjoy!

Nutrition Value: calories 100, fat 2, fiber 5, carbs 7, protein 3

529. Creamy Cauliflower Spread

Preparation time: 10 minutes
Cooking time: 15 minutes
Servings: 6

Ingredients:

1. 2 tablespoons olive oil
2. 8 garlic cloves, minced
3. ½ cup veggie stock
4. 6 cups cauliflower florets
5. Salt and black pepper to the taste
6. ½ cup coconut milk

Directions:

- In a dish that fits your air fryer, combine oil with garlic, stock, cauliflower, salt and pepper, toss, introduce in your air fryer and cook at 370 degrees F for 15 minutes.
- Transfer to your blender, add milk, blend well, divide into bowls and serve.
- Enjoy!

Nutrition Value: calories 129, fat 3, fiber 4, carbs 7, protein 4

530. Mango Dip

Preparation time: 10 minutes
Cooking time: 20 minutes
Servings: 4

Ingredients:

- 1 shallot, chopped
- 1 tablespoon vegetable oil
- ¼ teaspoon cardamom powder
- 2 tablespoons ginger, minced
- ½ teaspoon cinnamon powder
- 2 mangos, peeled and chopped
- 2 red hot chilies, chopped
- 1 apple, cored and chopped
- 1 and ¼ cup stevia
- 1 and ¼ apple cider vinegar

Directions:

1. In a pan that fits your air fryer, combine shallot with oil, cardamom, ginger, cinnamon, mangos, chilies, apple, stevia and vinegar, stir, introduce in the fryer and cook at 365 degrees F for 20 minutes.
2. Stir the dip really well, divide into bowls and serve.
3. Enjoy!

Nutrition Value: calories 100, fat 2, fiber 1, carbs 7, protein 2

531. Easy Tomato Chutney

Preparation time: 10 minutes
Cooking time: 10 minutes
Servings: 6

Ingredients:

- 3 pounds tomatoes, peeled and chopped
- 1 cup red wine vinegar
- 1 cup stevia
- 1-inch ginger piece, grated
- 3 garlic cloves, minced
- 2 yellow onions, chopped
- ¼ teaspoon cloves, ground
- ½ teaspoon coriander, ground
- ½ teaspoon sweet paprika
- 1 teaspoon chili powder

Directions:

1. Mix tomatoes and ginger in your blender, pulse well and transfer to a pan that fits your air fryer.
2. Add vinegar, stevia, garlic, onions, cloves, coriander, paprika and chili powder, stir, introduce in the fryer and cook at 365 degrees F for 10 minutes
3. Transfer to bowls and serve cold as a dip.
4. Enjoy!

Nutrition Value: calories 152, fat 3, fiber 5, carbs 14, protein 4

532. Turkish Tomato Dip

Preparation time: 10 minutes
Cooking time: 21 minutes
Servings: 14

Ingredients:

- 2 pounds tomatoes, peeled and chopped
- 1 apple, cored and chopped
- 1 yellow onion, chopped
- 6 ounces sultanas, chopped
- 3 ounces dates, chopped
- 3 teaspoons whole spice
- ½ pint vinegar
- ½ pound coconut sugar

Directions:

1. Put tomatoes in a pan that fits your air fryer, add apple, onion, sultanas, dates, whole spice and half of the vinegar, stir, introduce in the fryer

and cook at 360 degrees F for 15 minutes.
2. Add the rest of the vinegar and the sugar, stir, cook at 360 degrees F for 6 minutes more, whisk well, divide into bowls and serve cold.
3. Enjoy!

Nutrition Value: calories 100, fat 4, fiber 5, carbs 6, protein 2

533. Green Tomato and Currants Dip

Preparation time: 5 minutes
Cooking time: 15 minutes
Servings: 12

Ingredients:

- 2 pounds green tomatoes, chopped
- 1 white onion, chopped
- ¼ cup currants
- 1 Anaheim chili pepper, chopped
- 4 red chili peppers, chopped
- 2 tablespoons ginger, grated
- ¾ cup coconut sugar

Directions:

1. In a pan that fits your air fryer, mix green tomatoes with onion, currants, Anaheim pepper, chili pepper, ginger, sugar and vinegar, stir, introduce in the fryer and cook at 360 degrees F for 15 minutes.
2. Whisk the dip really well, divide it between bowls and serve cold.
3. Enjoy!

Nutrition Value: calories 80, fat 2, fiber 3, carbs 12, protein 3

534. Plum Spread

Preparation time: 10 minutes
Cooking time: 15 minutes
Servings: 20

Ingredients:

- 3 pounds plumps, pitted and chopped
- 2 onions, chopped
- 2 apples, cored and chopped
- 4 tablespoons ginger powder
- 4 tablespoons cinnamon powder
- 1-pint vinegar
- ¾ pound coconut sugar

Directions:

1. Put plumps, apples and onions in a pan that fits your air fryer, add ginger, cinnamon, sugar and vinegar, stir, introduce in the fryer and cook at 365 degrees F for 16 minutes.
2. Stir really well, divide into bowls and serve cold as a spread.
3. Enjoy!

Nutrition Value: calories 142, fat 4, fiber 6, carbs 17, protein 15

535. Broccoli Dip

Preparation time: 10 minutes
Cooking time: 16 minutes
Servings: 4

Ingredients:

- 1 cup water
- 3 cups broccoli florets
- 2 garlic cloves, minced
- Salt and black pepper to the taste
- 1/3 cup coconut milk
- 1 tablespoon white wine vinegar
- 1 tablespoons nutritional yeast
- 1 tablespoon olive oil

Directions:

1. In a pan that fits the fryer, combine, water with broccoli, garlic, salt and pepper, stir, introduce in the fryer and cook at 365 degrees F for 16 minutes.
2. Transfer broccoli mix to your blender, add coconut milk, vinegar, yeast and oil, pulse really well, divide into bowls and serve cold.
3. Enjoy!

Nutrition Value: calories 142, fat 8, fiber 4, carbs 8, protein 5

536. Easy Carrot Dip

Preparation time: 10 minutes
Cooking time: 15 minutes
Servings: 6

Ingredients:

- 4 tablespoons olive oil
- 2 cups carrot, grated
- ½ teaspoon cinnamon powder
- Salt and black pepper to the taste
- A pinch of cayenne pepper
- 1 tablespoon chives, chopped

Directions:

1. In a pan that fits the fryer, combine oil with carrots, cinnamon, salt, pepper and cayenne, stir, introduce in the fryer and cook at 365 degrees F for 15 minutes.
2. Add chives, stir really well, divide into bowls and serve cold as a dip
3. Enjoy!

Nutrition Value: calories 152, fat 3, fiber 3, carbs 14,

protein 3

537. Fennel and Cherry Tomatoes Spread

Preparation time: 10 minutes
Cooking time: 12 minutes
Servings: 6

Ingredients:

- 1 fennel bulb, cut into pieces
- 2 pints cherry tomatoes, halved
- ¼ cup veggie stock
- 5 thyme springs, chopped
- 1 tablespoons olive oil
- Salt and black pepper to the taste

Directions:

1. In a pan that fits the fryer, combine fennel with tomatoes, stock, thyme, oil, salt and pepper, toss, introduce in the fryer and cook at 365 degrees F for 12 minutes.
2. Mash the mixture a bit using a fork, stir well, divide into bowls and serve cold.
3. Enjoy!

Nutrition Value: calories 100, fat 2, fiber 4, carbs 5, protein 3

538. Leeks Spread

Preparation time: 5 minutes
Cooking time: 10 minutes
Servings: 8

Ingredients:

- 4 leeks, thinly sliced
- 1 tablespoon olive oil
- 1 cup coconut cream
- 3 tablespoons lemon juice
- Salt and black pepper to the taste

Directions:

1. In a pan that fits your air fryer, combine leeks with oil, lemon juice, salt and pepper, toss, introduce in the fryer and cook at 370 degrees F for 10 minutes.
2. Add coconut cream, stir really well, divide into bowls and serve cold.
3. Enjoy!

Nutrition Value: calories 142, fat 4, fiber 1, carbs 8, protein 2

539. Vegan Rolls

Preparation time: 10 minutes
Cooking time: 8 hours
Servings: 4

Ingredients:

- 1 cup brown lentils, cooked
- 1 green cabbage head, leaves separated
- ½ cup onion, chopped
- 1 cup brown rice, already cooked
- 2 ounces white mushrooms, chopped
- ¼ cup pine nuts, toasted
- ¼ cup raisins
- 2 garlic cloves, minced
- 2 tablespoons dill, chopped
- 1 tablespoon olive oil
- 25 ounces marinara sauce
- A pinch of salt and black pepper
- ¼ cup water

Directions:

1. In a bowl, mix lentils with onion, rice, mushrooms, pine nuts, raisins, garlic, dill, salt and pepper and whisk well.
2. Arrange cabbage leaves on a working surface, divide lentils mix and wrap them well.
3. Add marinara sauce and water to your slow cooker and stir.
4. Add cabbage rolls, cover and cook on Low for 8 hours.
5. Arrange cabbage rolls on a platter, drizzle sauce all over and serve.
6. Enjoy!

Nutrition Value: calories 261, fat 6, fiber 6, carbs 12, protein 3

540. Eggplant Appetizer

Preparation time: 10 minutes
Cooking time: 7 hours
Servings: 4

Ingredients:

- 1 and ½ cups tomatoes, chopped
- 3 cups eggplant, cubed
- 2 teaspoons capers
- 6 ounces green olives, pitted and sliced
- 4 garlic cloves, minced
- 2 teaspoons balsamic vinegar
- 1 tablespoon basil, chopped
- Salt and black pepper to the taste

Directions:

1. In your slow cooker, mix tomatoes with eggplant cubes, capers, green olives, garlic, vinegar, basil, salt and pepper, toss, cover and cook on Low for 7 hours.
2. Divide into small appetizer plates and serve as

an appetizer.
3. Enjoy!

Nutrition Value: calories 200, fat 6, fiber 5, carbs 9, protein 2

541. Vegan Veggie Dip

Preparation time: 10 minutes
Cooking time: 7 hours
Servings: 4

Ingredients:

- 1 cup carrots, sliced
- 1 and ½ cups cauliflower florets
- 1/3 cup cashews
- ½ cup turnips, chopped
- 2 and ½ cups water
- 1 cup almond milk
- 1 teaspoon garlic powder
- ¼ cup nutritional yeast
- ¼ teaspoon smoked paprika
- ¼ teaspoon mustard powder
- A pinch of salt

Directions:

1. In your slow cooker, mix carrots with cauliflower, cashews, turnips and water, stir, cover and cook on Low for 7 hours.
2. Drain, transfer to a blender, add almond milk, garlic powder, yeast, paprika, mustard powder and salt, blend well and serve as a snack.
3. Enjoy!

Nutrition Value: calories 291, fat 7, fiber 4, carbs 14, protein 3

542. Great Bolognese Dip

Preparation time: 10 minutes
Cooking time: 5 hours
Servings: 7

Ingredients:

- ½ cauliflower head, riced in your blender
- 54 ounces canned tomatoes, crushed
- 10 ounces white mushrooms, chopped
- 2 cups carrots, shredded
- 2 cups eggplant, cubed
- 6 garlic cloves, minced
- 2 tablespoons agave nectar
- 2 tablespoons balsamic vinegar
- 2 tablespoons tomato paste
- 1 tablespoon basil, chopped
- 1 and ½ tablespoons oregano, chopped
- 1 and ½ teaspoons rosemary, dried
- A pinch of salt and black pepper

Directions:

1. In your slow cooker, mix cauliflower rice with tomatoes, mushrooms, carrots, eggplant cubes, garlic, agave nectar, balsamic vinegar, tomato paste, rosemary, salt and pepper, stir, cover and cook on High for 5 hours.
2. Add basil and oregano, stir again, divide into bowls and serve as a dip.
3. Enjoy!

Nutrition Value: calories 251, fat 7, fiber 6, carbs 10, protein 6

543. Black Eyed Peas Pate

Preparation time: 10 minutes
Cooking time: 5 hours
Servings: 5

Ingredients:

- 1 and ½ cups black-eyed peas
- 3 cups water
- 1 teaspoon Cajun seasoning
- ½ cup pecans, toasted
- ½ teaspoon garlic powder
- ½ teaspoon jalapeno powder
- A pinch of salt and black pepper
- ¼ teaspoon liquid smoke
- ½ teaspoon Tabasco sauce

Directions:

1. In your slow cooker, mix black-eyed pea with Cajun seasoning, salt, pepper and water, stir, cover and cook on High for 5 hours.
2. Drain, transfer to a blender, add pecans, garlic powder, jalapeno powder, Tabasco sauce, liquid smoke, more salt and pepper, pulse well and serve as an appetizer.
3. Enjoy!

Nutrition Value: calories 221, fat 4, fiber 7, carbs 16, protein 4

544. Tofu Appetizer

Preparation time: 10 minutes
Cooking time: 7 hours
Servings: 6

Ingredients:

- ¼ cup yellow onions, sliced
- 1 cup carrot, sliced
- 14 ounces firm tofu, cubed
- For the sauce:
- ¼ cup soy sauce
- ½ cup water

- 3 tablespoons agave nectar
- 3 tablespoons nutritional yeast
- 1 teaspoon garlic, minced
- 1 tablespoon ginger, minced
- ½ tablespoon rice vinegar

Directions:
1. In your slow cooker, mix tofu with onion and carrots.
2. In a bowl, mix soy sauce with water, agave nectar, yeast, garlic, ginger and vinegar and whisk well.
3. Add this to slow cooker, cover and cook on Low for 7 hours.
4. Divide into appetizer bowls and serve.
5. Enjoy!

Nutrition Value: calories 251, fat 6, fiber 8, carbs 12, protein 3

545. Hummus

Preparation time: 10 minutes
Cooking time: 8 hours
Servings: 10

Ingredients:
- 1 cup chickpeas, dried
- 2 tablespoons olive oil
- 3 cups water
- A pinch of salt and black pepper
- 1 garlic clove, minced
- 1 tablespoon lemon juice

Directions:
1. In your slow cooker, mix chickpeas with water, salt and pepper, stir, cover and cook on Low for 8 hours.
2. Drain chickpeas, transfer to a blender, add oil, more salt and pepper, garlic and lemon juice, blend well, divide into bowls and serve.
3. Enjoy!

Nutrition Value: calories 211, fat 6, fiber 7, carbs 8, protein 4

546. Vegan Cashew Spread

Preparation time: 10 minutes
Cooking time: 3 hours
Servings: 10

Ingredients:
- 1 cup water
- 1 cup cashews
- 10 ounces vegan hummus
- ¼ teaspoon garlic powder
- ¼ teaspoon onion powder
- ¼ cup nutritional yeast
- A pinch of salt and black pepper
- ¼ teaspoon mustard powder
- 1 teaspoon apple cider vinegar

Directions:
1. In your slow cooker, mix water with cashews, yeast, salt and pepper, stir, cover and cook on High for 3 hours.
2. Transfer to your blender, add hummus, garlic powder, onion powder, mustard powder and vinegar, pulse well, divide into bowls and serve.
3. Enjoy!

Nutrition Value: calories 192, fat 7, fiber 7, carbs 12, protein 4

547. Spinach Dip

Preparation time: 10 minutes
Cooking time: 30 minutes
Servings: 4

Ingredients:
- ½ cup coconut cream
- ¾ cup coconut yogurt
- 10 ounces spinach leaves
- 8 ounces water chestnuts, chopped
- 1 garlic clove, minced
- Black pepper to the taste

Directions:
1. In your slow cooker, mix coconut cream with spinach, coconut yogurt, chestnuts, black pepper and garlic, stir, cover and cook on High for 30 minutes.
2. Blend using an immersion blender, divide into bowls and serve.
3. Enjoy!

Nutrition Value: calories 221, fat 5, fiber 7, carbs 12, protein 5

548. Chowder

Preparation time: 10 minutes
Cooking time: 8 hours
Servings: 8

Ingredients:
- 2 cups corn
- 2 cups potatoes, peeled and cubed
- 4 cups veggie stock
- 2 carrots, chopped
- 2 celery stalks, chopped
- 1 yellow onion, chopped
- A pinch of salt and black pepper

- 1 cup coconut cream
- 1 teaspoon thyme, dried
- 4 zucchinis, chopped
- ½ cup basil, chopped
- 3 tomatoes, chopped

Directions:
1. In your slow cooker, mix stock with corn, potatoes, carrot, celery, onion, salt, pepper, cream, zucchini and thyme, stir, cover and cook on Low for 8 hours.
2. Blend using an immersion blender, add basil and tomatoes, stir, divide into small bowls and serve as an appetizer.
3. Enjoy!

Nutrition Value: calories 311, fat 6, fiber 7, carbs 12, protein 4

549. Appetizer Potato Salad

Preparation time: 10 minutes
Cooking time: 8 hours
Servings: 6

Ingredients:
- 1 sweet onion, chopped
- ¼ cup white vinegar
- 2 tablespoons mustard
- A pinch of salt and black pepper
- 1 and ½ pounds gold potatoes, cut into medium chunks
- ¼ cup dill, chopped
- 1 cup celery, chopped
- Cooking spray

Directions:
1. Spray your slow cooker with cooking spray, add onion, vinegar, mustard, salt and pepper and whisk well.
2. Add celery and potatoes, toss them well, cover and cook on Low for 8 hours.
3. Divide salad into small bowls, sprinkle dill on top and serve as an appetizer.
4. Enjoy!

Nutrition Value: calories 251, fat 6, fiber 7, carbs 8, protein 7

550. Veggie Appetizer

Preparation time: 10 minutes
Cooking time: 3 hours
Servings: 4

Ingredients:
- 2 red bell peppers, cut into medium wedges
- 1 sweet potato, cut into medium wedges
- 3 zucchinis, sliced
- ½ cup garlic, minced
- 2 tablespoons olive oil
- A pinch of salt and black pepper
- 1 teaspoon Italian seasoning

Directions:
1. In your slow cooker, mix bell peppers with sweet potato, zucchinis, garlic, oil, salt, pepper and seasoning, toss, cover and cook on High for 3 hours.
2. Divide into small bowls and serve cold as an appetizer.
3. Enjoy!

Nutrition Value: calories 132, fat 3, fiber 3, carbs 4, protein 4

551. Black Bean Appetizer Salad

Preparation time: 10 minutes
Cooking time: 4 hours
Servings: 7

Ingredients:
- 1 tablespoon coconut aminos
- ½ teaspoon cumin, ground
- 1 cup canned black beans
- 1 cup salsa
- 6 cups romaine lettuce leaves
- ½ cup avocado, peeled, pitted and mashed

Directions:
In your slow cooker, mix black beans with salsa, cumin and aminos, stir, cover and cook on Low for 4 hours. In a salad bowl, mix lettuce leaves with black beans mix and mashed avocado, toss and serve as an appetizer. Enjoy!
Nutrition Value: calories 221, fat 4, fiber 7, carbs 12, protein 3

552. Colored Stuffed Bell Peppers

Preparation time: 10 minutes
Cooking time: 4 hours
Servings: 5

Ingredients:
- 1 yellow onion, chopped
- 2 teaspoons olive oil
- 2 celery ribs, chopped
- 1 tablespoon chili powder
- 3 garlic cloves, minced
- 2 teaspoon cumin, ground
- 1 and ½ teaspoon oregano, dried
- 2 cups white rice, already cooked

- 1 cup corn
- 1 tomato chopped
- 7 ounces canned pinto beans, drained
- 1 chipotle pepper in adobo
- A pinch of salt and black pepper
- 5 colored bell peppers, tops and insides scooped out
- ½ cup vegan enchilada sauce

Directions:
1. Heat up a pan with the oil over medium high heat, add onion and celery, stir and cook for 5 minutes.
2. Add garlic, stir, cook for 1 minute more, take off heat and mix with chili, cumin and oregano.
3. Also add rice, corn, beans, tomato, salt, pepper and chipotle pepper and stir well.
4. Stuff bell peppers with this mix and place them in your slow cooker.
5. Add enchilada sauce, cover and cook on Low for 4 hours.
6. Arrange stuffed bell peppers on a platter and serve them as an appetizer.
7. Enjoy!

Nutrition Value: calories 221, fat 5, fiber 4, carbs 19, protein 3

553. Corn Dip

Preparation time: 10 minutes
Cooking time: 2 hours
Servings: 8

Ingredients:
- 30 ounces canned corn, drained
- 2 green onions, chopped
- ½ cup coconut cream
- 8 ounces tofu, crumbled
- 1 jalapeno, chopped
- ½ teaspoon chili powder

Directions:
1. In your slow cooker, mix corn with green onions, coconut cream, tofu, chili powder and jalapeno, stir, cover and cook on Low for 2 hours.
2. Divide into bowls and serve as a dip.
3. Enjoy!

Nutrition Value: calories 332, fat 5, fiber 10, carbs 17, protein 4

554. Artichoke Spread

Preparation time: 10 minutes
Cooking time: 2 hours
Servings: 8

Ingredients:
- 28 ounces canned artichokes, drained and chopped
- 10 ounces spinach
- 8 ounces coconut cream
- 1 yellow onion, chopped
- 2 garlic cloves, minced
- ¾ cup coconut milk
- ½ cup tofu, pressed and crumbled
- 1/3 cup vegan avocado mayonnaise
- 1 tablespoon red vinegar
- A pinch of salt and black pepper

Directions:
1. In your slow cooker, mix artichokes with spinach, coconut cream, onion, garlic, coconut milk, tofu, avocado mayo, vinegar, salt and pepper, stir well, cover and cook on Low for 2 hours.
2. Divide into bowls and serve as an appetizer.
3. Enjoy!

Nutrition Value: calories 355, fat 24, fiber 4, carbs 19, protein 13

555. Mushroom Spread

Preparation time: 10 minutes
Cooking time: 4 hours
Servings: 6

Ingredients:
- 2 cups green bell peppers, chopped
- 1 cup yellow onion, chopped
- 3 garlic cloves, minced
- 1 pound mushrooms, chopped
- 28 ounces tomato sauce
- ½ cup tofu, pressed, drained and crumbled
- Salt and black pepper to the taste

Directions:
1. In your slow cooker, mix bell peppers with onion, garlic, mushrooms, tomato sauce, tofu, salt and pepper, stir, cover and cook on Low for 4 hours.
2. Divide into bowls and serve as a party spread.
3. Enjoy!

Nutrition Value: calories 245, fat 4, fiber 7, carbs 9, protein 3

556. Three Bean Dip

Preparation time: 10 minutes
Cooking time: 1 hour
Servings: 6

Ingredients:

- ½ cup salsa
- 2 cups canned refried beans
- 1 cup vegan nacho cheese
- 2 tablespoons green onions, chopped

Directions:
1. In your slow cooker, mix refried beans with salsa, vegan nacho cheese and green onions, stir, cover and cook on High for 1 hour.
2. Divide into bowls and serve as a party snack.
3. Enjoy!

Nutrition Value: calories 262, fat 5, fiber 10, carbs 20, protein 3

DESSERTS

557. Stewed Rhubarb
Preparation time: 10 minutes
Cooking time: 7 hours
Servings: 4

Ingredients:
- 5 cups rhubarb, chopped
- 2 tablespoons coconut butter
- 1/3 cup water
- 2/3 cup coconut sugar
- 1 teaspoon vanilla extract

Directions:
1. Put rhubarb in your slow cooker.
2. Add water and sugar, stir gently, cover and cook on Low for 7 hours.
3. Add coconut butter and vanilla extract, stir and keep in the fridge until it's cold.
4. Enjoy!

Nutrition Value: calories 120, fat 2, fiber 3, carbs 6, protein 1

558. Pudding Cake
Preparation time: 10 minutes
Cooking time: 2 hours and 30 minutes
Servings: 8

Ingredients:
- 1 and ½ cup stevia
- 1 cup flour
- ¼ cup baking cocoa+ 2 tablespoons
- ½ cup chocolate almond milk
- 2 teaspoons baking powder
- 2 tablespoons canola oil
- 1 teaspoon vanilla extract
- 1 and ½ cups hot water
- Cooking spray

Directions:
1. In a bowl, mix flour with 2 tablespoons cocoa, baking powder, almond milk, oil and vanilla extract, whisk well and spread on the bottom of the slow cooker after you've greased with cooking spray.
2. In a separate bowl, mix stevia with the rest of the cocoa and the water, whisk well and spread over the batter in your slow cooker.
3. Cover, cook your cake on High for 2 hours and 30 minutes.
4. Leave cake to cool down, slice and serve.
5. Enjoy!

Nutrition Value: calories 250, fat 4, fiber 3, carbs 40, protein 2

559. Sweet Peanut Butter Cake
Preparation time: 10 minutes
Cooking time: 2 hours and 30 minutes
Servings: 8

Ingredients:
- 1 cup coconut sugar
- 1 cup flour
- 3 tablespoons cocoa powder+ ½ cup
- 1 and ½ teaspoons baking powder
- ½ cup almond milk
- 2 tablespoons coconut oil
- 2 cups hot water
- 1 teaspoon vanilla extract
- ½ cup peanut butter
- Cooking spray

Directions:
1. In a bowl, mix half of the coconut sugar with 3 tablespoons cocoa, flour and baking powder and stir well.
2. Add coconut oil, vanilla and milk, stir well and pour into your slow cooker greased with cooking spray.
3. In another bowl, mix the rest of the sugar with the rest of the cocoa, peanut butter and hot water, stir well and pour over the batter in the slow cooker.
4. Cover pot, cook on High for 2 hours and 30 minutes, slice cake and serve.
5. Enjoy!

Nutrition Value: calories 242, fat 4, fiber 7, carbs 8, protein 4

560. Blueberry Cake
Preparation time: 10 minutes
Cooking time: 1 hour
Servings: 6

Ingredients:
- ½ cup whole wheat flour
- ¼ teaspoon baking powder
- ¼ teaspoon stevia
- ¼ cup blueberries
- 1/3 cup almond milk
- 1 teaspoon olive oil

- 1 teaspoon flaxseed, ground
- ½ teaspoon lemon zest, grated
- ¼ teaspoon vanilla extract
- ¼ teaspoon lemon extract
- Cooking spray

Directions:
1. In a bowl, mix flour with baking powder and stevia and stir.
2. Add blueberries, milk, oil, flaxseeds, lemon zest, vanilla extract and lemon extract and whisk well.
3. Spray your slow cooker with cooking spray, line it with parchment paper, pour cake batter, cover pot and cook on High for 1 hour.
4. Leave cake to cool down, slice and serve.
5. Enjoy!

Nutrition Value: calories 200, fat 4, fiber 4, carbs 10, protein 4

561. Peach Cobbler
Preparation time: 10 minutes
Cooking time: 4 hours
Servings: 4

Ingredients:
- 4 cups peaches, peeled and sliced
- ¼ cup coconut sugar
- ½ teaspoon cinnamon powder
- 1 and ½ cups vegan sweet crackers, crushed
- ¼ cup stevia
- ¼ teaspoon nutmeg, ground
- ½ cup almond milk
- 1 teaspoon vanilla extract
- Cooking spray

Directions:
1. In a bowl, mix peaches with coconut sugar and cinnamon and stir.
2. In a separate bowl, mix crackers with stevia, nutmeg, almond milk and vanilla extract and stir.
3. Spray your slow cooker with cooking spray and spread peaches on the bottom.
4. Add crackers mix, spread, cover and cook on Low for 4 hours.
5. Divide cobbler between plates and serve.
6. Enjoy!

Nutrition Value: calories 212, fat 4, fiber 4, carbs 7, protein 3

562. Apple Mix
Preparation time: 10 minutes
Cooking time: 4 hours
Servings: 6

Ingredients:
- 6 apples, cored, peeled and sliced
- 1 and ½ cups almond flour
- Cooking spray
- 1 cup coconut sugar
- 1 tablespoon cinnamon powder
- ¾ cup cashew butter, melted

Directions:
1. Add apple slices to your slow cooker after you've greased it with cooking spray
2. Add flour, sugar, cinnamon and coconut butter, stir gently, cover, cook on High for 4 hours, divide into bowls and serve cold.
3. Enjoy!

Nutrition Value: calories 200, fat 5, fiber 5, carbs 8, protein 4

563. Pears And Dried Fruits Bowls
Preparation time: 10 minutes
Cooking time: 4 hours
Servings: 12

Ingredients:
- 3 pears, cored and chopped
- ½ cup raisins
- 2 cups dried fruits
- 1 teaspoon ginger powder
- ¼ cup coconut sugar
- 1 teaspoon lemon zest, grated

Directions:
1. In your slow cooker, mix pears with raisins, dried fruits, ginger, sugar and lemon zest, stir, cover, cook on Low for 4 hours, divide into bowls and serve cold.
2. Enjoy!

Nutrition Value: calories 140, fat 3, fiber 4, carbs 6, protein 6

564. Strawberry Stew
Preparation time: 10 minutes
Cooking time: 3 hours
Servings: 10

Ingredients:
2 tablespoons lemon juice
2 pounds strawberries
4 cups coconut sugar
1 teaspoon cinnamon powder
1 teaspoon vanilla extract

Directions:
1. In your slow cooker, mix strawberries with

coconut sugar, lemon juice, cinnamon and vanilla, stir gently, cover and cook on Low for 3 hours.
2. Divide into bowls and serve cold.
3. Enjoy!

Nutrition Value: calories 100, fat 0, fiber 1, carbs 2, protein 2

565. Poached Plums

Preparation time: 10 minutes
Cooking time: 3 hours
Servings: 6

Ingredients:

- 14 plums, halved
- 1 and ¼ cups coconut sugar
- 1 teaspoon cinnamon powder
- ¼ cup water

Directions:

1. Arrange plums in your slow cooker, add sugar, cinnamon and water, stir, cover, cook on Low for 3 hours, divide into cups and serve cold.
2. Enjoy!

Nutrition Value: calories 150, fat 2, fiber 1, carbs 2, protein 3

566, Bananas And Agave Sauce

Preparation time: 10 minutes
Cooking time: 2 hours
Servings: 4

Ingredients:

- Juice of ½ lemon
- 3 tablespoons agave nectar
- 1 tablespoon coconut oil
- 4 bananas, peeled and sliced diagonally
- ½ teaspoon cardamom seeds

Directions:

1. Arrange bananas in your slow cooker, add agave nectar, lemon juice, oil and cardamom, cover and cook on Low for 2 hours.
2. Divide bananas on plates, drizzle agave sauce all over and serve.
3. Enjoy!

Nutrition Value: calories 120, fat 1, fiber 2, carbs 8, protein 3

567. Orange Cake

Preparation time: 10 minutes
Cooking time: 5 hours
Servings: 4

Ingredients:

- Cooking spray
- 1 teaspoon baking powder
- 1 cup almond flour
- 1 cup coconut sugar
- ½ teaspoon cinnamon powder
- 3 tablespoons coconut oil, melted
- ½ cup almond milk
- ½ cup pecans, chopped
- ¾ cup water
- ½ cup raisins
- ½ cup orange peel, grated
- ¾ cup orange juice

Directions:

1. In a bowl, mix flour with half of the sugar, baking powder, cinnamon, 2 tablespoons oil, milk, pecans and raisins, stir and pour this in your slow cooker after you've sprayed it with cooking spray.
2. Heat up a small pan over medium heat, add water, orange juice, orange peel, the rest of the oil and the rest of the sugar, stir, bring to a boil, pour over the mix in the slow cooker, cover and cook on Low for 5 hours.
3. Divide into dessert bowls and serve cold.
4. Enjoy!

Nutrition Value: calories 182, fat 3, fiber 1, carbs 4, protein 3

568. Stewed Apples

Preparation time: 10 minutes
Cooking time: 1 hour and 30 minutes
Servings: 5

Ingredients:

- 5 apples, tops cut off and cored
- 5 figs
- 1/3 cup coconut sugar
- ¼ cup pecans, chopped
- 2 teaspoons lemon zest, grated
- ½ teaspoon cinnamon powder
- 1 tablespoon lemon juice
- 1 tablespoon coconut oil
- ½ cup water

Directions:

1. Arrange apples in your slow cooker.
2. Add figs, coconut sugar, pecans, lemon zest, cinnamon, lemon juice, coconut oil and water, toss, cover and cook on High for 1 hour and 30 minutes.
3. Divide apples and sauce on plates and serve.
4. Enjoy!

Nutrition Value: calories 170, fat 1, fiber 2, carbs 6, protein 3

569. Pears And Orange Sauce

Preparation time: 10 minutes
Cooking time: 4 hours
Servings: 4

Ingredients:
- 4 pears, peeled and cored
- 2 cups orange juice
- ¼ cup maple syrup
- 2 teaspoons cinnamon powder
- 1 tablespoon ginger, grated

Directions:
1. In your slow cooker, mix pears with orange juice, maple syrup, cinnamon and ginger, cover and cook on Low for 4 hours.
2. Divide pears and orange sauce between plates and serve warm.
3. Enjoy!

Nutrition Value: calories 140, fat 1, fiber 2, carbs 3, protein 4

570. Almond Cookies

Preparation time: 10 minutes
Cooking time: 2 hours and 30 minutes
Servings: 12

Ingredients:
- 1 tablespoon flaxseed mixed with 2 tablespoons water
- ¼ cup coconut oil, melted
- 1 cup coconut sugar
- ½ teaspoon vanilla extract
- 1 teaspoon baking powder
- 1 and ½ cups almond meal
- ½ cup almonds, chopped

Directions:
1. In a bowl, mix oil with sugar, vanilla extract and flax meal and whisk.
2. Add baking powder, almond meal and almonds and stir well.
3. Line your slow cooker with parchment paper, spread cookie mix on the bottom of the pot, cover and cook on Low for 2 hours and 30 minutes.
4. Leave cookie sheet to cool down, cut into medium pieces and serve.
5. Enjoy!

Nutrition Value: calories 220, fat 2, fiber 1, carbs 3, protein 6

571. Pumpkin Cake

Preparation time: 10 minutes
Cooking time: 2 hours and 20 minutes
Servings: 10

Ingredients:
- 1 and ½ teaspoons baking powder
- Cooking spray
- 1 cup pumpkin puree
- 2 cups almond flour
- ½ teaspoon baking soda
- 1 and ½ teaspoons cinnamon, ground
- ¼ teaspoon ginger, ground
- 1 tablespoon coconut oil, melted
- 1 tablespoon flaxseed mixed with 2 tablespoons water
- 1 tablespoon vanilla extract
- 1/3 cup maple syrup
- 1 teaspoon lemon juice

Directions:
1. In a bowl, flour with baking powder, baking soda, cinnamon and ginger and stir.
2. Add flaxseed, coconut oil, vanilla, pumpkin puree, maple syrup and lemon juice, stir and pour in your slow cooker after you've sprayed it with cooking spray and lined with parchment paper.
3. Cover pot and cook on Low for 2 hours and 20 minutes.
4. Leave cake to cool down, slice and serve.
5. Enjoy!

Nutrition Value: calories 182, fat 3, fiber 2, carbs 3, protein 1

572. Strawberries Jam

Preparation time: 10 minutes
Cooking time: 4 hours
Servings: 10

Ingredients:
- 32 ounces strawberries, chopped
- 2 pounds coconut sugar
- Zest of 1 lemon, grated
- 4 ounces raisins
- 3 ounces water

Directions:
1. In your slow cooker, mix strawberries with coconut sugar, lemon zest, raisins and water, stir, cover and cook on High for 4 hours.
2. Divide into small jars and serve cold.
3. Enjoy!

Nutrition Value: calories 100, fat 3, fiber 2, carbs 2, protein 1

573. Lemon Jam

Preparation time: 10 minutes
Cooking time: 3 hours
Servings: 10

Ingredients:

- 2 pounds lemons, washed, peeled and sliced
- 2 pounds coconut sugar
- 1 tablespoon vinegar

Directions:

1. In your slow cooker, mix lemons with coconut sugar and vinegar, stir, cover and cook on High for 3 hours.
2. Divide into jars and serve cold.
3. Enjoy!

Nutrition Value: calories 100, fat 0, fiber 2, carbs 7, protein 4

574. Strawberries And Rhubarb Marmalade

Preparation time: 10 minutes
Cooking time: 3 hours
Servings: 8

Ingredients:

- 1/3 cup water
- 2 pounds rhubarb, chopped
- 2 pounds strawberries, chopped
- 1 cup coconut sugar
- 1 tablespoon mint, chopped

Directions:

1. In your slow cooker, mix water with rhubarb, strawberries, sugar and mint, stir, cover and cook on High for 3 hours.
2. Divide into cups and serve cold.
3. Enjoy!

Nutrition Value: calories 100, fat 1, fiber 4, carbs 10, protein 2

575. Sweet Potatoes Pudding

Preparation time: 10 minutes
Cooking time: 5 hours
Servings: 8

Ingredients:

- 1 cup water
- 1 tablespoon lemon peel, grated
- ½ cup coconut sugar
- 3 sweet potatoes peeled and sliced
- ¼ cup cashew butter
- ¼ cup maple syrup
- 1 cup pecans, chopped

Directions:

- In your slow cooker, mix water with lemon peel, coconut sugar, potatoes, cashew butter, maple syrup and pecans, stir, cover and cook on High for 5 hours.
- Divide sweet potato pudding into bowls and serve cold.
- Enjoy!

Nutrition Value: calories 200, fat 4, fiber 3, carbs 10, protein 4

576. Cherry Marmalade

Preparation time: 10 minutes
Cooking time: 3 hours
Servings: 6

Ingredients:

- 2 tablespoons lemon juice
- 3 tablespoons vegan gelatin
- 4 cups cherries, pitted
- 2 cups coconut sugar

Directions:

1. In your slow cooker, mix lemon juice with gelatin, cherries and coconut sugar, stir, cover and cook on High for 3 hours.
2. Divide into cups and serve cold.
3. Enjoy!

Nutrition Value: calories 211, fat 3, fiber 1, carbs 3, protein 3

577. Rice Pudding

Preparation time: 10 minutes
Cooking time: 5 hours
Servings: 4

Ingredients:

- 6 and ½ cups water
- 1 cup coconut sugar
- 2 cups white rice, washed and rinsed
- 2 cinnamon sticks
- ½ cup coconut, shredded

Directions:

1. In your slow cooker, mix water with coconut sugar, rice, cinnamon and coconut, stir, cover and cook on High for 5 hours.
2. Divide pudding into cups and serve cold.
3. Enjoy!

Nutrition Value: calories 213, fat 4, fiber 6, carbs 9, protein 4

578. Cinnamon Rice

Preparation time: 10 minutes
Cooking time: 35 minutes
Servings: 4

Ingredients:

- 3 and ½ cups water
- 1 cup coconut sugar
- 2 cups white rice, washed and rinsed
- 2 cinnamon sticks
- ½ cup coconut, shredded

Directions:

1. In your air fryer, mix water with coconut sugar, rice, cinnamon and coconut, stir, cover and cook at 365 degrees F for 35 minutes.
2. Divide pudding into cups and serve cold.
3. Enjoy!

Nutrition Value: calories 213, fat 4, fiber 6, carbs 9, protein 4

579. Cranberry Pudding

Preparation time: 10 minutes
Cooking time: 30 minutes
Servings: 4

Ingredients:

- 4 ounces dried cranberries, chopped
- A drizzle of olive oil
- 4 ounces dried apricots, chopped
- 1 cup white flour
- 3 teaspoons baking powder
- 1 cup coconut sugar
- 1 teaspoon ginger powder
- A pinch of cinnamon powder
- 15 tablespoons coconut butter
- 3 tablespoons maple syrup
- 3 tablespoons flax meal mixed with 3 tablespoons water
- 1 carrot, grated

Directions:

1. Grease a heatproof pudding pan with a drizzle of oil.
2. In a blender, mix flour with baking powder, sugar, cinnamon, ginger, butter, maple syrup and flax meal and pulse well.
3. Add dried fruits and carrot, fold them into the batter and spread this mix into the pudding mold.
4. Put the pudding in your air fryer and cook at 365 degrees F for 30 minutes.
5. Leave the pudding aside to cool down, slice and serve.
6. Enjoy!

Nutrition Value: calories 262, fat 7, fiber 4, carbs 12, protein 4

580. Chocolate and Coconut Bars

Preparation time: 10 minutes
Cooking time: 7 minutes
Servings: 12

Ingredients:

- 1 cup sugar free and vegan chocolate chips
- 2 tablespoons coconut butter
- 2/3 cup coconut cream
- 2 tablespoons stevia
- ¼ teaspoon vanilla extract

Directions:

1. Put the cream in a bowl, add stevia, butter and chocolate chips and stir
2. Leave aside for 5 minutes, stir well and mix the vanilla.
3. Transfer the mix into a lined baking sheet, introduce in your air fryer and cook at 356 degrees F for 7 minutes.
4. Leave the mix aside to cool down, slice and serve.
5. Enjoy!

Nutrition Value: calories 120, fat 5, fiber 4, carbs 6, protein 1

581. Raspberry Bars

Preparation time: 10 minutes
Cooking time: 6 minutes
Servings: 12

Ingredients:

- ½ cup coconut butter, melted
- ½ cup coconut oil
- ½ cup raspberries, dried
- ¼ cup swerve
- ½ cup coconut, shredded

Directions:

1. In your food processor, blend dried berries very well.
2. In a bowl that fits your air fryer, mix oil with butter, swerve, coconut and raspberries, toss well, introduce in the fryer and cook at 320 degrees F for 6 minutes.
3. Spread this on a lined baking sheet, keep in the fridge for an hour, slice and serve.
4. Enjoy!

Nutrition Value: calories 164, fat 22, fiber 2, carbs 4,

protein 2

582. Vanilla and Blueberry Squares

Preparation time: 10 minutes
Cooking time: 20 minutes
Servings: 8

Ingredients:

- 5 ounces coconut oil, melted
- ½ teaspoon baking powder
- 4 tablespoons stevia
- 1 teaspoon vanilla
- 4 ounces coconut cream
- 3 tablespoons flax meal combined with 3 tablespoons water
- ½ cup blueberries

Directions:

1. In a bowl, mix coconut oil with flax meal, coconut cream, vanilla, stevia and baking powder and blend using an immersion blender.
2. Fold blueberries, pour everything into a square baking dish that fits your air fryer, introduce in the fryer and cook at 320 degrees F for 20 minutes.
3. Slice into squares and serve cold.
4. Enjoy!

Nutrition Value: calories 150, fat 2, fiber 3, carbs 6, protein 4

583. Cocoa Brownies

Preparation time: 10 minutes
Cooking time: 20 minutes
Servings: 12

Ingredients:

- 6 ounces coconut oil, melted
- 3 tablespoons flax meal combined with 3 tablespoons water
- 3 ounces cocoa powder
- 2 teaspoons vanilla
- ½ teaspoon baking powder
- 4 ounces coconut cream
- 5 tablespoons stevia

Directions:

1. In a blender, mix flax meal with oil, cocoa powder, baking powder, vanilla, cream and stevia and stir using a mixer.
2. Pour this into a lined baking dish that fits your air fryer, introduce in the fryer and cook at 350 degrees F for 20 minutes.
3. Slice into rectangles and serve cold
4. Enjoy!

Nutrition Value: calories 208, fat 14, fiber 2, carbs 13, protein 5

584. Easy Blackberries Scones

Preparation time: 10 minutes
Cooking time: 10 minutes
Servings: 10

Ingredients:

- ½ cup coconut flour
- 1 cup blackberries
- 2 tablespoons flax meal combined with 2 tablespoons water
- ½ cup coconut cream
- ½ cup coconut butter
- ½ cup almond flour
- 5 tablespoons stevia
- 2 teaspoons vanilla extract
- 2 teaspoons baking powder

Directions:

1. In a bowl, mix almond flour with coconut flour, baking powder and blackberries and stir well.
2. In another bowl, mix cream with butter, vanilla extract, stevia and flax meal and stir well.
3. Combine the 2 mixtures, stir until you obtain your dough, shape 10 triangles from this mix, place them on a lined baking sheet, introduce in the air fryer and cook at 350 degrees F for 10 minutes.
4. Serve them cold.
5. Enjoy!

Nutrition Value: calories 170, fat 2, fiber 2, carbs 4, protein 3

585. Easy Buns

Preparation time: 10 minutes
Cooking time: 30 minutes
Servings: 8

Ingredients:

- ½ cup coconut flour
- 1/3 cup psyllium husks
- 2 tablespoons stevia
- 1 teaspoon baking powder
- ½ teaspoon cinnamon powder
- ½ teaspoon cloves, ground
- 3 tablespoons flax meal combined with 3 tablespoons water
- Some chocolate chips, unsweetened

Directions:

1. In a bowl, mix flour with psyllium husks, swerve, baking powder, salt, cinnamon, cloves

and chocolate chips and stir well.
2. Add water and flax meal, stir well until you obtain a dough, shape 8 buns and arrange them on a lined baking sheet.
3. Introduce in the air fryer and cook at 350 degrees for 30 minutes.
4. Serve these buns warm.

Nutrition Value: calories 140, fat 3, fiber 3, carbs 7, protein 6

586. Lemon Cream

Preparation time: 10 minutes
Cooking time: 30 minutes
Servings: 6

Ingredients:

- 1 and 1/3 pint almond milk
- 1 medium banana
- 4 tablespoons lemon zest, grated
- 3 tablespoons flax meal combined with 3 tablespoons water
- 5 tablespoons stevia
- 2 tablespoons lemon juice

Directions:

1. In a bowl, mix mashed banana with milk and swerve and stir very well.
2. Add lemon zest and lemon juice, whisk well, pour into ramekins, place them in your air fryer, cook at 360 degrees F for 30 minutes and serve cold.
3. Enjoy!

Nutrition Value: calories 180, fat 6, fiber 2, carbs 5, protein 7

587. Cocoa Berries Cream

Preparation time: 10 minutes
Cooking time: 10 minutes
Servings: 4

Ingredients:

- 3 tablespoons cocoa powder
- 14 ounces coconut cream
- 1 cup blackberries
- 1 cup raspberries
- 2 tablespoons stevia

Directions:

1. In a bowl, whisk cocoa powder with stevia and cream and stir.
2. Add raspberries and blackberries, toss gently, transfer to a pan that fits your air fryer, introduce in the fryer and cook at 350 degrees F for 10 minutes.
3. Divide into bowls and serve cold.

4. Enjoy!

Nutrition Value: calories 205, fat 34, fiber 2, carbs 6, protein 2

588. Easy Cocoa Pudding

Preparation time: 10 minutes
Cooking time: 20 minutes
Servings: 2

Ingredients:

- 2 tablespoons water
- ½ tablespoon agar
- 4 tablespoons stevia
- 4 tablespoons cocoa powder
- 2 cups coconut milk, hot

Directions:

1. In a bowl, mix milk with stevia and cocoa powder and stir well.
2. In a bowl, mix agar with water, stir well, add to the cocoa mix, stir and transfer to a pudding pan that fits your air fryer.
3. Introduce in the fryer and cook at 356 degrees F for 20 minutes.
4. Serve the pudding cold.
5. Enjoy!

Nutrition Value: calories 170, fat 2, fiber 1, carbs 4, protein 3

589. Blueberry Crackers

Preparation time: 10 minutes
Cooking time: 30 minutes
Servings: 12

Ingredients:

- ½ cup coconut butter
- ½ cup coconut oil, melted
- 1 cup blueberries
- 3 tablespoons coconut sugar

Directions:

1. In a pan that fits your air fryer, mix coconut butter with coconut oil, raspberries and sugar, toss, introduce in the fryer and cook at 367 degrees F for 30 minutes
2. Spread on a lined baking sheet, keep in the fridge for a few hours, slice crackers and serve.
3. Enjoy!

Nutrition Value: calories 174, fat 5, fiber 2, carbs 4, protein 7

590. Zucchini Bread

Preparation time: 10 minutes
Cooking time: 35 minutes
Servings: 6

Ingredients:
- 1 cup natural applesauce
- 1 ½ banana, mashed
- 1 tablespoon vanilla extract
- 4 tablespoons coconut sugar
- 2 cups zucchini, grated
- 2 and ½ cups coconut flour
- ½ cup baking cocoa powder
- 1 teaspoon baking soda
- ¼ teaspoon baking powder
- 1 teaspoon cinnamon powder
- ½ cup walnuts, chopped
- Cooking spray

Directions:
1. Grease a loaf pan with cooking spray, add zucchini, sugar, vanilla, banana, applesauce, flour, cocoa powder, baking soda, baking powder, cinnamon and walnuts, whisk well, introduce in the fryer and cook at 365 degrees F for 35 minutes.
2. Leave the bread to cool down, slice and serve.
3. Enjoy!

Nutrition Value: calories 192, fat 3, fiber 6, carbs 8, protein 3

591. Pear Pudding

Preparation time: 5 minutes
Cooking time: 30 minutes
Servings: 4

Ingredients:
- 2 cups pears, chopped
- 2 cups coconut milk
- 1 tablespoon coconut butter, melted
- 3 tablespoons stevia
- ½ teaspoon cinnamon powder
- 1 cup coconut flakes
- ½ cup walnuts, chopped

Directions:
1. In a pudding pan, mix milk with stevia, butter, coconut, cinnamon, pears and walnuts, stir, introduce in your air fryer and cook at 365 degrees F for 30 minutes.
2. Divide into bowls and serve cold.
3. Enjoy!

Nutrition Value: calories 202, fat 3, fiber 4, carbs 8, protein 7

592. Cauliflower Pudding

Preparation time: 10 minutes
Cooking time: 30 minutes
Servings: 4

Ingredients:
- 2 and ½ cups water
- 1 cup coconut sugar
- 2 cups cauliflower rice
- 2 cinnamon sticks
- ½ cup coconut, shredded

Directions:
1. In a pan that fits your air fryer, mix water with coconut sugar, cauliflower rice, cinnamon and coconut, stir, introduce in the fryer and cook at 365 degrees F for 30 minutes
2. Divide pudding into cups and serve cold.
3. Enjoy!

Nutrition Value: calories 203, fat 4, fiber 6, carbs 9, protein 4

593. Sweet Cauliflower Rice

Preparation time: 10 minutes
Cooking time: 30 minutes
Servings: 4

Ingredients:
- 1 and ½ cups cauliflower rice
- 1 and ½ teaspoons cinnamon powder
- 1/3 cup stevia
- 2 tablespoons coconut butter, melted
- 2 apples, peeled, cored and sliced
- 1 cup natural apple juice
- 3 cups almond milk
- ½ cup cherries, dried

Directions:
1. In a pan that fits your air fryer, combine rice with cinnamon, stevia, butter, apples, apple juice, almond milk and cherries, toss, introduce in your air fryer and cook at 365 degrees F for 30 minutes.
2. Divide between bowls and serve.
3. Enjoy!

Nutrition Value: calories 160, fat 3, fiber 3, carbs 7, protein 5

594. Espresso Vanilla Dessert

Preparation time: 10 minutes
Cooking time: 20 minutes
Servings: 4

Ingredients:
- 1 cup almond milk
- 4 tablespoons flax meal
- 2 tablespoons coconut flour

- 2 and ½ cups water
- 2 tablespoons stevia
- 1 teaspoon espresso powder
- 2 teaspoons vanilla extract
- Coconut cream for serving

Directions:
1. In a pan that fits your air fryer, mix flax meal with flour, water, stevia, milk, vanilla and espresso powder, stir, introduce in the fryer and cook at 365 degrees F for 20 minutes.
2. Divide into bowls and serve with coconut cream on top.
3. Enjoy!

Nutrition Value: calories 202, fat 2, fiber 1, carbs 6, protein 4

595. Sweet Rhubarb
Preparation time: 10 minutes
Cooking time: 10 minutes
Servings: 4

Ingredients:
- 5 cups rhubarb, chopped
- 2 tablespoons coconut butter, melted
- 1/3 cup water
- 1 tablespoon stevia
- 1 teaspoon vanilla extract

Directions:
1. Put rhubarb, ghee, water, stevia and vanilla extract in a pan that fits your air fryer, introduce in the fryer and cook at 365 degrees F for 10 minutes
2. Divide into small bowls and serve cold.
3. Enjoy!

Nutrition Value: calories 103, fat 2, fiber 1, carbs 6, protein 2

596. Pineapple and Apricots Delight
Preparation time: 10 minutes
Cooking time: 12 minutes
Servings: 10

Ingredients:
- 6 cups canned pineapple chunks, drained
- 4 cups canned apricots, halved and drained
- 3 cups natural applesauce
- 2 cups canned mandarin oranges, drained
- 2 tablespoons stevia
- 1 teaspoon cinnamon powder

Directions:
1. Put pineapples, apricots, applesauce, oranges, cinnamon and stevia in a pan that fits your air fryer, introduce in the fryer and cook at 360 degrees F for 12 minutes.
2. Divide into small bowls and serve cold.
3. Enjoy!

Nutrition Value: calories 130, fat 1, fiber 2, carbs 7, protein 2

597. Tantalizing Apple Pie Bites
Serving: 4
Preparation Time: 20 minutes
Cooking Time: 0 minutes

Ingredients
- 1 cup chopped walnuts
- ½ a cup of coconut oil
- ¼ cup of ground flaxseed
- ½ ounce of frozen dried apples
- 1 teaspoon of vanilla extract
- 1 teaspoon of cinnamon
- Liquid Stevia

Directions
1. Melt the coconut oil until it is liquid
2. Take your blender and add walnuts, coconut oil, and process well
3. Add flaxseeds, vanilla, and Stevia
4. Keep processing until a fine mixture form
5. Stop and add crumbled dried apples
6. Process until your desired texture appears
7. Portion the mixture amongst muffin molds and allow them to chill
8. Enjoy!

Nutrition Values:
Calories: 194
Fat: 19g
Carbs: 2g
Protein: 2.3g

598. Vegan Compliant Protein Balls
Serving: 8
Preparation Time: 20 minutes
Cooking Time: 0 minutes

Ingredients
- 1 cup of creamed coconut
- 2 scoops of Vega Sport Chocolate Protein (or any protein powder of your preference)
- ¼ cup of ground flax seed
- ½ a teaspoon of vanilla extract
- ½ a teaspoon of mint extract
- 1-2 tablespoon of cocoa powder

Directions

1. Take a large sized bowl and melt the creamed coconut
2. Add the vanilla extract and stir well
3. Stir in flax seed, protein powder and knead until the fine dough forms
4. Form 24 balls and allow the balls to chill for 10-15 minutes
5. Roll them up in some cocoa powder if you prefer and serve!

Nutrition Values:

Calories: 260
Fat: 20g
Carbs: 3g
Protein: 10g

T'

he Keto Lovers "Magical" Grain Free Granola

Serving: 10
Preparation Time: 10 minutes
Cooking Time: 75 minutes

Ingredients

- ½ a cup of raw sunflower seeds
- ½ a cup of raw hemp hearts
- ½ a cup of flaxseeds
- ¼ cup of chia seeds
- 2 tablespoon of Psyllium Husk powder
- 1 tablespoon of cinnamon
- Stevia
- ½ a teaspoon of baking powder
- ½ a teaspoon of salt
- 1 cup of water

Directions

1. Pre-heat your oven to 300 degrees Fahrenheit
2. Line up a baking sheet with parchment paper
3. Take your food processor and grind all the seeds
4. Add the dry ingredients and mix well
5. Stir in water until fully incorporated
6. Allow the mixture to sit for a while until it thickens up
7. Spread the mixture evenly on top of your baking sheet (giving a thickness of about ¼ inch)
8. Bake for 45 minutes
9. Break apart the granola and keep baking for another 30 minutes until the pieces are crunchy
10. Remove and allow them to cool
11. Enjoy!

Nutrition Values:

Calories: 292
Fat: 25g

Carbs: 12g
Protein: 8g

600. Pumpkin Butter Nut Cup

Serves: 5
Preparation Time: 135 minutes
Cooking Time: 0 minute

For Filing

- ½ a cup of organic pumpkin puree
- 1/2a cup of almond butter
- 4 tablespoon of organic coconut oil
- ¼ teaspoon of organic ground nutmeg
- ¼ teaspoon of organic ground ginger
- 1 teaspoon of organic ground cinnamon
- 1/8 teaspoon of organic ground clove
- 2 teaspoon of organic vanilla extract

For Topping

- 1 cup of organic raw cacao powder
- 1 cup of organic coconut oil

Directions

1. Take a medium-sized bowl and add all of the listed ingredients under pumpkin filling
2. Mix well until you have a creamy mixture
3. Take another bowl and add the topping mixture and mix well
4. Take a muffin cup and fill it up with 1/3 of the chocolate topping mix
5. Chill for 15 minutes
6. Add 1/3 of the pumpkin mix and layer out on top
7. Chill for 2 hours
8. Repeat until all the mixture has been used up
9. Enjoy!

Nutritional Values per Serving

Calories: 105
Fat: 10.1g
Carbohydrates: 3.3g
Protein: 2.9g

601 Unique Gingerbread Muffins

Serving: 12
Preparation Time: 15 minutes
Cooking Time: 30 minutes

Ingredients

- 1 tablespoon of ground flaxseed
- 6 tablespoon of coconut milk
- 1 tablespoon of apple cider vinegar
- ½ a cup of peanut butter
- 2 tablespoon of gingerbread spice blend
- 1 teaspoon of baking powder

- 1 teaspoon of vanilla extract
- 2-3 tablespoon of Swerve

Directions

1. Pre-heat your oven to a temperature of 350 degrees Fahrenheit
2. Take a bowl and add flaxseeds, sweetener, salt, vanilla, spices and coconut milk
3. Keep it on the side for a while
4. Add peanut butter, baking powder and keep mixing until combined well
5. Stir in peanut butter and baking powder
6. Mix well
7. Spoon the mixture into muffin liners
8. Bake for 30 minutes
9. Allow them to cool and enjoy!

Nutrition Values:
Calories:158
Fat: 13g
Carbs: 3g
Protein: 6g

602. The Vegan Pumpkin Spicy Fat Bombs

Serving: 12
Preparation Time: 100 minutes
Cooking Time: 0 minutes

Ingredients

- ¾ cup of pumpkin puree
- ¼ cup of hemp seeds
- ½ a cup of coconut oil
- 2 teaspoon of pumpkin pie spice
- 1 teaspoon of vanilla extract
- Liquid Stevia

Directions

1. Take a blender and add all of the ingredients
2. Blend them well and portion the mixture out into silicon molds
3. Allow them to chill and enjoy!

Nutrition Values:
Calories: 103
Fat: 10g
Carbs: 2g
Protein: 1g

603. The Low Carb "Matcha" Bombs

Serving: 12
Preparation Time: 100 minutes
Cooking Time: 0 minutes

Ingredients

- ¾ cup of hemp sees
- ½ a cup of coconut oil
- 2 tablespoon of coconut butter
- 1 teaspoon of matcha powder
- 2 tablespoon of vanilla extract
- ½ a teaspoon of mint extract
- Liquid Stevia

Directions

1. Take your blender and add hemp seeds, matcha, coconut oil, mint extract and Stevia
2. Blend well and divide the mixture into silicon molds
3. Melt the coconut butter and drizzle them on top of your cups
4. Allow the cups to chill and serve!

Nutrition Values:
Calories: 200
Fat: 20g
Carbs: 3g
Protein: 5g

604. The No-Bake Keto Cheese Cake

Serving: 4
Preparation Time: 120 minutes
Cooking Time: 0 minutes

Ingredients

For Crust

- 2 tablespoon of ground flaxseed
- 2 tablespoon of desiccated coconut
- 1 teaspoon of cinnamon

For Filling

- 4 ounce of vegan cream cheese
- 1 cup of soaked cashews
- ½ a cup of frozen blueberries
- 2 tablespoon of coconut oil
- 1 tablespoon of lemon juice
- 1 teaspoon of vanilla extract
- Liquid Stevia

Directions

1. Take a container and mix all of the crust ingredients
2. Mix them well and flatten them at the bottom to prepare the crust
3. Take a blender and mix all of the filling ingredients and blend until smooth
4. Distribute the filling on top of your crust and chill it in your freezer for about 2 hours
5. Enjoy!

Nutrition Values:
Calories: 182

Fat: 16g
Carbs: 6g
Protein: 3g

695. Raspberry Chocolate Cups

Serving: 12
Preparation Time: 60 minutes
Cooking Time: 0 minutes

Ingredients

- ½ a cup of cacao butter
- ½ a cup of coconut manna
- 4 tablespoon of powdered coconut milk
- 3 tablespoon of granulated sugar substitute
- 1 teaspoon of vanilla extract
- ¼ cup of dried and crushed frozen raspberries

Directions

1. Melt cacao butter and add coconut manna
2. Stir in vanilla extract
3. Take another dish and add coconut powder and sugar substitute
4. Stir the coconut mix into the cacao butter, 1 tablespoon at a time, making sure to keep mixing after each addition
5. Add the crushed dried raspberries
6. Mix well and portion it out into muffin tins
7. Chill for 60 minutes and enjoy!

Nutrition Values:

Calories: 158
Fat: 15g
Carbs: 1g
Protein: 3g

606. Exuberant Pumpkin Fudge

Serving: 25
Preparation Time: 120 minutes
Cooking Time: 0 minutes

Ingredients

- 1 and a ¾ cup of coconut butter
- 1 cup of pumpkin puree
- 1 teaspoon of ground cinnamon
- ¼ teaspoon of ground nutmeg
- 1 tablespoon of coconut oil

Directions

1. Take an 8x8 inch square baking pan and line it with aluminum foil to start with
2. Take a spoon of the coconut butter and add into a heated pan; let the butter melt over low heat
3. Toss in the spices and pumpkin and keep stirring it until a grainy texture has formed
4. Pour in the coconut oil and keep stirring it vigorously in order to make sure that everything is combined nicely
5. Scoop up the mixture into the previously prepared baking pan and distribute evenly
6. Place a piece of wax paper over the top of the mixture and press on the upper side to make evenly straighten up the topside
7. Remove the wax paper and throw it away
8. Place the mixture in your fridge and let it cool for about 1-2 hours
9. Take it out and cut it into slices, then eat

Nutrition Values:

Calories: 120
Protein: 1.2g
Carbs: 4.2g
Fats: 10.7g

1000 DAY DIET PLAN

Day	BREAKFAST	LUNCH/DINNER	DESSERT
1	Pear Oatmeal	Rich Chickpeas And Lentils Soup	Peach Cobbler
2	Pumpkin Oatmeal	Chard And Sweet Potato Soup	Blueberry Cake
3	Veggie Burrito	Chinese Soup And Ginger Sauce	Stewed Rhubarb
4	Apple Steel Cut Oats	Corn Cream Soup	Pudding Cake
5	Tofu Casserole	Veggie Medley	Sweet Peanut Butter Cake
6	Carrot Mix	Lentils Curry	Apple Mix
7	Blueberries Oats	Lentils Dal	Pears And Dried Fruits Bowls
8	Apple and Pears Mix	Rich Jackfruit Dish	Strawberry Stew
9	Bell Pepper Oatmeal	Vegan Gumbo	Poached Plums
10	Banana and Walnuts Oats	Chickpeas Delight	Sweet Rhubarb
11	Cool Tofu Breakfast Mix	Mediterranean Stew	Espresso Vanilla Dessert
12	Breakfast Broccoli and Tofu Bowls	Caribbean Dish	Sweet Cauliflower Rice
13	Strawberry Quinoa	Green Chili Soup	Cauliflower Pudding
14	Delicious Porridge	Special Minestrone Soup	Pear Pudding
15	Pumpkin Breakfast Muffins	Fresh Collard Greens Mix	Zucchini Bread
16	Mediterranean Chickpeas Breakfast	Endives Soup	Cocoa Brownies
17	Simple Granola	Fennel Soup	Blueberry Crackers
18	Breakfast Bowls	Asparagus Soup	Easy Cocoa Pudding
19	Sweet Potatoes Mix	Beets And Capers Mix	Cocoa Berries Cream
20	Simple Creamy Breakfast Potatoes	Mushroom Soup	Lemon Cream
21	Chia Pudding	Brussels Sprouts Delight	Easy Buns
22	Sweet Quinoa Mix	Artichoke Soup	Easy Blackberries Scones
23	Cranberry Coconut Quinoa	Intense Beet Soup	Lemon Jam
24	Zucchini Oatmeal	Chinese Carrot Cream	Pumpkin Cake
25	Cinnamon Oatmeal	Seitan Stew	Strawberries And Rhubarb Marmalade
26	Strawberry Choco shake	Spicy Carrot Stew	Strawberries Jam
27	Egg mayonnaise	Tomato Soup	Vanilla and Blueberry Squares
28	Coconut muffin	Collard Greens Mix	Raspberry Bars
29	Parsley Quiche	Classic Tomato Soup	Chocolate and Coconut Bars
30	Coconut Rice	Chinese Collard Greens Mix	Cranberry Pudding
31	Pear Oatmeal	Rich Chickpeas And Lentils Soup	Peach Cobbler
32	Pumpkin Oatmeal	Chard And Sweet Potato Soup	Blueberry Cake
33	Veggie Burrito	Chinese Soup And Ginger Sauce	Stewed Rhubarb
34	Apple Steel Cut Oats	Corn Cream Soup	Pudding Cake
35	Tofu Casserole	Veggie Medley	Sweet Peanut Butter Cake
36	Carrot Mix	Lentils Curry	Apple Mix
37	Blueberries Oats	Lentils Dal	Pears And Dried Fruits Bowls
38	Apple and Pears Mix	Rich Jackfruit Dish	Strawberry Stew
39	Bell Pepper Oatmeal	Vegan Gumbo	Poached Plums

40	Banana and Walnuts Oats	Chickpeas Delight	Sweet Rhubarb
41	Cool Tofu Breakfast Mix	Mediterranean Stew	Espresso Vanilla Dessert
42	Breakfast Broccoli and Tofu Bowls	Caribbean Dish	Sweet Cauliflower Rice
43	Strawberry Quinoa	Green Chili Soup	Cauliflower Pudding
44	Delicious Porridge	Special Minestrone Soup	Pear Pudding
45	Pumpkin Breakfast Muffins	Fresh Collard Greens Mix	Zucchini Bread
46	Mediterranean Chickpeas Breakfast	Endives Soup	Cocoa Brownies
47	Simple Granola	Fennel Soup	Blueberry Crackers
48	Breakfast Bowls	Asparagus Soup	Easy Cocoa Pudding
49	Sweet Potatoes Mix	Beets And Capers Mix	Cocoa Berries Cream
50	Simple Creamy Breakfast Potatoes	Mushroom Soup	Lemon Cream
51	Chia Pudding	Brussels Sprouts Delight	Easy Buns
52	Sweet Quinoa Mix	Artichoke Soup	Easy Blackberries Scones
53	Cranberry Coconut Quinoa	Intense Beet Soup	Lemon Jam
54	Zucchini Oatmeal	Chinese Carrot Cream	Pumpkin Cake
55	Cinnamon Oatmeal	Seitan Stew	Strawberries And Rhubarb Marmalade
56	Strawberry Choco shake	Spicy Carrot Stew	Strawberries Jam
57	Egg mayonnaise	Tomato Soup	Vanilla and Blueberry Squares
58	Coconut muffin	Collard Greens Mix	Raspberry Bars
59	Parsley Quiche	Classic Tomato Soup	Chocolate and Coconut Bars
60	Coconut Rice	Chinese Collard Greens Mix	Cranberry Pudding
61	Pear Oatmeal	Rich Chickpeas And Lentils Soup	Peach Cobbler
62	Pumpkin Oatmeal	Chard And Sweet Potato Soup	Blueberry Cake
63	Veggie Burrito	Chinese Soup And Ginger Sauce	Stewed Rhubarb
64	Apple Steel Cut Oats	Corn Cream Soup	Pudding Cake
65	Tofu Casserole	Veggie Medley	Sweet Peanut Butter Cake
66	Carrot Mix	Lentils Curry	Apple Mix
67	Blueberries Oats	Lentils Dal	Pears And Dried Fruits Bowls
68	Apple and Pears Mix	Rich Jackfruit Dish	Strawberry Stew
69	Bell Pepper Oatmeal	Vegan Gumbo	Poached Plums
70	Banana and Walnuts Oats	Chickpeas Delight	Sweet Rhubarb
71	Cool Tofu Breakfast Mix	Mediterranean Stew	Espresso Vanilla Dessert
72	Breakfast Broccoli and Tofu Bowls	Caribbean Dish	Sweet Cauliflower Rice
73	Strawberry Quinoa	Green Chili Soup	Cauliflower Pudding
74	Delicious Porridge	Special Minestrone Soup	Pear Pudding
75	Pumpkin Breakfast Muffins	Fresh Collard Greens Mix	Zucchini Bread
76	Mediterranean Chickpeas Breakfast	Endives Soup	Cocoa Brownies
77	Simple Granola	Fennel Soup	Blueberry Crackers
78	Breakfast Bowls	Asparagus Soup	Easy Cocoa Pudding
79	Sweet Potatoes Mix	Beets And Capers Mix	Cocoa Berries Cream
80	Simple Creamy Breakfast Potatoes	Mushroom Soup	Lemon Cream
81	Chia Pudding	Brussels Sprouts Delight	Easy Buns
82	Sweet Quinoa Mix	Artichoke Soup	Easy Blackberries Scones

83	Cranberry Coconut Quinoa	Intense Beet Soup	Lemon Jam
84	Zucchini Oatmeal	Chinese Carrot Cream	Pumpkin Cake
85	Cinnamon Oatmeal	Seitan Stew	Strawberries And Rhubarb Marmalade
86	Strawberry Choco shake	Spicy Carrot Stew	Strawberries Jam
87	Egg mayonnaise	Tomato Soup	Vanilla and Blueberry Squares
88	Coconut muffin	Collard Greens Mix	Raspberry Bars
89	Parsley Quiche	Classic Tomato Soup	Chocolate and Coconut Bars
90	Coconut Rice	Chinese Collard Greens Mix	Cranberry Pudding
91	Pear Oatmeal	Rich Chickpeas And Lentils Soup	Peach Cobbler
92	Pumpkin Oatmeal	Chard And Sweet Potato Soup	Blueberry Cake
93	Veggie Burrito	Chinese Soup And Ginger Sauce	Stewed Rhubarb
94	Apple Steel Cut Oats	Corn Cream Soup	Pudding Cake
95	Tofu Casserole	Veggie Medley	Sweet Peanut Butter Cake
96	Carrot Mix	Lentils Curry	Apple Mix
97	Blueberries Oats	Lentils Dal	Pears And Dried Fruits Bowls
98	Apple and Pears Mix	Rich Jackfruit Dish	Strawberry Stew
99	Bell Pepper Oatmeal	Vegan Gumbo	Poached Plums
100	Banana and Walnuts Oats	Chickpeas Delight	Sweet Rhubarb
101	Cool Tofu Breakfast Mix	Mediterranean Stew	Espresso Vanilla Dessert
102	Breakfast Broccoli and Tofu Bowls	Caribbean Dish	Sweet Cauliflower Rice
103	Strawberry Quinoa	Green Chili Soup	Cauliflower Pudding
104	Delicious Porridge	Special Minestrone Soup	Pear Pudding
105	Pumpkin Breakfast Muffins	Fresh Collard Greens Mix	Zucchini Bread
106	Mediterranean Chickpeas Breakfast	Endives Soup	Cocoa Brownies
107	Simple Granola	Fennel Soup	Blueberry Crackers
108	Breakfast Bowls	Asparagus Soup	Easy Cocoa Pudding
109	Sweet Potatoes Mix	Beets And Capers Mix	Cocoa Berries Cream
110	Simple Creamy Breakfast Potatoes	Mushroom Soup	Lemon Cream
111	Chia Pudding	Brussels Sprouts Delight	Easy Buns
112	Sweet Quinoa Mix	Artichoke Soup	Easy Blackberries Scones
113	Cranberry Coconut Quinoa	Intense Beet Soup	Lemon Jam
114	Zucchini Oatmeal	Chinese Carrot Cream	Pumpkin Cake
115	Cinnamon Oatmeal	Seitan Stew	Strawberries And Rhubarb Marmalade
116	Strawberry Choco shake	Spicy Carrot Stew	Strawberries Jam
117	Egg mayonnaise	Tomato Soup	Vanilla and Blueberry Squares
118	Coconut muffin	Collard Greens Mix	Raspberry Bars
119	Parsley Quiche	Classic Tomato Soup	Chocolate and Coconut Bars
120	Coconut Rice	Chinese Collard Greens Mix	Cranberry Pudding
121	Pear Oatmeal	Rich Chickpeas And Lentils Soup	Peach Cobbler
122	Pumpkin Oatmeal	Chard And Sweet Potato Soup	Blueberry Cake
123	Veggie Burrito	Chinese Soup And Ginger Sauce	Stewed Rhubarb
124	Apple Steel Cut Oats	Corn Cream Soup	Pudding Cake
125	Tofu Casserole	Veggie Medley	Sweet Peanut Butter Cake

126	Carrot Mix	Lentils Curry	Apple Mix
127	Blueberries Oats	Lentils Dal	Pears And Dried Fruits Bowls
128	Apple and Pears Mix	Rich Jackfruit Dish	Strawberry Stew
129	Bell Pepper Oatmeal	Vegan Gumbo	Poached Plums
130	Banana and Walnuts Oats	Chickpeas Delight	Sweet Rhubarb
131	Cool Tofu Breakfast Mix	Mediterranean Stew	Espresso Vanilla Dessert
132	Breakfast Broccoli and Tofu Bowls	Caribbean Dish	Sweet Cauliflower Rice
133	Strawberry Quinoa	Green Chili Soup	Cauliflower Pudding
134	Delicious Porridge	Special Minestrone Soup	Pear Pudding
135	Pumpkin Breakfast Muffins	Fresh Collard Greens Mix	Zucchini Bread
136	Mediterranean Chickpeas Breakfast	Endives Soup	Cocoa Brownies
137	Simple Granola	Fennel Soup	Blueberry Crackers
138	Breakfast Bowls	Asparagus Soup	Easy Cocoa Pudding
139	Sweet Potatoes Mix	Beets And Capers Mix	Cocoa Berries Cream
140	Simple Creamy Breakfast Potatoes	Mushroom Soup	Lemon Cream
141	Chia Pudding	Brussels Sprouts Delight	Easy Buns
142	Sweet Quinoa Mix	Artichoke Soup	Easy Blackberries Scones
143	Cranberry Coconut Quinoa	Intense Beet Soup	Lemon Jam
144	Zucchini Oatmeal	Chinese Carrot Cream	Pumpkin Cake
145	Cinnamon Oatmeal	Seitan Stew	Strawberries And Rhubarb Marmalade
146	Strawberry Choco shake	Spicy Carrot Stew	Strawberries Jam
147	Egg mayonnaise	Tomato Soup	Vanilla and Blueberry Squares
148	Coconut muffin	Collard Greens Mix	Raspberry Bars
149	Parsley Quiche	Classic Tomato Soup	Chocolate and Coconut Bars
150	Coconut Rice	Chinese Collard Greens Mix	Cranberry Pudding
151	Pear Oatmeal	Rich Chickpeas And Lentils Soup	Peach Cobbler
152	Pumpkin Oatmeal	Chard And Sweet Potato Soup	Blueberry Cake
153	Veggie Burrito	Chinese Soup And Ginger Sauce	Stewed Rhubarb
154	Apple Steel Cut Oats	Corn Cream Soup	Pudding Cake
155	Tofu Casserole	Veggie Medley	Sweet Peanut Butter Cake
156	Carrot Mix	Lentils Curry	Apple Mix
157	Blueberries Oats	Lentils Dal	Pears And Dried Fruits Bowls
158	Apple and Pears Mix	Rich Jackfruit Dish	Strawberry Stew
159	Bell Pepper Oatmeal	Vegan Gumbo	Poached Plums
160	Banana and Walnuts Oats	Chickpeas Delight	Sweet Rhubarb
161	Cool Tofu Breakfast Mix	Mediterranean Stew	Espresso Vanilla Dessert
162	Breakfast Broccoli and Tofu Bowls	Caribbean Dish	Sweet Cauliflower Rice
163	Strawberry Quinoa	Green Chili Soup	Cauliflower Pudding
164	Delicious Porridge	Special Minestrone Soup	Pear Pudding
165	Pumpkin Breakfast Muffins	Fresh Collard Greens Mix	Zucchini Bread
166	Mediterranean Chickpeas Breakfast	Endives Soup	Cocoa Brownies
167	Simple Granola	Fennel Soup	Blueberry Crackers
168	Breakfast Bowls	Asparagus Soup	Easy Cocoa Pudding

169	Sweet Potatoes Mix	Beets And Capers Mix	Cocoa Berries Cream
170	Simple Creamy Breakfast Potatoes	Mushroom Soup	Lemon Cream
171	Chia Pudding	Brussels Sprouts Delight	Easy Buns
172	Sweet Quinoa Mix	Artichoke Soup	Easy Blackberries Scones
173	Cranberry Coconut Quinoa	Intense Beet Soup	Lemon Jam
174	Zucchini Oatmeal	Chinese Carrot Cream	Pumpkin Cake
175	Cinnamon Oatmeal	Seitan Stew	Strawberries And Rhubarb Marmalade
176	Strawberry Choco shake	Spicy Carrot Stew	Strawberries Jam
177	Egg mayonnaise	Tomato Soup	Vanilla and Blueberry Squares
178	Coconut muffin	Collard Greens Mix	Raspberry Bars
179	Parsley Quiche	Classic Tomato Soup	Chocolate and Coconut Bars
180	Coconut Rice	Chinese Collard Greens Mix	Cranberry Pudding
181	Pear Oatmeal	Rich Chickpeas And Lentils Soup	Peach Cobbler
182	Pumpkin Oatmeal	Chard And Sweet Potato Soup	Blueberry Cake
183	Veggie Burrito	Chinese Soup And Ginger Sauce	Stewed Rhubarb
184	Apple Steel Cut Oats	Corn Cream Soup	Pudding Cake
185	Tofu Casserole	Veggie Medley	Sweet Peanut Butter Cake
186	Carrot Mix	Lentils Curry	Apple Mix
187	Blueberries Oats	Lentils Dal	Pears And Dried Fruits Bowls
188	Apple and Pears Mix	Rich Jackfruit Dish	Strawberry Stew
189	Bell Pepper Oatmeal	Vegan Gumbo	Poached Plums
190	Banana and Walnuts Oats	Chickpeas Delight	Sweet Rhubarb
191	Cool Tofu Breakfast Mix	Mediterranean Stew	Espresso Vanilla Dessert
192	Breakfast Broccoli and Tofu Bowls	Caribbean Dish	Sweet Cauliflower Rice
193	Strawberry Quinoa	Green Chili Soup	Cauliflower Pudding
194	Delicious Porridge	Special Minestrone Soup	Pear Pudding
195	Pumpkin Breakfast Muffins	Fresh Collard Greens Mix	Zucchini Bread
196	Mediterranean Chickpeas Breakfast	Endives Soup	Cocoa Brownies
197	Simple Granola	Fennel Soup	Blueberry Crackers
198	Breakfast Bowls	Asparagus Soup	Easy Cocoa Pudding
199	Sweet Potatoes Mix	Beets And Capers Mix	Cocoa Berries Cream
200	Simple Creamy Breakfast Potatoes	Mushroom Soup	Lemon Cream
201	Chia Pudding	Brussels Sprouts Delight	Easy Buns
202	Sweet Quinoa Mix	Artichoke Soup	Easy Blackberries Scones
203	Cranberry Coconut Quinoa	Intense Beet Soup	Lemon Jam
204	Zucchini Oatmeal	Chinese Carrot Cream	Pumpkin Cake
205	Cinnamon Oatmeal	Seitan Stew	Strawberries And Rhubarb Marmalade
206	Strawberry Choco shake	Spicy Carrot Stew	Strawberries Jam
207	Egg mayonnaise	Tomato Soup	Vanilla and Blueberry Squares
208	Coconut muffin	Collard Greens Mix	Raspberry Bars
209	Parsley Quiche	Classic Tomato Soup	Chocolate and Coconut Bars
210	Coconut Rice	Chinese Collard Greens Mix	Cranberry Pudding
211	Pear Oatmeal	Rich Chickpeas And Lentils Soup	Peach Cobbler

212	Pumpkin Oatmeal	Chard And Sweet Potato Soup	Blueberry Cake
213	Veggie Burrito	Chinese Soup And Ginger Sauce	Stewed Rhubarb
214	Apple Steel Cut Oats	Corn Cream Soup	Pudding Cake
215	Tofu Casserole	Veggie Medley	Sweet Peanut Butter Cake
216	Carrot Mix	Lentils Curry	Apple Mix
217	Blueberries Oats	Lentils Dal	Pears And Dried Fruits Bowls
218	Apple and Pears Mix	Rich Jackfruit Dish	Strawberry Stew
219	Bell Pepper Oatmeal	Vegan Gumbo	Poached Plums
220	Banana and Walnuts Oats	Chickpeas Delight	Sweet Rhubarb
221	Cool Tofu Breakfast Mix	Mediterranean Stew	Espresso Vanilla Dessert
222	Breakfast Broccoli and Tofu Bowls	Caribbean Dish	Sweet Cauliflower Rice
223	Strawberry Quinoa	Green Chili Soup	Cauliflower Pudding
224	Delicious Porridge	Special Minestrone Soup	Pear Pudding
225	Pumpkin Breakfast Muffins	Fresh Collard Greens Mix	Zucchini Bread
226	Mediterranean Chickpeas Breakfast	Endives Soup	Cocoa Brownies
227	Simple Granola	Fennel Soup	Blueberry Crackers
228	Breakfast Bowls	Asparagus Soup	Easy Cocoa Pudding
229	Sweet Potatoes Mix	Beets And Capers Mix	Cocoa Berries Cream
230	Simple Creamy Breakfast Potatoes	Mushroom Soup	Lemon Cream
231	Chia Pudding	Brussels Sprouts Delight	Easy Buns
232	Sweet Quinoa Mix	Artichoke Soup	Easy Blackberries Scones
233	Cranberry Coconut Quinoa	Intense Beet Soup	Lemon Jam
234	Zucchini Oatmeal	Chinese Carrot Cream	Pumpkin Cake
235	Cinnamon Oatmeal	Seitan Stew	Strawberries And Rhubarb Marmalade
236	Strawberry Choco shake	Spicy Carrot Stew	Strawberries Jam
237	Egg mayonnaise	Tomato Soup	Vanilla and Blueberry Squares
238	Coconut muffin	Collard Greens Mix	Raspberry Bars
239	Parsley Quiche	Classic Tomato Soup	Chocolate and Coconut Bars
240	Coconut Rice	Chinese Collard Greens Mix	Cranberry Pudding
241	Pear Oatmeal	Rich Chickpeas And Lentils Soup	Peach Cobbler
242	Pumpkin Oatmeal	Chard And Sweet Potato Soup	Blueberry Cake
243	Veggie Burrito	Chinese Soup And Ginger Sauce	Stewed Rhubarb
244	Apple Steel Cut Oats	Corn Cream Soup	Pudding Cake
245	Tofu Casserole	Veggie Medley	Sweet Peanut Butter Cake
246	Carrot Mix	Lentils Curry	Apple Mix
247	Blueberries Oats	Lentils Dal	Pears And Dried Fruits Bowls
248	Apple and Pears Mix	Rich Jackfruit Dish	Strawberry Stew
249	Bell Pepper Oatmeal	Vegan Gumbo	Poached Plums
250	Banana and Walnuts Oats	Chickpeas Delight	Sweet Rhubarb
251	Cool Tofu Breakfast Mix	Mediterranean Stew	Espresso Vanilla Dessert
252	Breakfast Broccoli and Tofu Bowls	Caribbean Dish	Sweet Cauliflower Rice
253	Strawberry Quinoa	Green Chili Soup	Cauliflower Pudding
254	Delicious Porridge	Special Minestrone Soup	Pear Pudding

255	Pumpkin Breakfast Muffins	Fresh Collard Greens Mix	Zucchini Bread
256	Mediterranean Chickpeas Breakfast	Endives Soup	Cocoa Brownies
257	Simple Granola	Fennel Soup	Blueberry Crackers
258	Breakfast Bowls	Asparagus Soup	Easy Cocoa Pudding
259	Sweet Potatoes Mix	Beets And Capers Mix	Cocoa Berries Cream
260	Simple Creamy Breakfast Potatoes	Mushroom Soup	Lemon Cream
261	Chia Pudding	Brussels Sprouts Delight	Easy Buns
262	Sweet Quinoa Mix	Artichoke Soup	Easy Blackberries Scones
263	Cranberry Coconut Quinoa	Intense Beet Soup	Lemon Jam
264	Zucchini Oatmeal	Chinese Carrot Cream	Pumpkin Cake
265	Cinnamon Oatmeal	Seitan Stew	Strawberries And Rhubarb Marmalade
266	Strawberry Choco shake	Spicy Carrot Stew	Strawberries Jam
267	Egg mayonnaise	Tomato Soup	Vanilla and Blueberry Squares
268	Coconut muffin	Collard Greens Mix	Raspberry Bars
269	Parsley Quiche	Classic Tomato Soup	Chocolate and Coconut Bars
270	Coconut Rice	Chinese Collard Greens Mix	Cranberry Pudding
271	Pear Oatmeal	Rich Chickpeas And Lentils Soup	Peach Cobbler
272	Pumpkin Oatmeal	Chard And Sweet Potato Soup	Blueberry Cake
273	Veggie Burrito	Chinese Soup And Ginger Sauce	Stewed Rhubarb
274	Apple Steel Cut Oats	Corn Cream Soup	Pudding Cake
275	Tofu Casserole	Veggie Medley	Sweet Peanut Butter Cake
276	Carrot Mix	Lentils Curry	Apple Mix
277	Blueberries Oats	Lentils Dal	Pears And Dried Fruits Bowls
278	Apple and Pears Mix	Rich Jackfruit Dish	Strawberry Stew
279	Bell Pepper Oatmeal	Vegan Gumbo	Poached Plums
280	Banana and Walnuts Oats	Chickpeas Delight	Sweet Rhubarb
281	Cool Tofu Breakfast Mix	Mediterranean Stew	Espresso Vanilla Dessert
282	Breakfast Broccoli and Tofu Bowls	Caribbean Dish	Sweet Cauliflower Rice
283	Strawberry Quinoa	Green Chili Soup	Cauliflower Pudding
284	Delicious Porridge	Special Minestrone Soup	Pear Pudding
285	Pumpkin Breakfast Muffins	Fresh Collard Greens Mix	Zucchini Bread
286	Mediterranean Chickpeas Breakfast	Endives Soup	Cocoa Brownies
287	Simple Granola	Fennel Soup	Blueberry Crackers
288	Breakfast Bowls	Asparagus Soup	Easy Cocoa Pudding
289	Sweet Potatoes Mix	Beets And Capers Mix	Cocoa Berries Cream
290	Simple Creamy Breakfast Potatoes	Mushroom Soup	Lemon Cream
291	Chia Pudding	Brussels Sprouts Delight	Easy Buns
292	Sweet Quinoa Mix	Artichoke Soup	Easy Blackberries Scones
293	Cranberry Coconut Quinoa	Intense Beet Soup	Lemon Jam
294	Zucchini Oatmeal	Chinese Carrot Cream	Pumpkin Cake
295	Cinnamon Oatmeal	Seitan Stew	Strawberries And Rhubarb Marmalade
296	Strawberry Choco shake	Spicy Carrot Stew	Strawberries Jam
297	Egg mayonnaise	Tomato Soup	Vanilla and Blueberry Squares

298	Coconut muffin	Collard Greens Mix	Raspberry Bars
299	Parsley Quiche	Classic Tomato Soup	Chocolate and Coconut Bars
300	Coconut Rice	Chinese Collard Greens Mix	Cranberry Pudding
301	Pear Oatmeal	Rich Chickpeas And Lentils Soup	Peach Cobbler
302	Pumpkin Oatmeal	Chard And Sweet Potato Soup	Blueberry Cake
303	Veggie Burrito	Chinese Soup And Ginger Sauce	Stewed Rhubarb
304	Apple Steel Cut Oats	Corn Cream Soup	Pudding Cake
305	Tofu Casserole	Veggie Medley	Sweet Peanut Butter Cake
306	Carrot Mix	Lentils Curry	Apple Mix
307	Blueberries Oats	Lentils Dal	Pears And Dried Fruits Bowls
308	Apple and Pears Mix	Rich Jackfruit Dish	Strawberry Stew
309	Bell Pepper Oatmeal	Vegan Gumbo	Poached Plums
310	Banana and Walnuts Oats	Chickpeas Delight	Sweet Rhubarb
311	Cool Tofu Breakfast Mix	Mediterranean Stew	Espresso Vanilla Dessert
312	Breakfast Broccoli and Tofu Bowls	Caribbean Dish	Sweet Cauliflower Rice
313	Strawberry Quinoa	Green Chili Soup	Cauliflower Pudding
314	Delicious Porridge	Special Minestrone Soup	Pear Pudding
315	Pumpkin Breakfast Muffins	Fresh Collard Greens Mix	Zucchini Bread
316	Mediterranean Chickpeas Breakfast	Endives Soup	Cocoa Brownies
317	Simple Granola	Fennel Soup	Blueberry Crackers
318	Breakfast Bowls	Asparagus Soup	Easy Cocoa Pudding
319	Sweet Potatoes Mix	Beets And Capers Mix	Cocoa Berries Cream
320	Simple Creamy Breakfast Potatoes	Mushroom Soup	Lemon Cream
321	Chia Pudding	Brussels Sprouts Delight	Easy Buns
322	Sweet Quinoa Mix	Artichoke Soup	Easy Blackberries Scones
323	Cranberry Coconut Quinoa	Intense Beet Soup	Lemon Jam
324	Zucchini Oatmeal	Chinese Carrot Cream	Pumpkin Cake
325	Cinnamon Oatmeal	Seitan Stew	Strawberries And Rhubarb Marmalade
326	Strawberry Choco shake	Spicy Carrot Stew	Strawberries Jam
327	Egg mayonnaise	Tomato Soup	Vanilla and Blueberry Squares
328	Coconut muffin	Collard Greens Mix	Raspberry Bars
329	Parsley Quiche	Classic Tomato Soup	Chocolate and Coconut Bars
330	Coconut Rice	Chinese Collard Greens Mix	Cranberry Pudding
331	Pear Oatmeal	Rich Chickpeas And Lentils Soup	Peach Cobbler
332	Pumpkin Oatmeal	Chard And Sweet Potato Soup	Blueberry Cake
333	Veggie Burrito	Chinese Soup And Ginger Sauce	Stewed Rhubarb
334	Apple Steel Cut Oats	Corn Cream Soup	Pudding Cake
335	Tofu Casserole	Veggie Medley	Sweet Peanut Butter Cake
336	Carrot Mix	Lentils Curry	Apple Mix
337	Blueberries Oats	Lentils Dal	Pears And Dried Fruits Bowls
338	Apple and Pears Mix	Rich Jackfruit Dish	Strawberry Stew
339	Bell Pepper Oatmeal	Vegan Gumbo	Poached Plums
340	Banana and Walnuts Oats	Chickpeas Delight	Sweet Rhubarb

341	Cool Tofu Breakfast Mix	Mediterranean Stew	Espresso Vanilla Dessert
342	Breakfast Broccoli and Tofu Bowls	Caribbean Dish	Sweet Cauliflower Rice
343	Strawberry Quinoa	Green Chili Soup	Cauliflower Pudding
344	Delicious Porridge	Special Minestrone Soup	Pear Pudding
345	Pumpkin Breakfast Muffins	Fresh Collard Greens Mix	Zucchini Bread
346	Mediterranean Chickpeas Breakfast	Endives Soup	Cocoa Brownies
347	Simple Granola	Fennel Soup	Blueberry Crackers
348	Breakfast Bowls	Asparagus Soup	Easy Cocoa Pudding
349	Sweet Potatoes Mix	Beets And Capers Mix	Cocoa Berries Cream
350	Simple Creamy Breakfast Potatoes	Mushroom Soup	Lemon Cream
351	Chia Pudding	Brussels Sprouts Delight	Easy Buns
352	Sweet Quinoa Mix	Artichoke Soup	Easy Blackberries Scones
353	Cranberry Coconut Quinoa	Intense Beet Soup	Lemon Jam
354	Zucchini Oatmeal	Chinese Carrot Cream	Pumpkin Cake
355	Cinnamon Oatmeal	Seitan Stew	Strawberries And Rhubarb Marmalade
356	Strawberry Choco shake	Spicy Carrot Stew	Strawberries Jam
357	Egg mayonnaise	Tomato Soup	Vanilla and Blueberry Squares
358	Coconut muffin	Collard Greens Mix	Raspberry Bars
359	Parsley Quiche	Classic Tomato Soup	Chocolate and Coconut Bars
360	Coconut Rice	Chinese Collard Greens Mix	Cranberry Pudding
361	Pear Oatmeal	Rich Chickpeas And Lentils Soup	Peach Cobbler
362	Pumpkin Oatmeal	Chard And Sweet Potato Soup	Blueberry Cake
363	Veggie Burrito	Chinese Soup And Ginger Sauce	Stewed Rhubarb
364	Apple Steel Cut Oats	Corn Cream Soup	Pudding Cake
365	Tofu Casserole	Veggie Medley	Sweet Peanut Butter Cake
366	Carrot Mix	Lentils Curry	Apple Mix
367	Blueberries Oats	Lentils Dal	Pears And Dried Fruits Bowls
368	Apple and Pears Mix	Rich Jackfruit Dish	Strawberry Stew
369	Bell Pepper Oatmeal	Vegan Gumbo	Poached Plums
370	Banana and Walnuts Oats	Chickpeas Delight	Sweet Rhubarb
371	Cool Tofu Breakfast Mix	Mediterranean Stew	Espresso Vanilla Dessert
372	Breakfast Broccoli and Tofu Bowls	Caribbean Dish	Sweet Cauliflower Rice
373	Strawberry Quinoa	Green Chili Soup	Cauliflower Pudding
374	Delicious Porridge	Special Minestrone Soup	Pear Pudding
375	Pumpkin Breakfast Muffins	Fresh Collard Greens Mix	Zucchini Bread
376	Mediterranean Chickpeas Breakfast	Endives Soup	Cocoa Brownies
377	Simple Granola	Fennel Soup	Blueberry Crackers
378	Breakfast Bowls	Asparagus Soup	Easy Cocoa Pudding
379	Sweet Potatoes Mix	Beets And Capers Mix	Cocoa Berries Cream
380	Simple Creamy Breakfast Potatoes	Mushroom Soup	Lemon Cream
381	Chia Pudding	Brussels Sprouts Delight	Easy Buns
382	Sweet Quinoa Mix	Artichoke Soup	Easy Blackberries Scones
383	Cranberry Coconut Quinoa	Intense Beet Soup	Lemon Jam

384	Zucchini Oatmeal	Chinese Carrot Cream	Pumpkin Cake
385	Cinnamon Oatmeal	Seitan Stew	Strawberries And Rhubarb Marmalade
386	Strawberry Choco shake	Spicy Carrot Stew	Strawberries Jam
387	Egg mayonnaise	Tomato Soup	Vanilla and Blueberry Squares
388	Coconut muffin	Collard Greens Mix	Raspberry Bars
389	Parsley Quiche	Classic Tomato Soup	Chocolate and Coconut Bars
390	Coconut Rice	Chinese Collard Greens Mix	Cranberry Pudding
391	Pear Oatmeal	Rich Chickpeas And Lentils Soup	Peach Cobbler
392	Pumpkin Oatmeal	Chard And Sweet Potato Soup	Blueberry Cake
393	Veggie Burrito	Chinese Soup And Ginger Sauce	Stewed Rhubarb
394	Apple Steel Cut Oats	Corn Cream Soup	Pudding Cake
395	Tofu Casserole	Veggie Medley	Sweet Peanut Butter Cake
396	Carrot Mix	Lentils Curry	Apple Mix
397	Blueberries Oats	Lentils Dal	Pears And Dried Fruits Bowls
398	Apple and Pears Mix	Rich Jackfruit Dish	Strawberry Stew
399	Bell Pepper Oatmeal	Vegan Gumbo	Poached Plums
400	Banana and Walnuts Oats	Chickpeas Delight	Sweet Rhubarb
401	Cool Tofu Breakfast Mix	Mediterranean Stew	Espresso Vanilla Dessert
402	Breakfast Broccoli and Tofu Bowls	Caribbean Dish	Sweet Cauliflower Rice
403	Strawberry Quinoa	Green Chili Soup	Cauliflower Pudding
404	Delicious Porridge	Special Minestrone Soup	Pear Pudding
405	Pumpkin Breakfast Muffins	Fresh Collard Greens Mix	Zucchini Bread
406	Mediterranean Chickpeas Breakfast	Endives Soup	Cocoa Brownies
407	Simple Granola	Fennel Soup	Blueberry Crackers
408	Breakfast Bowls	Asparagus Soup	Easy Cocoa Pudding
409	Sweet Potatoes Mix	Beets And Capers Mix	Cocoa Berries Cream
410	Simple Creamy Breakfast Potatoes	Mushroom Soup	Lemon Cream
411	Chia Pudding	Brussels Sprouts Delight	Easy Buns
412	Sweet Quinoa Mix	Artichoke Soup	Easy Blackberries Scones
413	Cranberry Coconut Quinoa	Intense Beet Soup	Lemon Jam
414	Zucchini Oatmeal	Chinese Carrot Cream	Pumpkin Cake
415	Cinnamon Oatmeal	Seitan Stew	Strawberries And Rhubarb Marmalade
416	Strawberry Choco shake	Spicy Carrot Stew	Strawberries Jam
417	Egg mayonnaise	Tomato Soup	Vanilla and Blueberry Squares
418	Coconut muffin	Collard Greens Mix	Raspberry Bars
419	Parsley Quiche	Classic Tomato Soup	Chocolate and Coconut Bars
420	Coconut Rice	Chinese Collard Greens Mix	Cranberry Pudding
421	Pear Oatmeal	Rich Chickpeas And Lentils Soup	Peach Cobbler
422	Pumpkin Oatmeal	Chard And Sweet Potato Soup	Blueberry Cake
423	Veggie Burrito	Chinese Soup And Ginger Sauce	Stewed Rhubarb
424	Apple Steel Cut Oats	Corn Cream Soup	Pudding Cake
425	Tofu Casserole	Veggie Medley	Sweet Peanut Butter Cake
426	Carrot Mix	Lentils Curry	Apple Mix

427	Blueberries Oats	Lentils Dal	Pears And Dried Fruits Bowls
428	Apple and Pears Mix	Rich Jackfruit Dish	Strawberry Stew
429	Bell Pepper Oatmeal	Vegan Gumbo	Poached Plums
430	Banana and Walnuts Oats	Chickpeas Delight	Sweet Rhubarb
431	Cool Tofu Breakfast Mix	Mediterranean Stew	Espresso Vanilla Dessert
432	Breakfast Broccoli and Tofu Bowls	Caribbean Dish	Sweet Cauliflower Rice
433	Strawberry Quinoa	Green Chili Soup	Cauliflower Pudding
434	Delicious Porridge	Special Minestrone Soup	Pear Pudding
435	Pumpkin Breakfast Muffins	Fresh Collard Greens Mix	Zucchini Bread
436	Mediterranean Chickpeas Breakfast	Endives Soup	Cocoa Brownies
437	Simple Granola	Fennel Soup	Blueberry Crackers
438	Breakfast Bowls	Asparagus Soup	Easy Cocoa Pudding
439	Sweet Potatoes Mix	Beets And Capers Mix	Cocoa Berries Cream
440	Simple Creamy Breakfast Potatoes	Mushroom Soup	Lemon Cream
441	Chia Pudding	Brussels Sprouts Delight	Easy Buns
442	Sweet Quinoa Mix	Artichoke Soup	Easy Blackberries Scones
443	Cranberry Coconut Quinoa	Intense Beet Soup	Lemon Jam
444	Zucchini Oatmeal	Chinese Carrot Cream	Pumpkin Cake
445	Cinnamon Oatmeal	Seitan Stew	Strawberries And Rhubarb Marmalade
446	Strawberry Choco shake	Spicy Carrot Stew	Strawberries Jam
447	Egg mayonnaise	Tomato Soup	Vanilla and Blueberry Squares
448	Coconut muffin	Collard Greens Mix	Raspberry Bars
449	Parsley Quiche	Classic Tomato Soup	Chocolate and Coconut Bars
450	Coconut Rice	Chinese Collard Greens Mix	Cranberry Pudding
451	Pear Oatmeal	Rich Chickpeas And Lentils Soup	Peach Cobbler
452	Pumpkin Oatmeal	Chard And Sweet Potato Soup	Blueberry Cake
453	Veggie Burrito	Chinese Soup And Ginger Sauce	Stewed Rhubarb
454	Apple Steel Cut Oats	Corn Cream Soup	Pudding Cake
455	Tofu Casserole	Veggie Medley	Sweet Peanut Butter Cake
456	Carrot Mix	Lentils Curry	Apple Mix
457	Blueberries Oats	Lentils Dal	Pears And Dried Fruits Bowls
458	Apple and Pears Mix	Rich Jackfruit Dish	Strawberry Stew
459	Bell Pepper Oatmeal	Vegan Gumbo	Poached Plums
460	Banana and Walnuts Oats	Chickpeas Delight	Sweet Rhubarb
461	Cool Tofu Breakfast Mix	Mediterranean Stew	Espresso Vanilla Dessert
462	Breakfast Broccoli and Tofu Bowls	Caribbean Dish	Sweet Cauliflower Rice
463	Strawberry Quinoa	Green Chili Soup	Cauliflower Pudding
464	Delicious Porridge	Special Minestrone Soup	Pear Pudding
465	Pumpkin Breakfast Muffins	Fresh Collard Greens Mix	Zucchini Bread
466	Mediterranean Chickpeas Breakfast	Endives Soup	Cocoa Brownies
467	Simple Granola	Fennel Soup	Blueberry Crackers
468	Breakfast Bowls	Asparagus Soup	Easy Cocoa Pudding
469	Sweet Potatoes Mix	Beets And Capers Mix	Cocoa Berries Cream

470	Simple Creamy Breakfast Potatoes	Mushroom Soup	Lemon Cream
471	Chia Pudding	Brussels Sprouts Delight	Easy Buns
472	Sweet Quinoa Mix	Artichoke Soup	Easy Blackberries Scones
473	Cranberry Coconut Quinoa	Intense Beet Soup	Lemon Jam
474	Zucchini Oatmeal	Chinese Carrot Cream	Pumpkin Cake
475	Cinnamon Oatmeal	Seitan Stew	Strawberries And Rhubarb Marmalade
476	Strawberry Choco shake	Spicy Carrot Stew	Strawberries Jam
477	Egg mayonnaise	Tomato Soup	Vanilla and Blueberry Squares
478	Coconut muffin	Collard Greens Mix	Raspberry Bars
479	Parsley Quiche	Classic Tomato Soup	Chocolate and Coconut Bars
480	Coconut Rice	Chinese Collard Greens Mix	Cranberry Pudding
481	Pear Oatmeal	Rich Chickpeas And Lentils Soup	Peach Cobbler
482	Pumpkin Oatmeal	Chard And Sweet Potato Soup	Blueberry Cake
483	Veggie Burrito	Chinese Soup And Ginger Sauce	Stewed Rhubarb
484	Apple Steel Cut Oats	Corn Cream Soup	Pudding Cake
485	Tofu Casserole	Veggie Medley	Sweet Peanut Butter Cake
486	Carrot Mix	Lentils Curry	Apple Mix
487	Blueberries Oats	Lentils Dal	Pears And Dried Fruits Bowls
488	Apple and Pears Mix	Rich Jackfruit Dish	Strawberry Stew
489	Bell Pepper Oatmeal	Vegan Gumbo	Poached Plums
490	Banana and Walnuts Oats	Chickpeas Delight	Sweet Rhubarb
491	Cool Tofu Breakfast Mix	Mediterranean Stew	Espresso Vanilla Dessert
492	Breakfast Broccoli and Tofu Bowls	Caribbean Dish	Sweet Cauliflower Rice
493	Strawberry Quinoa	Green Chili Soup	Cauliflower Pudding
494	Delicious Porridge	Special Minestrone Soup	Pear Pudding
495	Pumpkin Breakfast Muffins	Fresh Collard Greens Mix	Zucchini Bread
496	Mediterranean Chickpeas Breakfast	Endives Soup	Cocoa Brownies
497	Simple Granola	Fennel Soup	Blueberry Crackers
498	Breakfast Bowls	Asparagus Soup	Easy Cocoa Pudding
499	Sweet Potatoes Mix	Beets And Capers Mix	Cocoa Berries Cream
500	Simple Creamy Breakfast Potatoes	Mushroom Soup	Lemon Cream
501	Chia Pudding	Brussels Sprouts Delight	Easy Buns
502	Sweet Quinoa Mix	Artichoke Soup	Easy Blackberries Scones
503	Cranberry Coconut Quinoa	Intense Beet Soup	Lemon Jam
504	Zucchini Oatmeal	Chinese Carrot Cream	Pumpkin Cake
505	Cinnamon Oatmeal	Seitan Stew	Strawberries And Rhubarb Marmalade
506	Strawberry Choco shake	Spicy Carrot Stew	Strawberries Jam
507	Egg mayonnaise	Tomato Soup	Vanilla and Blueberry Squares
508	Coconut muffin	Collard Greens Mix	Raspberry Bars
509	Parsley Quiche	Classic Tomato Soup	Chocolate and Coconut Bars
510	Coconut Rice	Chinese Collard Greens Mix	Cranberry Pudding
511	Pear Oatmeal	Rich Chickpeas And Lentils Soup	Peach Cobbler
512	Pumpkin Oatmeal	Chard And Sweet Potato Soup	Blueberry Cake

513	Veggie Burrito	Chinese Soup And Ginger Sauce	Stewed Rhubarb
514	Apple Steel Cut Oats	Corn Cream Soup	Pudding Cake
515	Tofu Casserole	Veggie Medley	Sweet Peanut Butter Cake
516	Carrot Mix	Lentils Curry	Apple Mix
517	Blueberries Oats	Lentils Dal	Pears And Dried Fruits Bowls
518	Apple and Pears Mix	Rich Jackfruit Dish	Strawberry Stew
519	Bell Pepper Oatmeal	Vegan Gumbo	Poached Plums
520	Banana and Walnuts Oats	Chickpeas Delight	Sweet Rhubarb
521	Cool Tofu Breakfast Mix	Mediterranean Stew	Espresso Vanilla Dessert
522	Breakfast Broccoli and Tofu Bowls	Caribbean Dish	Sweet Cauliflower Rice
523	Strawberry Quinoa	Green Chili Soup	Cauliflower Pudding
524	Delicious Porridge	Special Minestrone Soup	Pear Pudding
525	Pumpkin Breakfast Muffins	Fresh Collard Greens Mix	Zucchini Bread
526	Mediterranean Chickpeas Breakfast	Endives Soup	Cocoa Brownies
527	Simple Granola	Fennel Soup	Blueberry Crackers
528	Breakfast Bowls	Asparagus Soup	Easy Cocoa Pudding
529	Sweet Potatoes Mix	Beets And Capers Mix	Cocoa Berries Cream
530	Simple Creamy Breakfast Potatoes	Mushroom Soup	Lemon Cream
531	Chia Pudding	Brussels Sprouts Delight	Easy Buns
532	Sweet Quinoa Mix	Artichoke Soup	Easy Blackberries Scones
533	Cranberry Coconut Quinoa	Intense Beet Soup	Lemon Jam
534	Zucchini Oatmeal	Chinese Carrot Cream	Pumpkin Cake
535	Cinnamon Oatmeal	Seitan Stew	Strawberries And Rhubarb Marmalade
536	Strawberry Choco shake	Spicy Carrot Stew	Strawberries Jam
537	Egg mayonnaise	Tomato Soup	Vanilla and Blueberry Squares
538	Coconut muffin	Collard Greens Mix	Raspberry Bars
539	Parsley Quiche	Classic Tomato Soup	Chocolate and Coconut Bars
540	Coconut Rice	Chinese Collard Greens Mix	Cranberry Pudding
541	Pear Oatmeal	Rich Chickpeas And Lentils Soup	Peach Cobbler
542	Pumpkin Oatmeal	Chard And Sweet Potato Soup	Blueberry Cake
543	Veggie Burrito	Chinese Soup And Ginger Sauce	Stewed Rhubarb
544	Apple Steel Cut Oats	Corn Cream Soup	Pudding Cake
545	Tofu Casserole	Veggie Medley	Sweet Peanut Butter Cake
546	Carrot Mix	Lentils Curry	Apple Mix
547	Blueberries Oats	Lentils Dal	Pears And Dried Fruits Bowls
548	Apple and Pears Mix	Rich Jackfruit Dish	Strawberry Stew
549	Bell Pepper Oatmeal	Vegan Gumbo	Poached Plums
550	Banana and Walnuts Oats	Chickpeas Delight	Sweet Rhubarb
551	Cool Tofu Breakfast Mix	Mediterranean Stew	Espresso Vanilla Dessert
552	Breakfast Broccoli and Tofu Bowls	Caribbean Dish	Sweet Cauliflower Rice
553	Strawberry Quinoa	Green Chili Soup	Cauliflower Pudding
554	Delicious Porridge	Special Minestrone Soup	Pear Pudding
555	Pumpkin Breakfast Muffins	Fresh Collard Greens Mix	Zucchini Bread

556	Mediterranean Chickpeas Breakfast	Endives Soup	Cocoa Brownies
557	Simple Granola	Fennel Soup	Blueberry Crackers
558	Breakfast Bowls	Asparagus Soup	Easy Cocoa Pudding
559	Sweet Potatoes Mix	Beets And Capers Mix	Cocoa Berries Cream
560	Simple Creamy Breakfast Potatoes	Mushroom Soup	Lemon Cream
561	Chia Pudding	Brussels Sprouts Delight	Easy Buns
562	Sweet Quinoa Mix	Artichoke Soup	Easy Blackberries Scones
563	Cranberry Coconut Quinoa	Intense Beet Soup	Lemon Jam
564	Zucchini Oatmeal	Chinese Carrot Cream	Pumpkin Cake
565	Cinnamon Oatmeal	Seitan Stew	Strawberries And Rhubarb Marmalade
566	Strawberry Choco shake	Spicy Carrot Stew	Strawberries Jam
567	Egg mayonnaise	Tomato Soup	Vanilla and Blueberry Squares
568	Coconut muffin	Collard Greens Mix	Raspberry Bars
569	Parsley Quiche	Classic Tomato Soup	Chocolate and Coconut Bars
570	Coconut Rice	Chinese Collard Greens Mix	Cranberry Pudding
571	Pear Oatmeal	Rich Chickpeas And Lentils Soup	Peach Cobbler
572	Pumpkin Oatmeal	Chard And Sweet Potato Soup	Blueberry Cake
573	Veggie Burrito	Chinese Soup And Ginger Sauce	Stewed Rhubarb
574	Apple Steel Cut Oats	Corn Cream Soup	Pudding Cake
575	Tofu Casserole	Veggie Medley	Sweet Peanut Butter Cake
576	Carrot Mix	Lentils Curry	Apple Mix
577	Blueberries Oats	Lentils Dal	Pears And Dried Fruits Bowls
578	Apple and Pears Mix	Rich Jackfruit Dish	Strawberry Stew
579	Bell Pepper Oatmeal	Vegan Gumbo	Poached Plums
580	Banana and Walnuts Oats	Chickpeas Delight	Sweet Rhubarb
581	Cool Tofu Breakfast Mix	Mediterranean Stew	Espresso Vanilla Dessert
582	Breakfast Broccoli and Tofu Bowls	Caribbean Dish	Sweet Cauliflower Rice
583	Strawberry Quinoa	Green Chili Soup	Cauliflower Pudding
584	Delicious Porridge	Special Minestrone Soup	Pear Pudding
585	Pumpkin Breakfast Muffins	Fresh Collard Greens Mix	Zucchini Bread
586	Mediterranean Chickpeas Breakfast	Endives Soup	Cocoa Brownies
587	Simple Granola	Fennel Soup	Blueberry Crackers
588	Breakfast Bowls	Asparagus Soup	Easy Cocoa Pudding
589	Sweet Potatoes Mix	Beets And Capers Mix	Cocoa Berries Cream
590	Simple Creamy Breakfast Potatoes	Mushroom Soup	Lemon Cream
591	Chia Pudding	Brussels Sprouts Delight	Easy Buns
592	Sweet Quinoa Mix	Artichoke Soup	Easy Blackberries Scones
593	Cranberry Coconut Quinoa	Intense Beet Soup	Lemon Jam
594	Zucchini Oatmeal	Chinese Carrot Cream	Pumpkin Cake
595	Cinnamon Oatmeal	Seitan Stew	Strawberries And Rhubarb Marmalade
596	Strawberry Choco shake	Spicy Carrot Stew	Strawberries Jam
597	Egg mayonnaise	Tomato Soup	Vanilla and Blueberry Squares
598	Coconut muffin	Collard Greens Mix	Raspberry Bars

599	Parsley Quiche	Classic Tomato Soup	Chocolate and Coconut Bars
600	Coconut Rice	Chinese Collard Greens Mix	Cranberry Pudding
601	Pear Oatmeal	Rich Chickpeas And Lentils Soup	Peach Cobbler
602	Pumpkin Oatmeal	Chard And Sweet Potato Soup	Blueberry Cake
603	Veggie Burrito	Chinese Soup And Ginger Sauce	Stewed Rhubarb
604	Apple Steel Cut Oats	Corn Cream Soup	Pudding Cake
605	Tofu Casserole	Veggie Medley	Sweet Peanut Butter Cake
606	Carrot Mix	Lentils Curry	Apple Mix
607	Blueberries Oats	Lentils Dal	Pears And Dried Fruits Bowls
608	Apple and Pears Mix	Rich Jackfruit Dish	Strawberry Stew
609	Bell Pepper Oatmeal	Vegan Gumbo	Poached Plums
610	Banana and Walnuts Oats	Chickpeas Delight	Sweet Rhubarb
611	Cool Tofu Breakfast Mix	Mediterranean Stew	Espresso Vanilla Dessert
612	Breakfast Broccoli and Tofu Bowls	Caribbean Dish	Sweet Cauliflower Rice
613	Strawberry Quinoa	Green Chili Soup	Cauliflower Pudding
614	Delicious Porridge	Special Minestrone Soup	Pear Pudding
615	Pumpkin Breakfast Muffins	Fresh Collard Greens Mix	Zucchini Bread
616	Mediterranean Chickpeas Breakfast	Endives Soup	Cocoa Brownies
617	Simple Granola	Fennel Soup	Blueberry Crackers
618	Breakfast Bowls	Asparagus Soup	Easy Cocoa Pudding
619	Sweet Potatoes Mix	Beets And Capers Mix	Cocoa Berries Cream
620	Simple Creamy Breakfast Potatoes	Mushroom Soup	Lemon Cream
621	Chia Pudding	Brussels Sprouts Delight	Easy Buns
622	Sweet Quinoa Mix	Artichoke Soup	Easy Blackberries Scones
623	Cranberry Coconut Quinoa	Intense Beet Soup	Lemon Jam
624	Zucchini Oatmeal	Chinese Carrot Cream	Pumpkin Cake
625	Cinnamon Oatmeal	Seitan Stew	Strawberries And Rhubarb Marmalade
626	Strawberry Choco shake	Spicy Carrot Stew	Strawberries Jam
627	Egg mayonnaise	Tomato Soup	Vanilla and Blueberry Squares
628	Coconut muffin	Collard Greens Mix	Raspberry Bars
629	Parsley Quiche	Classic Tomato Soup	Chocolate and Coconut Bars
630	Coconut Rice	Chinese Collard Greens Mix	Cranberry Pudding
631	Pear Oatmeal	Rich Chickpeas And Lentils Soup	Peach Cobbler
632	Pumpkin Oatmeal	Chard And Sweet Potato Soup	Blueberry Cake
633	Veggie Burrito	Chinese Soup And Ginger Sauce	Stewed Rhubarb
634	Apple Steel Cut Oats	Corn Cream Soup	Pudding Cake
635	Tofu Casserole	Veggie Medley	Sweet Peanut Butter Cake
636	Carrot Mix	Lentils Curry	Apple Mix
637	Blueberries Oats	Lentils Dal	Pears And Dried Fruits Bowls
638	Apple and Pears Mix	Rich Jackfruit Dish	Strawberry Stew
639	Bell Pepper Oatmeal	Vegan Gumbo	Poached Plums
640	Banana and Walnuts Oats	Chickpeas Delight	Sweet Rhubarb
641	Cool Tofu Breakfast Mix	Mediterranean Stew	Espresso Vanilla Dessert

642	Breakfast Broccoli and Tofu Bowls	Caribbean Dish	Sweet Cauliflower Rice
643	Strawberry Quinoa	Green Chili Soup	Cauliflower Pudding
644	Delicious Porridge	Special Minestrone Soup	Pear Pudding
645	Pumpkin Breakfast Muffins	Fresh Collard Greens Mix	Zucchini Bread
646	Mediterranean Chickpeas Breakfast	Endives Soup	Cocoa Brownies
647	Simple Granola	Fennel Soup	Blueberry Crackers
648	Breakfast Bowls	Asparagus Soup	Easy Cocoa Pudding
649	Sweet Potatoes Mix	Beets And Capers Mix	Cocoa Berries Cream
650	Simple Creamy Breakfast Potatoes	Mushroom Soup	Lemon Cream
651	Chia Pudding	Brussels Sprouts Delight	Easy Buns
652	Sweet Quinoa Mix	Artichoke Soup	Easy Blackberries Scones
653	Cranberry Coconut Quinoa	Intense Beet Soup	Lemon Jam
654	Zucchini Oatmeal	Chinese Carrot Cream	Pumpkin Cake
655	Cinnamon Oatmeal	Seitan Stew	Strawberries And Rhubarb Marmalade
656	Strawberry Choco shake	Spicy Carrot Stew	Strawberries Jam
657	Egg mayonnaise	Tomato Soup	Vanilla and Blueberry Squares
658	Coconut muffin	Collard Greens Mix	Raspberry Bars
659	Parsley Quiche	Classic Tomato Soup	Chocolate and Coconut Bars
660	Coconut Rice	Chinese Collard Greens Mix	Cranberry Pudding
661	Pear Oatmeal	Rich Chickpeas And Lentils Soup	Peach Cobbler
662	Pumpkin Oatmeal	Chard And Sweet Potato Soup	Blueberry Cake
663	Veggie Burrito	Chinese Soup And Ginger Sauce	Stewed Rhubarb
664	Apple Steel Cut Oats	Corn Cream Soup	Pudding Cake
665	Tofu Casserole	Veggie Medley	Sweet Peanut Butter Cake
666	Carrot Mix	Lentils Curry	Apple Mix
667	Blueberries Oats	Lentils Dal	Pears And Dried Fruits Bowls
668	Apple and Pears Mix	Rich Jackfruit Dish	Strawberry Stew
669	Bell Pepper Oatmeal	Vegan Gumbo	Poached Plums
670	Banana and Walnuts Oats	Chickpeas Delight	Sweet Rhubarb
671	Cool Tofu Breakfast Mix	Mediterranean Stew	Espresso Vanilla Dessert
672	Breakfast Broccoli and Tofu Bowls	Caribbean Dish	Sweet Cauliflower Rice
673	Strawberry Quinoa	Green Chili Soup	Cauliflower Pudding
674	Delicious Porridge	Special Minestrone Soup	Pear Pudding
675	Pumpkin Breakfast Muffins	Fresh Collard Greens Mix	Zucchini Bread
676	Mediterranean Chickpeas Breakfast	Endives Soup	Cocoa Brownies
677	Simple Granola	Fennel Soup	Blueberry Crackers
678	Breakfast Bowls	Asparagus Soup	Easy Cocoa Pudding
679	Sweet Potatoes Mix	Beets And Capers Mix	Cocoa Berries Cream
680	Simple Creamy Breakfast Potatoes	Mushroom Soup	Lemon Cream
681	Chia Pudding	Brussels Sprouts Delight	Easy Buns
682	Sweet Quinoa Mix	Artichoke Soup	Easy Blackberries Scones
683	Cranberry Coconut Quinoa	Intense Beet Soup	Lemon Jam
684	Zucchini Oatmeal	Chinese Carrot Cream	Pumpkin Cake

685	Cinnamon Oatmeal	Seitan Stew	Strawberries And Rhubarb Marmalade
686	Strawberry Choco shake	Spicy Carrot Stew	Strawberries Jam
687	Egg mayonnaise	Tomato Soup	Vanilla and Blueberry Squares
688	Coconut muffin	Collard Greens Mix	Raspberry Bars
689	Parsley Quiche	Classic Tomato Soup	Chocolate and Coconut Bars
690	Coconut Rice	Chinese Collard Greens Mix	Cranberry Pudding
691	Pear Oatmeal	Rich Chickpeas And Lentils Soup	Peach Cobbler
692	Pumpkin Oatmeal	Chard And Sweet Potato Soup	Blueberry Cake
693	Veggie Burrito	Chinese Soup And Ginger Sauce	Stewed Rhubarb
694	Apple Steel Cut Oats	Corn Cream Soup	Pudding Cake
695	Tofu Casserole	Veggie Medley	Sweet Peanut Butter Cake
696	Carrot Mix	Lentils Curry	Apple Mix
697	Blueberries Oats	Lentils Dal	Pears And Dried Fruits Bowls
698	Apple and Pears Mix	Rich Jackfruit Dish	Strawberry Stew
699	Bell Pepper Oatmeal	Vegan Gumbo	Poached Plums
700	Banana and Walnuts Oats	Chickpeas Delight	Sweet Rhubarb
701	Cool Tofu Breakfast Mix	Mediterranean Stew	Espresso Vanilla Dessert
702	Breakfast Broccoli and Tofu Bowls	Caribbean Dish	Sweet Cauliflower Rice
703	Strawberry Quinoa	Green Chili Soup	Cauliflower Pudding
704	Delicious Porridge	Special Minestrone Soup	Pear Pudding
705	Pumpkin Breakfast Muffins	Fresh Collard Greens Mix	Zucchini Bread
706	Mediterranean Chickpeas Breakfast	Endives Soup	Cocoa Brownies
707	Simple Granola	Fennel Soup	Blueberry Crackers
708	Breakfast Bowls	Asparagus Soup	Easy Cocoa Pudding
709	Sweet Potatoes Mix	Beets And Capers Mix	Cocoa Berries Cream
710	Simple Creamy Breakfast Potatoes	Mushroom Soup	Lemon Cream
711	Chia Pudding	Brussels Sprouts Delight	Easy Buns
712	Sweet Quinoa Mix	Artichoke Soup	Easy Blackberries Scones
713	Cranberry Coconut Quinoa	Intense Beet Soup	Lemon Jam
714	Zucchini Oatmeal	Chinese Carrot Cream	Pumpkin Cake
715	Cinnamon Oatmeal	Seitan Stew	Strawberries And Rhubarb Marmalade
716	Strawberry Choco shake	Spicy Carrot Stew	Strawberries Jam
717	Egg mayonnaise	Tomato Soup	Vanilla and Blueberry Squares
718	Coconut muffin	Collard Greens Mix	Raspberry Bars
719	Parsley Quiche	Classic Tomato Soup	Chocolate and Coconut Bars
720	Coconut Rice	Chinese Collard Greens Mix	Cranberry Pudding
721	Pear Oatmeal	Rich Chickpeas And Lentils Soup	Peach Cobbler
722	Pumpkin Oatmeal	Chard And Sweet Potato Soup	Blueberry Cake
723	Veggie Burrito	Chinese Soup And Ginger Sauce	Stewed Rhubarb
724	Apple Steel Cut Oats	Corn Cream Soup	Pudding Cake
725	Tofu Casserole	Veggie Medley	Sweet Peanut Butter Cake
726	Carrot Mix	Lentils Curry	Apple Mix
727	Blueberries Oats	Lentils Dal	Pears And Dried Fruits Bowls

728	Apple and Pears Mix	Rich Jackfruit Dish	Strawberry Stew
729	Bell Pepper Oatmeal	Vegan Gumbo	Poached Plums
730	Banana and Walnuts Oats	Chickpeas Delight	Sweet Rhubarb
731	Cool Tofu Breakfast Mix	Mediterranean Stew	Espresso Vanilla Dessert
732	Breakfast Broccoli and Tofu Bowls	Caribbean Dish	Sweet Cauliflower Rice
733	Strawberry Quinoa	Green Chili Soup	Cauliflower Pudding
734	Delicious Porridge	Special Minestrone Soup	Pear Pudding
735	Pumpkin Breakfast Muffins	Fresh Collard Greens Mix	Zucchini Bread
736	Mediterranean Chickpeas Breakfast	Endives Soup	Cocoa Brownies
737	Simple Granola	Fennel Soup	Blueberry Crackers
738	Breakfast Bowls	Asparagus Soup	Easy Cocoa Pudding
739	Sweet Potatoes Mix	Beets And Capers Mix	Cocoa Berries Cream
740	Simple Creamy Breakfast Potatoes	Mushroom Soup	Lemon Cream
741	Chia Pudding	Brussels Sprouts Delight	Easy Buns
742	Sweet Quinoa Mix	Artichoke Soup	Easy Blackberries Scones
743	Cranberry Coconut Quinoa	Intense Beet Soup	Lemon Jam
744	Zucchini Oatmeal	Chinese Carrot Cream	Pumpkin Cake
745	Cinnamon Oatmeal	Seitan Stew	Strawberries And Rhubarb Marmalade
746	Strawberry Choco shake	Spicy Carrot Stew	Strawberries Jam
747	Egg mayonnaise	Tomato Soup	Vanilla and Blueberry Squares
748	Coconut muffin	Collard Greens Mix	Raspberry Bars
749	Parsley Quiche	Classic Tomato Soup	Chocolate and Coconut Bars
750	Coconut Rice	Chinese Collard Greens Mix	Cranberry Pudding
751	Pear Oatmeal	Rich Chickpeas And Lentils Soup	Peach Cobbler
752	Pumpkin Oatmeal	Chard And Sweet Potato Soup	Blueberry Cake
753	Veggie Burrito	Chinese Soup And Ginger Sauce	Stewed Rhubarb
754	Apple Steel Cut Oats	Corn Cream Soup	Pudding Cake
755	Tofu Casserole	Veggie Medley	Sweet Peanut Butter Cake
756	Carrot Mix	Lentils Curry	Apple Mix
757	Blueberries Oats	Lentils Dal	Pears And Dried Fruits Bowls
758	Apple and Pears Mix	Rich Jackfruit Dish	Strawberry Stew
759	Bell Pepper Oatmeal	Vegan Gumbo	Poached Plums
760	Banana and Walnuts Oats	Chickpeas Delight	Sweet Rhubarb
761	Cool Tofu Breakfast Mix	Mediterranean Stew	Espresso Vanilla Dessert
762	Breakfast Broccoli and Tofu Bowls	Caribbean Dish	Sweet Cauliflower Rice
763	Strawberry Quinoa	Green Chili Soup	Cauliflower Pudding
764	Delicious Porridge	Special Minestrone Soup	Pear Pudding
765	Pumpkin Breakfast Muffins	Fresh Collard Greens Mix	Zucchini Bread
766	Mediterranean Chickpeas Breakfast	Endives Soup	Cocoa Brownies
767	Simple Granola	Fennel Soup	Blueberry Crackers
768	Breakfast Bowls	Asparagus Soup	Easy Cocoa Pudding
769	Sweet Potatoes Mix	Beets And Capers Mix	Cocoa Berries Cream
770	Simple Creamy Breakfast Potatoes	Mushroom Soup	Lemon Cream

771	Chia Pudding	Brussels Sprouts Delight	Easy Buns
772	Sweet Quinoa Mix	Artichoke Soup	Easy Blackberries Scones
773	Cranberry Coconut Quinoa	Intense Beet Soup	Lemon Jam
774	Zucchini Oatmeal	Chinese Carrot Cream	Pumpkin Cake
775	Cinnamon Oatmeal	Seitan Stew	Strawberries And Rhubarb Marmalade
776	Strawberry Choco shake	Spicy Carrot Stew	Strawberries Jam
777	Egg mayonnaise	Tomato Soup	Vanilla and Blueberry Squares
778	Coconut muffin	Collard Greens Mix	Raspberry Bars
779	Parsley Quiche	Classic Tomato Soup	Chocolate and Coconut Bars
780	Coconut Rice	Chinese Collard Greens Mix	Cranberry Pudding
781	Pear Oatmeal	Rich Chickpeas And Lentils Soup	Peach Cobbler
782	Pumpkin Oatmeal	Chard And Sweet Potato Soup	Blueberry Cake
783	Veggie Burrito	Chinese Soup And Ginger Sauce	Stewed Rhubarb
784	Apple Steel Cut Oats	Corn Cream Soup	Pudding Cake
785	Tofu Casserole	Veggie Medley	Sweet Peanut Butter Cake
786	Carrot Mix	Lentils Curry	Apple Mix
787	Blueberries Oats	Lentils Dal	Pears And Dried Fruits Bowls
788	Apple and Pears Mix	Rich Jackfruit Dish	Strawberry Stew
789	Bell Pepper Oatmeal	Vegan Gumbo	Poached Plums
790	Banana and Walnuts Oats	Chickpeas Delight	Sweet Rhubarb
791	Cool Tofu Breakfast Mix	Mediterranean Stew	Espresso Vanilla Dessert
792	Breakfast Broccoli and Tofu Bowls	Caribbean Dish	Sweet Cauliflower Rice
793	Strawberry Quinoa	Green Chili Soup	Cauliflower Pudding
794	Delicious Porridge	Special Minestrone Soup	Pear Pudding
795	Pumpkin Breakfast Muffins	Fresh Collard Greens Mix	Zucchini Bread
796	Mediterranean Chickpeas Breakfast	Endives Soup	Cocoa Brownies
797	Simple Granola	Fennel Soup	Blueberry Crackers
798	Breakfast Bowls	Asparagus Soup	Easy Cocoa Pudding
799	Sweet Potatoes Mix	Beets And Capers Mix	Cocoa Berries Cream
800	Simple Creamy Breakfast Potatoes	Mushroom Soup	Lemon Cream
801	Chia Pudding	Brussels Sprouts Delight	Easy Buns
802	Sweet Quinoa Mix	Artichoke Soup	Easy Blackberries Scones
803	Cranberry Coconut Quinoa	Intense Beet Soup	Lemon Jam
804	Zucchini Oatmeal	Chinese Carrot Cream	Pumpkin Cake
805	Cinnamon Oatmeal	Seitan Stew	Strawberries And Rhubarb Marmalade
806	Strawberry Choco shake	Spicy Carrot Stew	Strawberries Jam
807	Egg mayonnaise	Tomato Soup	Vanilla and Blueberry Squares
808	Coconut muffin	Collard Greens Mix	Raspberry Bars
809	Parsley Quiche	Classic Tomato Soup	Chocolate and Coconut Bars
810	Coconut Rice	Chinese Collard Greens Mix	Cranberry Pudding
811	Pear Oatmeal	Rich Chickpeas And Lentils Soup	Peach Cobbler
812	Pumpkin Oatmeal	Chard And Sweet Potato Soup	Blueberry Cake
813	Veggie Burrito	Chinese Soup And Ginger Sauce	Stewed Rhubarb

814	Apple Steel Cut Oats	Corn Cream Soup	Pudding Cake
815	Tofu Casserole	Veggie Medley	Sweet Peanut Butter Cake
816	Carrot Mix	Lentils Curry	Apple Mix
817	Blueberries Oats	Lentils Dal	Pears And Dried Fruits Bowls
818	Apple and Pears Mix	Rich Jackfruit Dish	Strawberry Stew
819	Bell Pepper Oatmeal	Vegan Gumbo	Poached Plums
820	Banana and Walnuts Oats	Chickpeas Delight	Sweet Rhubarb
821	Cool Tofu Breakfast Mix	Mediterranean Stew	Espresso Vanilla Dessert
822	Breakfast Broccoli and Tofu Bowls	Caribbean Dish	Sweet Cauliflower Rice
823	Strawberry Quinoa	Green Chili Soup	Cauliflower Pudding
824	Delicious Porridge	Special Minestrone Soup	Pear Pudding
825	Pumpkin Breakfast Muffins	Fresh Collard Greens Mix	Zucchini Bread
826	Mediterranean Chickpeas Breakfast	Endives Soup	Cocoa Brownies
827	Simple Granola	Fennel Soup	Blueberry Crackers
828	Breakfast Bowls	Asparagus Soup	Easy Cocoa Pudding
829	Sweet Potatoes Mix	Beets And Capers Mix	Cocoa Berries Cream
830	Simple Creamy Breakfast Potatoes	Mushroom Soup	Lemon Cream
831	Chia Pudding	Brussels Sprouts Delight	Easy Buns
832	Sweet Quinoa Mix	Artichoke Soup	Easy Blackberries Scones
833	Cranberry Coconut Quinoa	Intense Beet Soup	Lemon Jam
834	Zucchini Oatmeal	Chinese Carrot Cream	Pumpkin Cake
835	Cinnamon Oatmeal	Seitan Stew	Strawberries And Rhubarb Marmalade
836	Strawberry Choco shake	Spicy Carrot Stew	Strawberries Jam
837	Egg mayonnaise	Tomato Soup	Vanilla and Blueberry Squares
838	Coconut muffin	Collard Greens Mix	Raspberry Bars
839	Parsley Quiche	Classic Tomato Soup	Chocolate and Coconut Bars
840	Coconut Rice	Chinese Collard Greens Mix	Cranberry Pudding
841	Pear Oatmeal	Rich Chickpeas And Lentils Soup	Peach Cobbler
842	Pumpkin Oatmeal	Chard And Sweet Potato Soup	Blueberry Cake
843	Veggie Burrito	Chinese Soup And Ginger Sauce	Stewed Rhubarb
844	Apple Steel Cut Oats	Corn Cream Soup	Pudding Cake
845	Tofu Casserole	Veggie Medley	Sweet Peanut Butter Cake
846	Carrot Mix	Lentils Curry	Apple Mix
847	Blueberries Oats	Lentils Dal	Pears And Dried Fruits Bowls
848	Apple and Pears Mix	Rich Jackfruit Dish	Strawberry Stew
849	Bell Pepper Oatmeal	Vegan Gumbo	Poached Plums
850	Banana and Walnuts Oats	Chickpeas Delight	Sweet Rhubarb
851	Cool Tofu Breakfast Mix	Mediterranean Stew	Espresso Vanilla Dessert
852	Breakfast Broccoli and Tofu Bowls	Caribbean Dish	Sweet Cauliflower Rice
853	Strawberry Quinoa	Green Chili Soup	Cauliflower Pudding
854	Delicious Porridge	Special Minestrone Soup	Pear Pudding
855	Pumpkin Breakfast Muffins	Fresh Collard Greens Mix	Zucchini Bread
856	Mediterranean Chickpeas Breakfast	Endives Soup	Cocoa Brownies

857	Simple Granola	Fennel Soup	Blueberry Crackers
858	Breakfast Bowls	Asparagus Soup	Easy Cocoa Pudding
859	Sweet Potatoes Mix	Beets And Capers Mix	Cocoa Berries Cream
860	Simple Creamy Breakfast Potatoes	Mushroom Soup	Lemon Cream
861	Chia Pudding	Brussels Sprouts Delight	Easy Buns
862	Sweet Quinoa Mix	Artichoke Soup	Easy Blackberries Scones
863	Cranberry Coconut Quinoa	Intense Beet Soup	Lemon Jam
864	Zucchini Oatmeal	Chinese Carrot Cream	Pumpkin Cake
865	Cinnamon Oatmeal	Seitan Stew	Strawberries And Rhubarb Marmalade
866	Strawberry Choco shake	Spicy Carrot Stew	Strawberries Jam
867	Egg mayonnaise	Tomato Soup	Vanilla and Blueberry Squares
868	Coconut muffin	Collard Greens Mix	Raspberry Bars
869	Parsley Quiche	Classic Tomato Soup	Chocolate and Coconut Bars
870	Coconut Rice	Chinese Collard Greens Mix	Cranberry Pudding
871	Pear Oatmeal	Rich Chickpeas And Lentils Soup	Peach Cobbler
872	Pumpkin Oatmeal	Chard And Sweet Potato Soup	Blueberry Cake
873	Veggie Burrito	Chinese Soup And Ginger Sauce	Stewed Rhubarb
874	Apple Steel Cut Oats	Corn Cream Soup	Pudding Cake
875	Tofu Casserole	Veggie Medley	Sweet Peanut Butter Cake
876	Carrot Mix	Lentils Curry	Apple Mix
877	Blueberries Oats	Lentils Dal	Pears And Dried Fruits Bowls
878	Apple and Pears Mix	Rich Jackfruit Dish	Strawberry Stew
879	Bell Pepper Oatmeal	Vegan Gumbo	Poached Plums
880	Banana and Walnuts Oats	Chickpeas Delight	Sweet Rhubarb
881	Cool Tofu Breakfast Mix	Mediterranean Stew	Espresso Vanilla Dessert
882	Breakfast Broccoli and Tofu Bowls	Caribbean Dish	Sweet Cauliflower Rice
883	Strawberry Quinoa	Green Chili Soup	Cauliflower Pudding
884	Delicious Porridge	Special Minestrone Soup	Pear Pudding
885	Pumpkin Breakfast Muffins	Fresh Collard Greens Mix	Zucchini Bread
886	Mediterranean Chickpeas Breakfast	Endives Soup	Cocoa Brownies
887	Simple Granola	Fennel Soup	Blueberry Crackers
888	Breakfast Bowls	Asparagus Soup	Easy Cocoa Pudding
889	Sweet Potatoes Mix	Beets And Capers Mix	Cocoa Berries Cream
890	Simple Creamy Breakfast Potatoes	Mushroom Soup	Lemon Cream
891	Chia Pudding	Brussels Sprouts Delight	Easy Buns
892	Sweet Quinoa Mix	Artichoke Soup	Easy Blackberries Scones
893	Cranberry Coconut Quinoa	Intense Beet Soup	Lemon Jam
894	Zucchini Oatmeal	Chinese Carrot Cream	Pumpkin Cake
895	Cinnamon Oatmeal	Seitan Stew	Strawberries And Rhubarb Marmalade
896	Strawberry Choco shake	Spicy Carrot Stew	Strawberries Jam
897	Egg mayonnaise	Tomato Soup	Vanilla and Blueberry Squares
898	Coconut muffin	Collard Greens Mix	Raspberry Bars
899	Parsley Quiche	Classic Tomato Soup	Chocolate and Coconut Bars

1000 Day Diet Plan

900	Coconut Rice	Chinese Collard Greens Mix	Cranberry Pudding
901	Pear Oatmeal	Rich Chickpeas And Lentils Soup	Peach Cobbler
902	Pumpkin Oatmeal	Chard And Sweet Potato Soup	Blueberry Cake
903	Veggie Burrito	Chinese Soup And Ginger Sauce	Stewed Rhubarb
904	Apple Steel Cut Oats	Corn Cream Soup	Pudding Cake
905	Tofu Casserole	Veggie Medley	Sweet Peanut Butter Cake
906	Carrot Mix	Lentils Curry	Apple Mix
907	Blueberries Oats	Lentils Dal	Pears And Dried Fruits Bowls
908	Apple and Pears Mix	Rich Jackfruit Dish	Strawberry Stew
909	Bell Pepper Oatmeal	Vegan Gumbo	Poached Plums
910	Banana and Walnuts Oats	Chickpeas Delight	Sweet Rhubarb
911	Cool Tofu Breakfast Mix	Mediterranean Stew	Espresso Vanilla Dessert
912	Breakfast Broccoli and Tofu Bowls	Caribbean Dish	Sweet Cauliflower Rice
913	Strawberry Quinoa	Green Chili Soup	Cauliflower Pudding
914	Delicious Porridge	Special Minestrone Soup	Pear Pudding
915	Pumpkin Breakfast Muffins	Fresh Collard Greens Mix	Zucchini Bread
916	Mediterranean Chickpeas Breakfast	Endives Soup	Cocoa Brownies
917	Simple Granola	Fennel Soup	Blueberry Crackers
918	Breakfast Bowls	Asparagus Soup	Easy Cocoa Pudding
919	Sweet Potatoes Mix	Beets And Capers Mix	Cocoa Berries Cream
920	Simple Creamy Breakfast Potatoes	Mushroom Soup	Lemon Cream
921	Chia Pudding	Brussels Sprouts Delight	Easy Buns
922	Sweet Quinoa Mix	Artichoke Soup	Easy Blackberries Scones
923	Cranberry Coconut Quinoa	Intense Beet Soup	Lemon Jam
924	Zucchini Oatmeal	Chinese Carrot Cream	Pumpkin Cake
925	Cinnamon Oatmeal	Seitan Stew	Strawberries And Rhubarb Marmalade
926	Strawberry Choco shake	Spicy Carrot Stew	Strawberries Jam
927	Egg mayonnaise	Tomato Soup	Vanilla and Blueberry Squares
928	Coconut muffin	Collard Greens Mix	Raspberry Bars
929	Parsley Quiche	Classic Tomato Soup	Chocolate and Coconut Bars
930	Coconut Rice	Chinese Collard Greens Mix	Cranberry Pudding
931	Pear Oatmeal	Rich Chickpeas And Lentils Soup	Peach Cobbler
932	Pumpkin Oatmeal	Chard And Sweet Potato Soup	Blueberry Cake
933	Veggie Burrito	Chinese Soup And Ginger Sauce	Stewed Rhubarb
934	Apple Steel Cut Oats	Corn Cream Soup	Pudding Cake
935	Tofu Casserole	Veggie Medley	Sweet Peanut Butter Cake
936	Carrot Mix	Lentils Curry	Apple Mix
937	Blueberries Oats	Lentils Dal	Pears And Dried Fruits Bowls
938	Apple and Pears Mix	Rich Jackfruit Dish	Strawberry Stew
939	Bell Pepper Oatmeal	Vegan Gumbo	Poached Plums
940	Banana and Walnuts Oats	Chickpeas Delight	Sweet Rhubarb
941	Cool Tofu Breakfast Mix	Mediterranean Stew	Espresso Vanilla Dessert
942	Breakfast Broccoli and Tofu Bowls	Caribbean Dish	Sweet Cauliflower Rice

943	Strawberry Quinoa	Green Chili Soup	Cauliflower Pudding
944	Delicious Porridge	Special Minestrone Soup	Pear Pudding
945	Pumpkin Breakfast Muffins	Fresh Collard Greens Mix	Zucchini Bread
946	Mediterranean Chickpeas Breakfast	Endives Soup	Cocoa Brownies
947	Simple Granola	Fennel Soup	Blueberry Crackers
948	Breakfast Bowls	Asparagus Soup	Easy Cocoa Pudding
949	Sweet Potatoes Mix	Beets And Capers Mix	Cocoa Berries Cream
950	Simple Creamy Breakfast Potatoes	Mushroom Soup	Lemon Cream
951	Chia Pudding	Brussels Sprouts Delight	Easy Buns
952	Sweet Quinoa Mix	Artichoke Soup	Easy Blackberries Scones
953	Cranberry Coconut Quinoa	Intense Beet Soup	Lemon Jam
954	Zucchini Oatmeal	Chinese Carrot Cream	Pumpkin Cake
955	Cinnamon Oatmeal	Seitan Stew	Strawberries And Rhubarb Marmalade
956	Strawberry Choco shake	Spicy Carrot Stew	Strawberries Jam
957	Egg mayonnaise	Tomato Soup	Vanilla and Blueberry Squares
958	Coconut muffin	Collard Greens Mix	Raspberry Bars
959	Parsley Quiche	Classic Tomato Soup	Chocolate and Coconut Bars
960	Coconut Rice	Chinese Collard Greens Mix	Cranberry Pudding
961	Pear Oatmeal	Rich Chickpeas And Lentils Soup	Peach Cobbler
962	Pumpkin Oatmeal	Chard And Sweet Potato Soup	Blueberry Cake
963	Veggie Burrito	Chinese Soup And Ginger Sauce	Stewed Rhubarb
964	Apple Steel Cut Oats	Corn Cream Soup	Pudding Cake
965	Tofu Casserole	Veggie Medley	Sweet Peanut Butter Cake
966	Carrot Mix	Lentils Curry	Apple Mix
967	Blueberries Oats	Lentils Dal	Pears And Dried Fruits Bowls
968	Apple and Pears Mix	Rich Jackfruit Dish	Strawberry Stew
969	Bell Pepper Oatmeal	Vegan Gumbo	Poached Plums
970	Banana and Walnuts Oats	Chickpeas Delight	Sweet Rhubarb
971	Cool Tofu Breakfast Mix	Mediterranean Stew	Espresso Vanilla Dessert
972	Breakfast Broccoli and Tofu Bowls	Caribbean Dish	Sweet Cauliflower Rice
973	Strawberry Quinoa	Green Chili Soup	Cauliflower Pudding
974	Delicious Porridge	Special Minestrone Soup	Pear Pudding
975	Pumpkin Breakfast Muffins	Fresh Collard Greens Mix	Zucchini Bread
976	Mediterranean Chickpeas Breakfast	Endives Soup	Cocoa Brownies
977	Simple Granola	Fennel Soup	Blueberry Crackers
978	Breakfast Bowls	Asparagus Soup	Easy Cocoa Pudding
979	Sweet Potatoes Mix	Beets And Capers Mix	Cocoa Berries Cream
980	Simple Creamy Breakfast Potatoes	Mushroom Soup	Lemon Cream
981	Chia Pudding	Brussels Sprouts Delight	Easy Buns
982	Sweet Quinoa Mix	Artichoke Soup	Easy Blackberries Scones
983	Cranberry Coconut Quinoa	Intense Beet Soup	Lemon Jam
984	Zucchini Oatmeal	Chinese Carrot Cream	Pumpkin Cake
985	Cinnamon Oatmeal	Seitan Stew	Strawberries And Rhubarb Marmalade

986	Strawberry Choco shake	Spicy Carrot Stew	Strawberries Jam
987	Egg mayonnaise	Tomato Soup	Vanilla and Blueberry Squares
988	Coconut muffin	Collard Greens Mix	Raspberry Bars
989	Parsley Quiche	Classic Tomato Soup	Chocolate and Coconut Bars
990	Coconut Rice	Chinese Collard Greens Mix	Cranberry Pudding
991	Pear Oatmeal	Rich Chickpeas And Lentils Soup	Peach Cobbler
992	Pumpkin Oatmeal	Chard And Sweet Potato Soup	Blueberry Cake
993	Veggie Burrito	Chinese Soup And Ginger Sauce	Stewed Rhubarb
994	Apple Steel Cut Oats	Corn Cream Soup	Pudding Cake
995	Tofu Casserole	Veggie Medley	Sweet Peanut Butter Cake
996	Carrot Mix	Lentils Curry	Apple Mix
997	Blueberries Oats	Lentils Dal	Pears And Dried Fruits Bowls
998	Apple and Pears Mix	Rich Jackfruit Dish	Strawberry Stew
999	Bell Pepper Oatmeal	Vegan Gumbo	Poached Plums
1000	Banana and Walnuts Oats	Chickpeas Delight	Sweet Rhubarb

10-TIPS FOR SUCCESS

1. It is essential to easily maintain a proper exercise routine to easily make sure that your whole body is in tip-top shape all throughout the regime.
2. People often get confused regarding the fact of how a lot of carbs they can consume per day. The basic standard carb count is that you should simply keep your carb intake somewhere around 20-50g with such a maximum intake of 100-150g at best.
3. It is essential that you simply keep your protein intake in check. Too much protein will cause the whole body to start burning up protein instead of Fat! So, try to easily keep a balance.
4. A grave mistake which people makes is that they sometimes try just to lower down the Fat intake as well, thinking that it will double the effectiveness of a Ketogenic Diet. However, that is completely wrong, & you should never skip out on your fat intake.
5. Make sure to really go for as much water as you can. While you're on a Ketogenic Diet, the whole body will start just to flush away electrolytes which will make you weak. To tackle this effect, it is essential to simply keep your whole body fully hydrated at all time & have a good amount of salt as well.
6. To lose weight, it is easy to be tempted by some diets. One of these variations is a high-fat diet. It is generally recommended for carbs, high-fat foods, such as the Atkins diet, consuming a high percentage of calories from fat to control blood sugar levels and trigger fat burning. Although a high-fat diet may have some weight loss benefits, it also presents serious risks to consider.
7. The high-fat diet usually involves limiting the consumption of high fiber foods such as fruits and cereals. Without fiber to maintain digestive health, also you can quickly constipate and undergo abdominal augmentation. Nutrition experts such as Mauro Di Pasquale, author of The Metabolic Diet, recommend high-fat diets as a fiber supplement, such as a psyllium husk.
8. No matter what any diet you follow, you still need to consume fewer calories than you burn to lose weight. Fats contain more than thrice as much calories as protein and carbohydrates, which makes it easy to consume too many calories. Although the consumption of high-fat foods may be saturated, protein-rich foods will allow you to eat much more than a high-fat diet.
9. Heart disease is the most severe dietary risk, with high-fat content. High-fat foods often recommend foods high in saturated fats such as beef, bacon, and brown fowl. Source from the American Heart Association, a diet high in saturated fats can dramatically increase cholesterol, increasing the risk of heart disease. The AHA recommends limiting total fat consumption to 25-35% of total calories, only 7% of saturated fat.

10. A diet high in fat can cause ketosis if it is taken to the extreme, a process in which fat breaks down due to lack of glucose in carbohydrates. Ketosis is a catabolic disease that consumes muscles quickly, slowing metabolism. The slow metabolism makes losing weight more difficult, which compromises your efforts to lose fat. High-fat diets are all the rage. But they also are dangerous; Although children are rich in high-fat foods such as meat, cheese, butter, dairy products, and egg yolks, they generally have no consequences. New research has provided more information on what is happening in the human body when a person eats a high-fat meal. Greasy foods can take many forms, from traditional fats to unhealthy foods such as smoothies, hamburgers, and fries, as well as adding butter to morning coffee for your health. It is therefore worth asking how much dietary fat, especially from animal sources, is your health.

CONCLUSION

Thanks for downloading this book. Once you've gotten the okay to start a Keto vegetarian diet, don't be afraid to ask questions. Sometimes, side effects of the Keto diet like dizziness, intense fatigue, and mental fogginess can be scary if you don't know how to combat them. A medical professional will always give you the best advice, but these sneaky ways of maximizing your body's potential will definitely increase the odds of success with a vegetarian Keto diet.

Happy Keto-Vegetarian Lifestyle!

Made in the USA
Middletown, DE
08 February 2020